COVID-19 AND SOCIAL DETERMINANTS OF HEALTH

Wicked Issues and Relationalism

Edited by
Adrian Bonner

With a foreword by
Richard Smith

P

First published in Great Britain in 2023 by

Policy Press, an imprint of
Bristol University Press
University of Bristol
1–9 Old Park Hill
Bristol
BS2 8BB
UK
t: +44 (0)117 374 6645
e: bup-info@bristol.ac.uk

Details of international sales and distribution partners are available at
policy.bristoluniversitypress.co.uk

© Bristol University Press 2023

British Library Cataloguing in Publication Data
A catalogue record for this book is available from the British Library

ISBN 978-1-4473-6494-8 hardcover
ISBN 978-1-4473-6495-5 paperback
ISBN 978-1-4473-6496-2 ePub
ISBN 978-1-4473-6497-9 ePdf

The right of Adrian Bonner to be identified as editor of this work has been asserted by him in
accordance with the Copyright, Designs and Patents Act 1988.

Cover design: Andrew Corbett
Bristol University Press and Policy Press use environmentally responsible
print partners.
Printed and bound in Great Britain by CMP, Poole

The initial planning of this book began in December 2019. On 31 January 2020 the first case of COVID-19 was recorded in the UK. The World Health Organization (WHO) declared that COVID-19 infection had reached the level of a pandemic in March. On 26 March 2020 The Health Protection (Coronavirus Restrictions, England) Regulations came into effect. During the following two years three waves of COVID-19 variants resulted in extreme pressures in the health services of the UK and other countries. Many people and families have been adversely affected directly by COVID-19, and suffered unintended consequences, including health, financial and relational stressors, and locking down of schools and workplaces.

On 10 May 2022, WHO reported 515,192,979 confirmed cases of COVID-19, and 6,254,140 deaths globally, including 177,000 deaths in the UK which were attributed to COVID-19.

This book is dedicated to:

Those who have lost loved ones

Health and social care workers

Members of the community who have worked voluntarily to support those in need

As world communities begin to recover from the COVID-19 pandemic, the world order is undergoing a major threat from the invasion of Ukraine by Russia, impacting on the economic stability of Europe and increasing the possibility of a third world war.

In the conclusion to this publication the concepts of wicked issues and relationalism, applied to COVID-19 and climate change, will, hopefully, inform responses to this major social determinant of life and death.

At this time the invasion of Ukraine by Russia the Office of the United Nations High Commission has verified the deaths of 3,459 civilians including 238 children (figures considered to be significant under-representations of actual deaths).

Adrian Bonner

29 September 2022

Contents

List of figures and tables   viii
Notes on contributors   x
Foreword by Richard Smith   xxvi

Introduction   1
Adrian Bonner

PART I   **Wicked issues and relationalism**   **17**
       Adrian Bonner
1   Using relationalism to navigate wicked issues: investing for a   21
       'relational dividend'?
       Richard Simmons
2   Relationalism, wicked issues and social determinants of health   41
       Adrian Bonner
3   Responding to the COVID-19 pandemic: a sociopolitical perspective   56
       David J. Hunter
4   Giving children the best start in life?   70
       Edward Kunonga, Victoria Cooling, Brighton Chireka and
       Tsitsi Chawatama

PART II   **Regionalism and geopolitical environments**   **83**
       Adrian Bonner
5   Levelling up in the North and North-East England: complex   87
       and fragmented governance and the new National Health
       Service and local government partnerships
       John Shutt
6   UK local council strategies post-COVID-19: the local   100
       economy, climate change and community wellbeing
       Manuel Abellan
7.1   Case study: Racism and xenophobia – America's deadly   114
       pre-existing conditions during the COVID-19
       pandemic's first year
       Joanna Sharpless and Annie Dell
7.2   Case study: Safe at home? Exploring intersecting   125
       vulnerabilities under COVID-19 and the role of faith
       actors in the South African context
       Selina Palm

7.3   Case study: COVID-19 and increased vulnerabilities to human   133
        trafficking and modern slavery – perspectives from
        India and Nepal
        Tribeni Gurung, Nishan Lo, Lallian Kunga and Vijaya Lama
7.4   Case study: COVID-19 and governing for health and wellbeing   143
        in New Zealand – putting communities at the centre
        Peter McKinlay and Anna Matheson

PART III Public sector, COVID-19 and culture change   **151**
        Michael Bennett
8   The changing context of public governance and the need for   155
        innovation and creating public value
        Joyce Liddle
9   The effect of COVID-19 on the financial sustainability of local   170
        government
        Aileen Murphie
10   UN sustainability goals and social value: local authority   192
        perspectives
        Rob Whiteman, Tim Reade and Dave Ayre
11   Housing policy and provision after COVID-19   210
        Peter Murphy
12   Employment and support   230
        Elizabeth Taylor, Andrew Morton and Annie Dell

PART IV The third sector   **241**
        Claire Bonham
13   Relational collaboration and innovation in responding to need   245
        and austerity: food banks
        Alex Murdock
14   Volunteering and small charities   258
        Chris O'Leary and Rita Chadha
15   Creating added value: the third sector, local and national   268
        government working together to address domestic abuse
        Emily Hodge
16   Wicked issues: a faith-based perspective   282
        Drew McCombe and Dean Pallant

PART V The case for relationalism   **307**
        Richard Smith
17.1   Case study: A relationalism exemplar   309
        Richard Smith
17.2   Case study: Housing and homelessness   312
        Adam Cunnington

17.3	Case study: Environmental planning in a post-COVID-19 world *Nigel Saunders*	319
17.4	Case study: Central England Co-operative society *Luke Olly and Hannah Gallimore*	326
PART VI	**Engagement and proposed changes** *Richard Smith*	**333**
18	Soft and hard measures in optimising wellbeing through procurement, commissioning and partnering *Mark Cook*	338
19	Relational procurement: translating lessons learned from large infrastructural projects *Mike Bresnen, Sarah-Jane Lennie and Nick Marshall*	351
20	The impact of 'the lost decade' on developing a relational culture in public–private partnering *Michael Burton*	366
21	When the politically impossible becomes the politically inevitable: has the moment arrived for the wholesale adoption of relationism? *Nigel Ball*	376
	Conclusion *Adrian Bonner*	392
	Appendix	402
	Index	407

List of figures and tables

Figures

I.1	Number of deaths in WHO regions from 1 January 2020 to 8 May 2020	6
I.2	Five elements of a framework to assess England's response to COVID-19	9
I.3	Social determinants of health: Policy Press publications reflecting the impact of socioeconomic change on health and wellbeing	12
1.1	Trust-based relationships and relational work	32
5.1	Combined Authorities in England and the North East region	89
5.2	Integrated care systems were being constructed and operated in the region as COVID-19 progressed	93
6.1	Taxes collected at the federal and local level as a percentage of total tax revenue	103
8.1	Share of UK gross domestic product at current prices	156
8.2	Social and public value	157
9.1	Changes in components of spending power in English local authorities, 2010–2011 to 2020–2021	172
9.2	Level of deprivation and gross rates payable per capita by billing authority	173
9.3	Commercial property purchases by English local authorities, 2010–2011 to 2018–2019	175
9.4	Debt servicing costs as a share of spending power in English local authorities, 2010–2011 to 2018–2019	176
9.5	Change in demand in key local authority service areas in England	178
9.6	Year on year changes in prices	179
9.7	Change in service spend by English local authorities, gross of sales, fees and charges, 2010–2011 to 2018–2019	180
9.8	Social care as a share of service spend	181
9.9	Cost pressures in local authorities	183
9.10	Cost pressures in district councils, metropolitan districts, London Boroughs and County Councils	185
9.11	Great Manchester Combined Authority's geographical boundaries with Clinical Commissioning Groups, Fire and Rescue Authorities, Sustainability and Transformation Plan footprints and Police force boundaries	189
10.1	The difference in carbon emissions between the leading emitters and the rest of the world	196
11.1a	New homes, 1969–2020: yearly	213
11.1b	New homes, 1969–2020: every three years	214

11.1c	New homes, 1969–2020: every five years	215
11.2	Affordable homes, 1991–2020	218
15.1	Standing Together Against Domestic Abuse, 2020	272
16.1	The Malachi Project, a pop-up hostel	291
16.2	Nationalities of potential victims who entered support managed by The Salvation Army in 2019–2020	298
17.1	Centre for Partnering exemplar showing relational dividend	310
17.2	UK nominal house prices, 1991–2015	313
VI.1	The types of projects forming part of the Exemplar Initiative and the need for new types of partners to deliver a relational dividend	335
VI.2	The major impact of a relational partnering environment compared with a more traditional approach, with a particular focus on the need for equal partners balancing social and commercial value	336
19.1	Summary model of public–private commissioning and contracting	360
A.1	The five aims of the Centre for Partnering	404
A.2	Evolution of the Centre for Partnering and relationalism	405
A.3	The Centre for Partnering: a 'facilitating' organisation	406

Tables

I.1	Ten criteria which could be ascribed to the term 'wicked issue'	3
I.2	Responses from authors who responded to the editor's request to rate the content of their chapters against the ten criteria which could be ascribed to the term 'wicked issue'	4
1.1	Competing/complementary forms of knowledge	25
10.1	The 21 highest emitters of carbon by nation-state, 2018	197
10.2	The 21 per capita highest emitters of carbon by nation-state, 2018	198
10.3	Cumulative CO_2 emissions, 1900–2004	199
11.1	Housing tenure, 2007 and 2017	219
13.1	Levels of social innovation	249
13.2	Framework for examples of collaboration and innovation	250
16.1	The current provision of The Salvation Army's Homelessness Services Unit services in the UK	287
16.2	The Salvation Army's Homelessness Services Unit services in Dublin	288
16.3a	User satisfaction survey of service users in November 2020 indicating very satisfied or satisfied	289
16.3b	User satisfaction survey February/March 2021	290

Notes on contributors

Editor

Adrian Bonner's current research focuses on the impact of economic austerity policies on health, social care and housing strategies, reflected in the publications *Social Determinants of Health: An Interdisciplinary Approach to Social Inequality and Wellbeing* (Policy Press, 2018) and *Local Authorities and Social Determinants of Health* (Policy Press, 2020). A key theme emerging from these books is the recognition of the need for relationships at an individual level, and partnerships between the public, private and third sectors in addressing the range of complex issues (wicked issues) related to the social determinants of health. *Local Authorities and Social Determinants of Health*, the second book in the social determinants series, has provided a platform for the development of the Centre for Partnering (CfP), co-founded by Adrian and other contributors in this book. CfP is a network of universities working with the public, private and third sectors.

Adrian's early research was concerned with neurobiological aspects of alcohol, as reflected in publications and teaching activities in the 1990s at the Universities of Surrey and Kent. At this time, he became Chairman of the Congress of the European Society for Biomedical Research into Alcohol (Bonner, 2005). *Social Exclusion and the Way Out: An Individual and Community Response to Human Social Dysfunction* (Bonner, 2006) provided the basis for research into *The Seeds of Exclusion* (Bonner et al, 2008), a major report that continues to influence Salvation Army strategic planning. These activities were undertaken while he was a Reader in the Centre for Health Service Studies, University of Kent, and was Director of the Addictive Behaviour Group, which facilitated the development of undergraduate and postgraduate teaching and research activities.

From 2010 to 2012, he was seconded from the University of Kent to become the Director of the Institute of Alcohol Studies. This involved participating in the UK government's Responsibility Deal and membership of the European Alcohol Health Forum, an advisory group supporting the work of the European Commission. These insights into UK and European policy development have influenced his current activities, which include interdisciplinary research into health inequalities, membership of HealthWatch and the Joint Mental Health and Wellbeing Clinical Commissioning Group in the London Borough of Sutton. He is an honorary Professor in the Faculty of Social Sciences, University of Stirling, and Director for Communities, Health and Wellbeing, Centre for Partnering.

- Bonner, A. (ed) (2020) *Local Authorities and Social Determinants of Health*, Bristol: Policy Press.
- Bonner, A. (ed) (2018) *Social Determinants of Health: An Interdisciplinary Approach to Social Inequality and Wellbeing*, Bristol: Policy Press.
- Bonner, A. and Gilmore, I. (2012) 'The UK Responsibility Deal and its Implications for Effective Alcohol Policy in the UK and Internationally'. *Addiction*, 107: 2063–2065.
- Bonner, A., Luscombe, C., van den Bree, M. and Taylor P.J. (2008) *The Seeds of Exclusion*, London: The Salvation Army.
- Bonner A. (2006) *Social Exclusion and the Way Out: An Individual and Community Response to Human Social Dysfunction*, John Wiley & Sons, Chichester, UK..
- Bonner, A. (ed) (2005) *10th Congress of the European Society for Biomedical Research into Alcohol*, Canterbury 4–7 September 2005, Oxford: Oxford University Press.
- Bonner, A. and Waterhouse, J. (eds) (1996) *Addictive Behaviour: Molecules to Mankind*, Macmillan, Basingstoke, UK

Contributors

Manuel Abellan has been a councillor since 2014 in the London Borough of Sutton. He was Vice-Chair of the Environment and Neighbourhood Committee in Sutton from 2016 to 2018 and then appointed as Chair of the Environment and Sustainable Transport Committee in 2018 and Deputy Leader in 2020. He has also been Vice-Chair of the Transport and Environment Committee at London Councils since 2018. Manuel also worked for Tom Brake MP, Liberal Democrat for Carshalton and Wallington, between 2012 and 2019 in various capacities including as his Head of Office.

Dave Ayre is Property Networks Manager for the Chartered Institute of Public Finance and Accountancy and advises on asset management, partnering and wider property issues throughout the UK. He is a qualified public service manager with extensive experience in the development, procurement and implementation of innovative public/private partnerships. He has considerable local government experience and has also worked as a consultant to public and private sector organisations delivering public services. He has contributed at a national level to the development of successive government performance management regimes for planning, property and construction through the Planning Officers Society, the Local Government Construction Taskforce and Constructing Excellence, and written guidance on collaboration between public sector organisations. He is a regular contributor to articles in the local government and housing media. He is author of CIPFA's 'Guide to Local Authority and Public Sector Asset Management'.

Nigel Ball is Executive Director of the Government Outcomes Lab (GO Lab), which is based in Oxford University's Blavatnik School of Government. Nigel leads the work of engaging with decision-makers in government and beyond who are involved in efforts to improve social outcomes through cross-sector partnering. Prior to joining the GO Lab, Nigel was part of the founding team of West London Zone for Children and Young People, leveraging multiple public and private sources of funding towards a partnership of mainly local charities to support at-risk children to achieve better outcomes. Nigel's previous roles include being Head of Innovation at Teach First, the leading education charity, and supporting social entrepreneurship in East Africa. He is a qualified teacher, having learnt his craft in a secondary school in Eccles, Manchester. He holds a first class BA in English and Linguistics from the University of York.

Michael Bennett is Director of the Centre for Partnering and of Public Intelligence. He is an advisor to a range of public and governmental organisations as well as to private companies. Previously he was Director of the Society of Local Authority Chief Executives where he held a number of senior policy roles.

Claire Bonham is Chief Executive of the IARS International Institute, a youth-focused international research organisation. She has 20 years' experience working in the voluntary sector, having worked in national strategic roles for various organisations championing the causes of children, the elderly, victims of crime, homelessness and poverty around the world. Claire regularly delivers training across the sector and is a regular guest speaker on a Policy Officer Apprenticeships programme. Claire holds a PhD in International Relations and a Masters in Critical Global Studies. She has contributed book chapters and journal articles on various aspects of her work, including criminal justice and working with marginalised communities.

Mike Bresnen is Professor of Organisation Studies at Manchester Metropolitan University Business School, having worked previously at the universities of Manchester, Leicester, Warwick, Cardiff and Loughborough. He has researched and published widely on healthcare managers, on the organisation and management of projects (with particular reference to the construction industry) and on learning and innovation in project-based settings. His most recent funded research has been on healthcare management and leadership in the National Health Service, project-based learning in construction, manufacturing and services (Engineering and Physical Sciences

Research Council) and biomedical innovation processes in the UK and US (Economic and Social Research Council).

Michael Burton has spent over 30 years as a journalist and editor covering the public sector. After training on local newspapers he was for 20 years editor of *The Municipal Journal* (*MJ*), the market-leading weekly title for UK local government and then editorial director of *The MJ* and its events business where among other duties he arranged conference agendas with senior civil servants and public and private sector senior executives. He is also a board director of *The MJ*'s parent publishing and events company the Hemming Group and is the author of three books, *The Politics of Public Sector Reform from Thatcher to the Coalition* (Palgrave Macmillan, 2013), *The Politics of Austerity: A Recent History* (Palgrave Macmillan, 2016) and *The Lost Decade: Britain from Broke to Brexit* (Palgrave Macmillan, 2022).

Rita Chadha was Chief Executive Officer of the Small Charities Coalition and has spent more than 30 years working with charities and not-for-profits. She has led charities working locally and nationally and is in her spare time an active volunteer in her local community, and a trustee of three other charities. Rita has particular specialisms in governance, localism, equality and diversity as they relate to the intersection between the not-for-profit sector and public sector.

Tsitsi Chawatama is Consultant Paediatrician in London. She has specialist interests in Global Health and medical education and has been a Royal College of Paediatrics and Child Health Deputy College Tutor. She is passionate about empowering others to care for the world's most vulnerable children through capacity building, training and programme development and has worked extensively in the non-governmental organisation and development sector. Her board appointments have included UK-Med, AFRUCA-Safeguarding Children, Sentebale, and Chair of Trustees at Save the Children UK.

Brighton Chireka is General Practitioner (GP) and a Certified Lifestyle Physician in Kent and Medway Clinical Commissioning Group at NHS Kent, where he is the named GP for Safeguarding. His initial training was at the University of Zimbabwe. He is an international health consultant and has an award in the NHS Leadership Academy, in Executive Healthcare Leadership. He is a Founding Fellow of the Faculty of Medical Leadership and Management and he is also an Honorary Fellow at Teesside University.

Mark Cook is Partner at Anthony Collins Solicitors, having advised on procurement and public–private partnerships for 30 years. He is the lawyer who has most contributed to the inclusion of community benefits at the core of public contracts in the United Kingdom. He contributed to the drafting of the Public Services (Social Value) Act 2012 and the content of the Procurement Reform (Scotland) Act 2014. He also contributed to the Can Do Toolkits in Wales. He is company secretary to catalytic do-tank Collaborate, and he is deeply committed to creating alternatives to the commissioner–contractor dynamic.

Victoria Cooling is a specialty registrar in public health based in North East England. She is passionate about improving population health outcomes and reducing health inequalities and has 20 years' experience working in a diverse range of health and care organisation's at a local and regional level. Working across traditional organisational boundaries to tackle complex public health challenges and deliver system-wide transformation, improve healthcare quality and improve the health and wellbeing of the population. Victoria has a Master's in Public Health, an MSc in Healthcare Management, a Diploma in Reflective Practice and is a graduate of the NHS Management Training Scheme.

Adam Cunnington was, most recently, Chief Executive of Public Sector Plc, a proponent of relational partnering through its strategic property partnerships with councils across the country. Together these partnerships have delivered substantial financial, economic and social value to the communities in which they operate. Prior to joining Public Sector Plc, Adam was a Development Director at Land Securities, the country's largest listed property company and was responsible for the 17 million sq ft new settlement being developed at Ebbsfleet Valley in Kent.

Tony Daniels' working background and experience for the last 15 years has comprised of performance management and senior management roles including: working for Milton Keynes Council as a Senior Strategic Implementation Manager delivering the National Sure Start Programme, as a Senior Programme Manager for Bedfordshire YMCA Hostels, as a Divisional Director of Community Services for The Salvation Army. All of the aforementioned roles have been related to driving up quality, delivery and overall service performance, as well as shaping and writing strategy. Tony is also a professionally qualified Youth and Community Worker, who worked as an Area Youth Worker for Northamptonshire County Council, as a paid Volunteer Development Officer for Northampton University, as a visiting lecturer at Leicester University (as a consultant on behalf of the National Youth Agency) and as a visiting lecturer at Bedfordshire University on their Youth and Community Degree Course.

Annie Dell holds a Masters in Public Policy from Kings College London, and was Policy Adviser for The Salvation Army UK and Ireland. She specialises in social policy, particularly around employment and welfare.

Anne-Marie Douglas is the contract manager of the Home Office Victim Care Contract awarded to The Salvation Army, which she has directed since the operational delivery on 1 July 2011. Anne-Marie manages the prime contract, which has provided wide ranging support to many thousands of potential and confirmed victims of human trafficking and modern slavery, via 12 subcontracting organisations. A former civil servant, Ann-Marie was employed by the equivalent of the Department for Work and Pensions for 21 years before moving on to the NHS Business Services Authority, where she spent 11 years and played a significant role in the restructuring of the Authority. Ann-Marie is a solutions focused leader with extensive experience in operational management and strategic leadership.

Hannah Gallimore is Corporate Responsibility Manager and Social Change Manager at Central England Co-operative. She gained a postgraduate degree in legal practice from the University of Birmingham. Hannah is committed to community development as demonstrated by the innovative project to use corporate funding to support the rehabilitation of people in contact with the criminal justice system into the community.

Anne Gregora is a registered social worker, graduating at the University of Queensland, Australia. She has worked in direct practice to support people from a refugee background to resettle and survivors of trafficking in a safe house context. For the past eight years, she has worked with The Salvation Army in the United Kingdom, coordinating the organisation's international modern slavery and human trafficking response. She is a trustee for a charity working with women in London who have survived trafficking and sexual exploitation. Anne is deeply passionate about human rights and social justice so that everyone can experience life in all its fullness.

Tribeni Gurung is International Projects Advisor, specialising in modern slavery and anti-human trafficking projects, at The Salvation Army UK. Working across Europe, Africa, South Asia and South East Asia, Tribeni has extensive project management experience and works alongside Salvation Army UK partners in providing technical support to develop context-specific anti-trafficking responses. Tribeni has a background in research and has an MSc in Social Research Methodology from the London School of Economics. She is passionate about seeking justice and bringing change using a research and evidence-based approach. More recently, Tribeni co-led a research piece commissioned by the International Anti-Human Trafficking

Network and Joint Learning Initiative that focused on how the international anti-trafficking response has adapted to COVID-19.

Emily Hodge is Commissioning Manager and Domestic Abuse Lead, London Borough of Sutton and Geographic Lead for London/South East England, Practice and Partnerships Team, Domestic Abuse Commissioner's Office. Prior to this role, Emily worked in strategic operations roles for an advocacy charity and before that for a local Volunteer Centre, delivering non-statutory support services as part of the prevention and early intervention agenda. Emily has led a number of change agendas in various organisations, and was a co-producer in the development of Sutton's developmental assets model that was adopted by the borough to measure added social value. Rooted in her local area and committed to seeing people's lives improve, Emily is deeply involved in community development where she lives and the community sponsorship of a Syrian family who are resettling in the UK (UNHCR programme).

David J. Hunter is Professor of Health Policy and Management, Institute of Health and Society, Newcastle University. David graduated in political science from Edinburgh University. His academic career spans over 40 years researching complex health systems with a focus on how health policy is formed and implemented. Between 1999 and July 2017, David was Director of the Centre for Public Policy and Health at Durham University. The Centre was designated a WHO Collaborating Centre in Complex Health Systems Research, Knowledge and Action in 2014. In August 2017 he transferred to the Institute of Health and Society, Newcastle University and became an Emeritus Professor in August 2018. Recent former positions include being a non-executive director of the National Institute of Health and Care Excellence (2008–2016); an Appointed Governor of South Tees Hospitals NHS Foundation Trust (2009–2017); and a special advisor to the UK Parliamentary Health Committee. He is an Honorary Member of the UK Faculty of Public Health, and Fellow of the Royal College of Physicians (Edinburgh).

Edward Kunonga is Director for Population Health Management for the North of England Commissioning Support as well as a consultant in public health working for Tees Esk and Wear Valley Mental Health NHS Foundation Trust and County Durham and Darlington Acute NHS Foundation Trust. Edward spent nine years as Director of Public Health and Public Protection for Middlesbrough Council, with the last three years of that tenure being the joint director of public health across Middlesbrough and Redcar and Cleveland Borough Councils (the first joint public health service in the North East). As part of this arrangement Edward was instrumental in the development of the joint health and wellbeing board across these two local authorities, chief officer for emergency preparedness and response for the council as well as taking a regional lead role for public mental health. Edward has Honorary Professorship at Teesside University and contributes to a wide range of teaching and research activities.

Lallian Kunga is Secretary for Programme Administration and Territorial Contact Person for Modern Slavery and Human Trafficking for The Salvation Army India East Territory. In 2018, Lieutenant Colonel Lallian Kunga was Director of the territories' anti-human trafficking project which involved creating awareness in communities and supporting the repatriation of trafficked survivors. As one of the only anti-trafficking responses in Mizoram state, Lieutenant Colonel Lallian Kunga mobilised more than 100 volunteers to respond to modern slavery and human trafficking in their local communities. He has worked closely with many partners including the police in Mizoram state and government at various levels to address the problem and to respond to vulnerabilities faced by people during the COVID-19 pandemic. Today Lieutenant Colonel Lallian Kunga is recognised as one of the focal persons in driving the anti-trafficking agenda in Mizoram state.

Vijaya Lama is President of The LightHouse Foundation, Nepal, and has been working closely with vulnerable and discriminated communities, especially those who are at risk of exploitation. The Christian Community School is also an affiliation of the LightHouse Foundation where Vijaya holds the position of Chief Executive Officer. At this school victims who have been rescued from trafficking or exploitation are given education, healthcare and accommodation. In addition to this, Vijaya is the Sub-Coordinator of Gokarneshwor Municipality under the Government of Nepal and within this position he works closely with local organisations to help children and women who are at risk of trafficking to India and other countries. Vijaya has always been passionate about helping the most vulnerable communities in Nepal.

Sarah-Jane Lennie is Lecturer in the Police, Organisation and Policy Department of the Open University Business School. She is a chartered psychologist and was previously Research Associate in Organisational Studies and Behaviour at Manchester Metropolitan University. Sarah-Jane lectures in business psychology, specialising in emotions in the work place and mental health and well-being. Prior to returning to academia Sarah-Jane served for 18 years as a police officer, to the rank of detective inspector. Sarah-Jane is an associate to the College of Policing as a subject matter expert. She is also an ambassador for Police Care UK, a charity supporting police officers and their families, and committee member of the Association of Business Psychology, North West Branch.

Joyce Liddle is Professor of Public Leadership and Enterprise, Director of Research and KE, Newcastle BS, Northumbria. Joyce was formerly Professor of Public Leadership and Management at Institute de Management Public et Gouvernance, Aix-Marseille Université, France. A graduate of the University of Durham, Joyce has a doctorate from the University of Warwick and has held previous senior academic roles at Nottingham Business School, University of Nottingham, University of Durham, Sunderland and Teesside Business Schools. Previously Honorary Chair of the UK Joint University Council, Fellow of UK Academy of Social Sciences, Fellow of Regional Studies Association and Fellow of Joint University Council, Joyce holds (or has held) Visiting Professorships at the Universities of Eastern Finland, Tor Vergata, Rome, Paul Cezanne, France, Northumbria, Edge Hill and Glasgow Caledonian. Joyce has published over 200 articles, 25 book chapters and 14 books, co-edits an Annual Book series on Critical Perspectives on International Public Management, chairs the Editorial Advisory Board for the *International Journal of Public Sector Management* (Joyce was Editor in Chief and Book Review Editor for 14 years), and is consulting editor or Education Technology, Services and Research member on six other international journals in public management and leadership, regional and local governance and development.

Nishan Lo is an officer, pastor and one of the founding members at The Salvation Mission in Nepal. Since its establishment in 2009, Captain Nishan has been involved in various community development work such as working with vulnerable groups and responding to emergencies. In 2013, Captain Nishan had a prominent role in implementing the Salvation Mission's anti-trafficking project that focused on preventing and protecting vulnerable women and survivors of trafficking. Captain Nishan is also leading the Salvation Mission's COVID-19 response in Nepal. His main role in this response is to coordinate with the government and other stakeholders to assist hospitals and communities by distributing materials, medical equipment and food packages as well as establishing isolation facilities for people who have tested positive for the virus.

Nick Marshall is Senior Research Fellow in the Centre for Change, Entrepreneurship, and Innovation Management (CENTRIM) at the University of Brighton. He is academic lead for CENTRIM's research group on Organisational Change and Renewal. His research focuses on organisational knowledge, learning, and innovation. He is particularly interested in the social and political practices of producing, negotiating, and using knowledge within varied organisational settings, but especially project-based, network, and temporary forms of organising. He is the Chair of the Special Interest Group on Innovation of the British Academy of Management. He holds an MA in geography from St. Peter's College, Oxford and a PhD in economic geography from King's College, London.

Anna Matheson is Senior Lecturer in Health Policy in the School of Health, Te Herenga Waka, Victoria University of Wellington, New Zealand. She has a background in public health with a focus on understanding the nature of health inequality and the effectiveness of approaches to intervention. Much of her work has examined the policy/community relationship as a key contributor to enabling communities to act effectively on their own needs. Anna currently leads the Evaluation of Healthy Families NZ, a multicommunity health and wellbeing initiative, and is a Principal Investigator with Te Pūnaha Matatini – New Zealand's Centre of Research Excellence for Complex Systems.

Drew McCombe is Secretary for Mission with responsibilities for the oversight of Salvation Army operations across the UK and Ireland. In this senior national leadership role, Drew oversees the extensive range of church and community-focused services, examples of which are presented in Case studies 16.1–16.4. Drew is a Salvation Army officer working in local churches prior to moving into regional and national leadership roles. He has an MA in evangelism and mission.

Peter McKinlay has more than 30 years' experience as a researcher and adviser on local governance and local government. As well as New Zealand, he has worked extensively in Australia, including NSW, Victoria and South Australia. He has been an active member of the Research Advisory Group of the Commonwealth Local Government Forum, and co-edited for it the book *New Century Local Government* (Commonwealth Secretariat) in 2020. He has published widely on aspects of local government and local governance, presented at numerous conferences both in New Zealand and internationally, and maintains an extensive network of international researchers and practitioners on local governance. His present focus is on reorienting New Zealand's local government sector so that it is able to play a much more substantial role in the governance of its communities, including working with central government on developing an effective wellbeing policy.

Andrew Morton is Labour Market Policy Officer at the Employment Related Services Association (ERSA). Andrew graduated with a Doctorate in political economy from the University of Leeds in 2019 and currently holds in Research Fellowship in Global Health Policy, also at the University of Leeds. Andrew has pursued research in various social policy, employment and healthcare subjects and started working at ERSA in 2021.

Alex Murdock is Professor Emeritus, London South Bank University, Business School, and has board level and organisational development experience (including two Chair roles) in charities and social business enterprises. Alex has authored or co-authored six books and numerous other publications, and is the co-editor of *International Public Management Review*. Alex is on the Editorial Board of various journals and currently co-editor of a special issue of *Voluntas* (a leading management journal), with residential academic roles in the US, Denmark, France and Germany, Potsdam University, Institute for Public Management, Berlin. Alex is a Visiting Professor (2012–Current) Universities of Cagliari and Turin, Italy, Visiting Professor 2019 and 2020, and University of Rennes, Laboratoire interdisciplinaire de Recherche en Innovations Sociétales LiRIS (2016–current), Arizona State University, Center for Organizational Research and Design USA, Visiting Fellow (2014–current).

Aileen Murphie has been Director of Ministry for Housing, Communities and Local Government and local government value for money at the National Audit Office from 2013 to March 2021. She has published reports to parliament on the financial sustainability of local authorities, most recently a ground-breaking report on local authority commercial investments. She has also reported regularly on adult social care, most recently on the effect of the COVID-19 pandemic on the social system, readying the NHS and adult social care for the pandemic, highlighting that the public sector response was hampered by long-standing issues including lack of integration locally. On housing, she has published 'Housing in England: an overview, homelessness, planning for new homes' and a progress review of the government's biggest housing initiative, help to buy. A regular commentator on live issues in local government, including local economic growth and devolution, she is also honorary professor at Durham University Business School.

Peter Murphy is Professor of Public Policy and Management and Director of the Public Policy and Management Research Group at Nottingham Business School, Nottingham Trent University. Prior to joining the Business School in 2009, he was a Senior Civil Servant in four Whitehall departments between 2000 and 2009 and spent 23 years in local government most recently as Chief Executive of Melton Borough Council in Leicestershire. His research focuses on public policy and public service delivery, and in particular the performance management, governance, scrutiny, public assurance, and value-for-money arrangements of public services. Peter specialises in practically based and applied research. Between 2010 and 2020 he was Vice Chair of the Leaned Society for Public Administration, and Vice Chair (Research) of the Public Administration Committee of the Joint Universities Council.

Chris O'Leary is a public policy specialist and Deputy Director of the Policy Evaluation and Research Unit at Manchester Metropolitan University. He has written and commented on issues around commissioning and procurement, particularly on the barriers faced by local charities and small businesses. His empirical research focuses on social innovation, particularly where different parts of social provision interact. Much of his published research is around housing/homelessness and its interaction with health and social care, and the criminal justice system

Luke Olly spends his days looking for problems to solve such as high fuel bills, waste and getting people living more sustainably as Energy and Environment Manager at Central England Co-operative, a regional convenience food retailer and funeral provider, and as Chair of Ecobirmingham, a West Midlands based sustainability charity. He currently leads on the creation and delivery of a business wide sustainability strategy, including carbon reduction programs across the built environment and refrigeration, and the development innovative ways to deal with traditional waste streams such as food waste and plastics. He is a Full member of the Institute of Environmental Management and Assessment and a Chartered Environmentalist with ten years' experience working in the sustainability sector.

Dean Pallant is Secretary for Communications at The Salvation Army and was previously Director of The Salvation Army's International Social Justice Commission based in New York City. Born and bred in Zimbabwe, his doctoral studies at King's College London resulted in the publication of his first book, *Keeping Faith in Faith-Based Organisations* in 2012. Dean was a founding member of the Joint Learning Initiative on Faith and Local Communities (www.jliflc.com).

Selina Palm is an interdisciplinary researcher-activist based at the Unit for Religion and Development Research at Stellenbosch University, South Africa. She has delivered research or projects work in 15 countries across four continents with over 15 years of community development experience in sub-Saharan Africa around HIV and AIDS and vulnerable populations. She has published in the fields of human rights, practice-based knowledge, violence against women, children and queer bodies, reproductive justice, disability, and the role of hope in social transformation. She holds a PhD in the intersections between religion, culture and human rights. She specialises in ending violence against women and children and the complex roles of religion and has delivered a webinar series on the impact of COVID-19 on women and children and the roles of local faith actors.

Jenny Pattinson gained her experience of what it means to deliver outstanding care during her time managing regulatory Inspection teams for the Care Quality Commission and previously the Healthcare Commission. Jenny is also a local councillor for Watford Borough Council, Leader of the Liberal Democrat Group and a Cabinet member, holding the Portfolio for Wellbeing and Mental Health. Jenny was Director of Older People's Services at The Salvation Army until 2022, where she led the teams delivering care that is 'Rooted in Love' to older vulnerable adults living in The Salvation Army's residential care homes.

Tim Reade is a professionally qualified chartered surveyor and leads the Chartered Institute of Public Finance and Accountancy's (CIPFA) Property Advisory Team delivering network activity and consultancy to multiple public sector clients. Tim joined CIPFA in October 2017 from Savills where he specialised in property and asset management. Having qualified with DTZ Investments and later moved to Savills, Tim brings a wealth of private sector property and asset management experience to the Property Advisory Services (PAS) team, which he leads. In addition to his employment with CIPFA as head of PAS, Tim is a Lieutenant Colonel in the Army Reserve. As a proven team leader and manager, Tim ensures the PAS team provides well informed, concise and timely public sector network events which are supplemented, where required, with support and consultancy on a client by client basis.

Nicholas Redmore is Director of The Salvation Army Homeless Services unit. This extensive management role provides overall strategic and operational responsibility of The Salvation Army's Homelessness Services across the United Kingdom and Republic of Ireland. Prior to this role Nick was Director of the Research and Development Unit. Graduating in addiction studies at the University of Kent, he has over 30 years of extensive experience in leading and managing homelessness services locally and regionally in England and Wales.

Nigel Saunders is an Institute of Directors qualified board director at Pozzoni Architecture, with extensive expertise in delivering architectural services across the public, private and third sectors. While much of his work is within the housing sector, he also works with schools, colleges and universities, together with healthcare providers. He has a particular expertise in designing for our ageing population, being passionate about intergenerational living and its role in delivering social benefits. He has been one of the driving forces behind Pozzoni's designs for a theoretical mixed use urban community, with senior and general needs living alongside care, leisure, learning and other supporting facilities. Nigel is a contributor to the All-Party Parliamentary Group on Housing and Care for Older People and is an active member of Greater Manchester Combined Authority's, Ageing Hub 'Housing and Planning Group', which aims to address the city region's housing options for older people. Nigel has a passion for building strong long-term relationships by understanding the needs of clients, community and stakeholders. A significant proportion of his work is secured via competitive procurement routes, whether via framework agreements or project tenders.

Joanna Sharpless is a palliative care physician at Beth Israel Deaconess Medical Center (BIDMC) and an Instructor of Medicine at Harvard Medical School in Boston, Massachusetts, US. She received her bachelor's degree in English literature and her medical degree from Brown University. After graduating from residency in Family and Social Medicine at Montefiore Medical Center in the Bronx, New York, she continued on to the Harvard Interprofessional Palliative Care Fellowship Program at Massachusetts General Hospital and Dana-Farber Cancer Institute. Since 2019, she has been full-time faculty at BIDMC, where she is committed to providing outstanding palliative care to hospitalised patients with serious illnesses, including COVID-19, and to educating future palliative care leaders. Her other interests include narrative medicine and advocating for social justice in medicine. Her writing has appeared in *Time Magazine*, *Academic Medicine*, *The Journal of Pain and Symptom Management* and *The Journal of Palliative Medicine*, among others.

John Shutt is Professor of Public Policy and Management at Newcastle Business School, Northumbria University, United Kingdom. He is a Visiting Professor to the Amsterdam University of Applied Sciences and the Amsterdam Campus of Northumbria University. John works in the public sector and has research interests in urban and regional economic development and regional and urban governance. Previously employed at Leeds Beckett University and Manchester University John directed the European Research Institute in Leeds and prior to that worked at Manchester University in the Department of Geography. Between 1989 and 1994 he was Deputy Director of the Centre for Local Economic Strategies, the local authority economic think tank based in Manchester and he has worked in policy roles for both Sheffield and Birmingham City Councils. John is interested in leadership for change in the public sector and leadership in economic development and regeneration and is an active member of the Regional Studies Association.

Richard Simmons is Professor in Public and Social Policy and Co-Director of the Mutuality Research Programme at the University of Stirling. Over the last decade or so he has led an extensive programme of research on voice and cooperation in public policy. This includes four studies funded by the Economic and Social Research Council/Arts and Humanities Research Council, a Single Regeneration Budget-funded study, and work for the National Health Service, Scottish Executive, National Consumer Council, Carnegie Trust, Organisation for Economic Co-operation and Development, World Bank, Co-operatives UK, Nesta and the Care Inspectorate. He is currently working on an EU (H2020) project working with local municipal governments and schools to improve the quality of primary school meals through better procurement. He writes widely on these issues for academic, policy and practitioner audiences. His book, *The Consumer in Public Services*, is published by the Policy Press. As well as a series of journal articles in high-quality international journals such as *Social Policy and Administration*, *Policy and Politics*, *Annals of Public and Co-operative Economics* and *Public Policy and Administration*, Richard has written a number of policy-oriented publications and professional journal articles for a practitioner audience. His research interests are broadly in the field of user voice, the governance, delivery and innovation of public services and the role of mutuality and co-operation in public policy. The Mutuality Research Programme has acquired an international reputation as a centre of excellence for research, knowledge exchange and consultancy on these issues.

Richard Smith has enjoyed various senior management positions in both public and private sectors. Qualifying as a barrister in 1978 he initially worked within GEC-Marconi and then was appointed as director of Contract Services (1988) and Head of Businesses (1991) for Portsmouth City Council where he was instrumental in the introduction of the council's internal market (1991–1995). He founded Public Sector Plc in 2006, a private sector organisation utilising a new and innovative legal framework based on a cultural relationship between partners forming in advance of formal legal commitments. In 2019, he established the Centre for Partnering (CfP), in partnership with Adrian Bonner, as a new organisation initially bringing together five universities. CfP is focused on developing and introducing the idea of relationalism and in evidencing the relational dividend that arises from its application. An aim of CfP will be to accredit organisations and individuals in the use of relationalism utilising a knowledge base compiled from the CfP's Exemplar Projects Initiative. Richard is an honorary professor at the University of Stirling and chairman of the CfP.

Elizabeth Taylor is Chief Executive of the Employment Related Services Association (ERSA). Coming from the employment support sector, she secured her first job as an advisor in 1983. She soon became involved in national and international policy work. Elizabeth spoke at the World

Conference for Youth on Employment Strategies on Vancouver Island in 1986 and has continued to contribute, network and share. From 1989 to 2019 Elizabeth managed the delivery of employment support, enterprise support (including social enterprise) and training programmes, delivered with 23 different funding streams including- local authorities, Training Agency, Training and Enterprise Councils, Urban Programme, ESF, ERDF, City Challenge, Single Regeneration Budget, Employment Services, Jobcentre Plus, Department for Work and Pensions (DWP), City Strategy Pathfinder, DWP District Managers Flexible Support Fund, Primary Care Trust, Care Trust Plus, Department of Health, the Future Jobs Fund, National Lottery Building Better Opportunities, Esme Fairbairn, Tudor Trust and the Lloyds TSB Foundation. Elizabeth became ERSA's Chief Executive in 2018.

Wendy Wasels has over 27 years' volunteering and working experience in the third sector. At the Royal Society for the Prevention of Cruelty to Animals (RSPCA) she managed the Community Fundraising function facilitating the raising of over £4 million through partnership working with a major supermarket chain for local animal welfare work. Working as a project manager she was responsible for implementing a number of major projects to harness the involvement of volunteers including the RSPCA's wildlife casualty first-responder scheme, animal befriender programme. She is now enjoying the challenge of supporting volunteerism across The Salvation Army and managing the piloting and implementation of their new volunteer data and engagement system. In her spare time Wendy runs a 90-strong community choir that entertains and raises funds in the Sussex area as well as a small acapella group to help people gain confidence through singing. Wendy has a BSc in Psychology from University College London and in 2020 obtained the ILM L5 Diploma in Leadership in Management.

Rob Whiteman is Chief Executive of the Chartered Institute of Public Finance and Accountancy (CIPFA). CIPFA is the only professional accountancy body in the world exclusively dedicated to public finance, working with donors, partner governments, accountancy bodies and the public sector to advance public finance and support better public services. Rob was previously a senior civil servant in the Home Office as Chief Executive of the UK Border Agency responsible for border security and immigration. Before that he worked as Managing Director of the Improvement and Development Agency, Chief Executive of the London Borough of Barking and Dagenham and Director of Resources at the London Borough of Lewisham. Rob is a well-known international speaker and commentator on public financial management and good governance.

Foreword

Richard Smith

When it comes to relationalism and the contribution it can make to the future of partnering of different organisations, there is a huge opportunity ahead of us. If we look back on the history of public and private sectors, there have been notable failures.

In the previous publication dealing with the subject of *Local Authorities and the Social Determinants of Health* there was concern expressed over local government's ability to continue to support their communities post-Brexit. Now with the advent of COVID-19 and the cost of living crisis, this concern must be multiplied and perhaps a predominant wicked issue for the foreseeable future.

In the UK and other countries the capacity of the public sector has never been more sorely tested through, in particular, the National Health Service and local authorities needing to support the care of the community and disadvantaged people. The notion of a relational approach was posed at the conclusion of *Local Authorities and the Social Determinants of Health*. This book evolves this thinking, particularly in the context of a relational cultural environment. The pandemic has brought about a seismic shock to national and global economies, leading to financial challenges which threaten the health and wellbeing of people and communities. It is now even more imperative that the partnering of the public, private and third sectors combine effectively to deliver enhanced public and social value, and address key social determinants of health. This book addresses the importance of relationalism. It also addresses some of the wicked issues raised hitherto in the previous volumes in the context of improving the partnering culture. In other words, in the context of more transparency and joint working, finding solutions and trust are crucially important. What beneficial effects can arise in the current environment through relationalism and how many of those complex wicked issues can more satisfactorily be dealt with?

A future partnership of equals facilitated within a regime promoting open dialogue can provide the necessary trust between contracting partners. It means re-skilling and training. The goals set within the UN Sustainability agenda (the 17th Goal) support this view.

The danger in a future partnering framework is an overemphasis on compliance with rules and regulation, especially related to commissioning and procurement. If the regime is too complex with too many regulations, this will lead to a stifling of innovation. On the other hand, too few rules will often lead to ambiguity and a tendency towards the status quo in order to resist challenge. On balance, the imposition of regulations should promote a new culture based upon relationships. This is to facilitate a culture of partnering equals. The regime should encourage both sides to offer a solution which is more heavily focused on outcomes than on contractual transactions.

From a procurement perspective, one important consideration is a recognition of the differing procurement functions within the Client role. The function of Commissioner, as specifier, should be differentiated from the more methodological client procurement process involving selection, appointment and implementation of partnerships. This goes to the essence of partnering culture and facilitates greater opportunity to introduce the idea of relationalism.

A wide network of individuals and organisations have come together in this publication to offer thoughts and ideas through their contributions on understanding the different cultural, social, economic, geopolitical and environmental perspectives of the public, private and third sectors. One of the objectives that is hoped will come from this collection of contributions is a set of recommendations affecting legal (procurement), and financial (accounting), rules and procedures.

This publication and the contributions within it are unique in that the ideas that are put forward are supported on an ongoing developmental basis through a number of intersectoral discussion groups made up of academics, practitioners, clients and commissioners, including senior experienced individuals from public, private and third sector organisations. Collectively they are represented within the Centre for Partnering.

In order to give some practical focus to the issue of relationalism and the social and commercial dividend that can arise from it, the Centre for Partnering has proposed the establishment of an 'Exemplar' programme. This initiative involves the creation of a relational environment through which a number of projects can be evolved. Through these projects it will be possible to develop a knowledge base based upon the differences that a relational culture can make to the public, private and third sectors. The longer term objective will be to disseminate the results of the Exemplar Projects Initiative through a form of accreditation involving re-skilling and change to behaviour of partners. The Exemplar Projects Initiative is presented in Part V.

An outcome from this initiative is the evidencing of the Relational Dividend in terms of the Functional, Financial, Social and Emotional value and then, through compilation of the knowledge base, to accredit organisations and individuals with an understanding of how to apply relationalism within public, third and private sectors.

Introduction

Adrian Bonner

This book focuses on the challenges of the COVID-19 pandemic currently dominating the agenda of global, national and local policymakers, from the perspective of the UK. This major public health crisis presents a threat which is impacting adversely on global economic structures, and exacerbating a number of pre-existing **wicked issues** ('difficult or impossible to solve because of incomplete, contradictory, and changing requirements, and not resolved by traditional "technical" managerial approaches to the provision of public services'; Rittel and Webber, 1973). These interlinked issues include climate change, racial justice, austerity, housing and homelessness, employment, domestic abuse, human trafficking and modern slavery.

'The pandemic is unequal in three ways: it has killed unequally, been experienced unequally and will impoverish unequally' (Bambra et al, 2021). Climate change, another wicked issue, identified as a major global threat to human existence, impacts disproportionately on these socioeconomic challenges, across countries and communities. The additive adverse consequences of the two global challenges of COVID-19 and climate change present significant challenges at local, national and global levels, within the geopolitical context of inequalities.

The interconnectivity and interdependence of the domains of the rainbow model of social determinants of health as described by Dahlgren and Whitehead (1991) can be used to examine the response and impact of the COVID-19 pandemic and climate change, affecting people and communities around the world. The rainbow model of health described by Dahlgren and Whitehead was explored in *Social Determinants of Health: Social Inequality and Wellbeing*, published in 2018 by Policy Press (Bonner, 2018). In that first volume of the social determinants of health series, poor nutrition, alcohol-related harm, homelessness, mental health, learning disabilities, health and wellbeing in the digital society were reviewed by practitioners, service managers and academics from a range of life and social sciences disciplines. The health and wellbeing of people at the lower end of the social gradient was viewed from psycho-socio-geopolitical perspectives in 2018, nine years into UK austerity policies launched after the global economic downturn in 2008. An important set of indicators of social inequalities in the UK, at that time, was presented in the Marmot Review (Marmot, 2010).

The second Marmot Review (2020) indicated that, within a decade, there had been a significant increase in social and health inequalities experienced by many individuals and families being precariously situated in socially deprived and forgotten communities. This was reflected in the second volume in the social determinants of health series, *Local Authorities and Social Determinants of Health*, published in October 2020 (Bonner, 2020). That publication was developed during Brexit, the process of the UK leaving the EU. During the period, 2010 to 2020, the UK was suffering the consequences of a decade of austerity budgets. The sociopolitical issues discussed in *Local Authorities and Social Determinants of Health*, and the previous volume, include the health and wellbeing of people and communities which have been undermined by ongoing funding reductions in health and social care and local authorities, exacerbated by problems in implementing the Care Act (2014), and reorganisation of the National Health Service (NHS). There had been limited progress in integration of the NHS and the social care sector.

During the writing of *Local Authorities and Social Determinants of Health,* the COVID-19 pandemic began to generate immense pressures on the health systems, care homes for the elderly, social care and the homeless. Stresses within some families, related to lockdown, included reductions in family finances, due to unemployment (particularly in the hospitality and non-essential retailing businesses), loss of access to outside activities, homeschooling of children (sometimes without access to online support), loss of family support structures due to shielding of older relatives, and the loss of community assets and structures linked to the closure of churches, other places of worship and the hospitality industry. Locking down communities and COVID-19-related changes in the previous patterns of behaviour were associated with stress-related mental health associated with COVID-19 issues, increased chances of domestic abuse, and increased health and economic vulnerability in some households. Increased vulnerability to human trafficking and modern slavery (due to closure of businesses resulting in loss of personal and family income) was noted in the UK and other countries. In the UK, the higher levels of social and health inequalities in 2020, compared to 2010, left many people at the lower end of the social gradient with less resilience to cope with the pandemic than others. This was apparent in the age-related mortality data, which showed higher incidences of mortality in the lower socioeconomic groups, particularly in people who were elderly, homeless, Black, Asian and Minority Ethnic (BAME) groups, and people who lived and worked in less safe COVID-19 environments (see Case studies 7.1, 7.2, 16.1, 16.2, 16.3). The indirect impact of these challenges on children in the community is reviewed in Chapter 4.

Strategic planners at local and national levels have developed various approaches to tackling these apparently intractable problems, including a

Table I.1: Ten criteria which could be ascribed to the term 'wicked issue'

1	It does not have a definitive formulation
2	It does not have a 'stopping rule', that is, it does not have an inherent logic that signals when it is solved
3	There is no way to test the solution to this wicked problem
4	It cannot be studied by trial and error. The solutions are irreversible, every trial counts
5	The solutions are not true or false, only good or bad
6	There is no end to the number of solutions or approaches to this wicked problem
7	This wicked issue is essentially unique
8	This wicked problem can always be described as the symptoms of other wicked problems
9	The way this problem is described determines its possible solutions
10	Planners, who present solutions to this problems, should not be wrong. They are liable for the consequences of the solutions which they generate; the effects can significantly affect people touched by these actions

Source: Rittel and Webber (1973)

'system-based' approach, which included social and technical perspectives. Rittel and Webber pointed to the inappropriateness and lack of acceptance and lack of confidence, by society, of these strategic approaches. These planning approaches are inappropriate because: there can be no planning theory which is relevant to the whole of society; each problem has its own intrinsic quality; and because of the tension across society to address equality. The wickedness of these problems is identified by the ten characteristics listed in Table I.1. From these criteria both the COVID-19 pandemic and possibly climate change could be described as quintessential wicked issues (see Chapter 1). Table I.2 shows the responses from authors of this volume when asked to complete the checklist.

The progression of COVID-19

On 10 May 2022 the World Health Organization (WHO) reported 515,192,979 confirmed cases of COVID-19, and 6,254,140 deaths, globally. A total of 3,886,112,928 vaccine doses had been administered. Total global deaths has not yet approached the magnitude of previous viral pandemics such as the Black Death (1347–1351: 200 million deaths), Spanish Flu (1918–1919: 40–50 million deaths) and Aids/HIV (1981–present: 25–35 million deaths) (LePan, 2020). According to WHO reports, there is significant regional variation in number of deaths due to COVID-19 (see Figure I.1).

Table I.2: Responses from authors who responded to the editor's request to rate the content of their chapters against the ten criteria which could be ascribed to the term 'wicked issue'

	Wicked issue criteria	Yes	No	Unknown
1	It does not have a definitive formulation	HH LAF GBFV IJ TMS DA	HP	RX
2	It does not have a 'stopping rule', that is, it does not have an inherent logic that signals when it is solved	HH RX LAF TMS HP DA IJ		GBF GBFV
3	There is no way to test the solution to this wicked problem	DA IJ	HP GBFV RX LAF GBF TMS	HH
4	It cannot be studied by trial and error. The solutions are irreversible, every trial counts	HH DA GBFV IJ HP RX LAF TMS		
5	The solutions are not true or false, only good or bad	DA HP IJ RX LAF TMS	HH	GBFV
6	There is no end to the number of solutions or approaches to this wicked problem	RX DA LAF GBFV IJ	HH HP TMS	
7	This wicked issue is essentially unique	DA GBFV IJ HH LAF TMS	HP	

Table I.2: Responses from authors who responded to the editor's request to rate the content of their chapters against the ten criteria which could be ascribed to the term 'wicked issue' (continued)

	Wicked issue criteria	Yes	No	Unknown
8	This wicked problem can always be described as the symptoms of other wicked problems	HH HP DA GBFV IJ LAF TMS DA	RX	
9	The way this problem is described determines its possible solutions	HH HP DA RX LAF TMS GBFV IJ		
10	Planners, who present solutions to this problems, should not be wrong. They are liable for the consequences of the solutions which they generate; the effects can significantly affect people touched by these actions	HH RX LAF TMS HP DA GBFV IJ		

Note: HP: Housing Policy (Chapter 11); HH: housing and homelessness (Chapter 11, Case studies 16.1 and 17.2); DA: domestic abuse (Chapter 15); GBFV: gender-based family violence (Case study 7.2); IJ: intergenerational justice (Chapter 4); TMS: trafficking and modern slavery (Case studies 7.3 and 16.3); LAF: local authority funding (Chapter 9); RX: relationalism (Chapter 2)
Source: Rittel and Webber (1973)

A timeline of the progression of COVID-19 in the UK, from December 2019 to July 2020, was presented in Appendix A of *Local Authorities and Social Determinants of Health*, published in October 2020 (pp 427–8).

An important step in reducing COVID-19 in the world population is mass vaccinations. In recognising the need for vaccinations, governments have funded the research and development of vaccines.

Despite apparent progress in reducing COVID-19 infections and deaths by September 2020, a third wave of infections was spreading across the globe. From November mutations of the virus arose from an increasing number of countries, including South Africa and Brazil, and more recently from India (the Delta variant). These COVID-19 variants threaten to challenge the effectiveness of the newly developed vaccines, losing their effectiveness over time (Russell, 2021). An immediate response to this was to restrict

Figure I.1: Number of deaths in WHO regions from 1 January 2020 to 8 May 2020

Situation by WHO Region

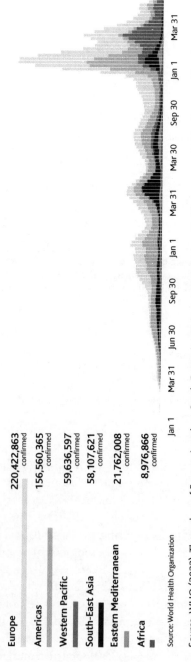

Europe
220,422,863
confirmed

Americas
156,560,365
confirmed

Western Pacific
59,636,597
confirmed

South-East Asia
58,107,621
confirmed

Eastern Mediterranean
21,762,008
confirmed

Africa
8,976,866
confirmed

Source: World Health Organization

Source: WHO (2022). The regions of Europe, Americas, South-East Asia, Western Pacific, Eastern Mediterranean and Africa have provided the underlying data.

movements between countries. The unequal availability of vaccines across the world is not only a social justice issue; 'No one is safe until all are safe' highlights the need to provide vaccinations to all people across the social gradient and across the global community. Problems with unequal access to supplies of vaccines have led to major inequalities in vaccine availability across developed and less well developed countries.

By 7 May 2022, 66.1 per cent (5,159,358,123 people) of the world's population had received one dose, 60 per cent (4,681,355,166 people) had been fully vaccinated and 24.3 per cent (1,893,755,335 people) had received a booster vaccination (Anon, 2022a).

As in other countries, the UK government was faced with balancing the protection of the NHS, controlling the spread of the virus by closing down communities, and protecting the economy. In an attempt to protect the economy, the UK Chancellor, Rishi Sunak, launched a multibillion-pound scheme in April 2020, which allowed employees to be furloughed with 80 per cent of their pre-COVID-19 pay made available from the exchequer. Despite this financial support, by 1 July 2020 a significant number of businesses had closed and several thousand people had been made redundant. The furlough scheme, which aimed at supporting people laid off from businesses forced to close during lockdown, ended on 30 September 2021 (BBC, 2021).

Further closures and redundancies were expected: '7.6 million, 24% of the UK workforce, are at risk of COVID-19 related Lockdown. People and places with the lowest income are the most vulnerable' (Allas et al, 2020). In the spring of 2021, the UK government published a roadmap, *COVID-19 Response: Autumn and Winter 2021* (HMG, 2021a).

The government response to COVID-19 was updated in winter 2021, reporting progress in the procurement of vaccines, vaccinating more of its population than any other country in Europe, and that the link between increased infections and severe disease had been significantly weakened. However, it was noted that 'cases [of infection] are still rising, as are hospitalisations … vigilance must be maintained and people will be asked to make informed decisions and act carefully and proportionally … the dominant Delta variant is estimated to be 40-80% more transmissible than the previously dominant Alpha variant' (HMG, 2021b).

A number of agencies and research groups have been monitoring infection rates, these include the Office for National Statistics (ONS, 2021), and the Oxford COVID-19 Government Response Tracker (Hale et al, 2021). Since January 2020, the Oxford COVID-19 Government Response Tracker has systematically collected information on policy measures taken by governments to address COVID-19, covering 180 countries. The data collected included information on school closures, travel restrictions and vaccination policies.

On 1 January 2022 in excess of 100 million case of COVID-19 were recorded due to an upsurge in the Omicron variant (ONS 2021). The Institute for Health Metric Evaluation model indictated that 57 per cent of the world had been infected by COVID-19 on 24 February 2022 (IHME, 2022).

The use of lockdowns has been a key public health measure intended to reduce the transmission of COVID-19. The frequent policy changes or U-turns of the UK government have been described as classic behavioural traps resulting from political short-termism. An explanation for this political decision making has been attributed to information gaps, risk methodologies, mis-sequencing, behavioural tendencies and political (and human) desire for quick wins. The increased information from healthcare and the socioeconomic impact, for example, of closing down schools, and the consequences of unequal access to online education in lockdown, has led to the management of the pandemic from the perspectives of 'risk budgets' (El-Erian, 2021).

The impact of lockdown on the health and wellbeing of children has been of great concern during the progression of COVID-19, in relation to adverse effects on educational attainment with the additive effects of being locked down, in many cases in limited accommodation, with a lack of green space, the economic stress of loss of family income and impact on the family diet and mental health issues, has led to increased stress within the family unit (see Chapter 4). The social and economic impact of three waves of the COVID-19 pandemic have been reviewed by Fisayo and Tsukagoshi (Fisayo and Tsukagoshi, 2021).

In addition to the large number of deaths and ill health, the exacerbation of adversity in childhood due to the COVID-19 pandemic, disruption of daily life and livelihoods, there have been major shocks to local and to national economies, and some communities have been disproportionately impacted. From the perspective of COVID-19-related deaths, England compares poorly in comparison to other socioeconomically equivalent countries. In August 2021, England had the highest accumulated number of deaths in the world. There are many lessons to be learned, including the need to act swiftly in locking down, and the need for an *effective* 'protective ring around social care', a failure which contributed to the deaths of 26,000 excess deaths in care home residents in 2020.

A positive aspect of the government response was the procurement and rollout of vaccinations, however, the early implementation of lockdowns and a *functional* 'protective ring around social care' would have added to the success of this public health measure.

Lessons have been learned in understanding the strengths and weaknesses of health, care and public health systems in the UK and other countries (see Chapter 3 and Case study 7.4). The King's Fund has proposed a framework to assess England's response to COVID-19 (see Figure I.2).

Figure I.2: Five elements of a framework to assess England's response to COVID-19, with comments indicating the key consequences of the UK's policy response to the pandemic

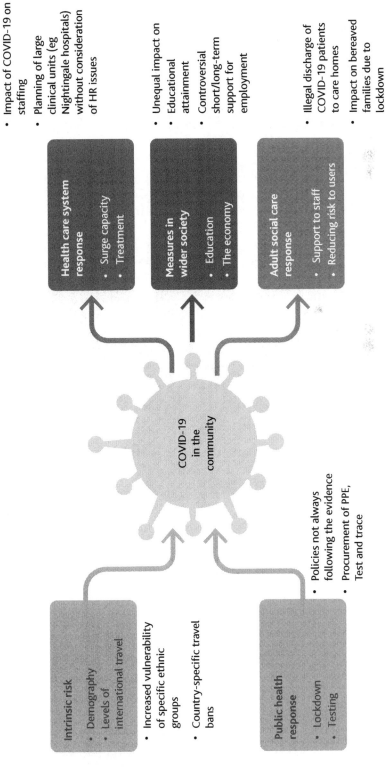

Source: Adapted from Warren and Murray (2021)

Climate change

The COVID-19 pandemic has brought widespread global concerns from both public health and political–economic perspectives, as already discussed. Paradoxically, lockdown has refocused people's attention on green spaces and the environment. The renewed quality of life of those who could work from home made it preferable to commuting to and working in city workplaces. This change in public attitude has been seen as a politically opportune time to address the major threats of climate change and its wide-ranging effects on health and wellbeing across the world. Addressing climate change and the need to prepare for future pandemics was the issue for leaders of the seven most economically developed countries at the G7 conference, held in Cornwall in June 2021.

At the COP26 conference (HMG, 2022), held in Glasgow in November 2021, over 100 leaders pledged to 'endeavour to work together in each sector, including public-private collaborations, end deforestation. ... Economic development globally for clean technologies and sustainable solutions ... support UN Sustainable Development Goals, strength climate resilience ... and realise multiple co-benefits such as cleaner air, water and better health' (HMG, 2022).

Climate change requires a global response from all sectors of society, as discussed in Chapter 10. Both the climate change crisis and COVID-19 have irreversible changes, social and geographical inequalities, weakening of international solidarity, high momentum trends, and are less costly to prevent than to cure (Manzanedo and Manning, 2020). COVID-19 has highlighted the importance of environmental sustainability (Markard and Rosenbloom, 2020).

Understanding how to react to future shocks and stressors

Mitigating against risk is important from health, social justice and economic perspectives. These wicked issues present important lessons for governments, businesses and organisations. The interrelated impact and responses to these major challenges can be summarised by: *reaction-resilience-recover-new reality* (KPMG, 2020).

From the perspective of national and local governments, addressing the wicked issues of COVID-19 and climate change are complex issues which appeared to be 'difficult or impossible to solve because of incomplete, contradictory, and changing requirements, and not resolved by traditional "technical" managerial approaches to the provision of public services' (Rittel and Webber, 1973; see Chapter 1).

At the time of finalising this publication, the invasion by Russia of Ukraine is a new emerging threat to global stability and world peace. The wicked issues listed in Table I.2 will all be impacted by this illegal aggressive activity by one of the world's most powerful nuclear powers. In May 2022 more than 3,381 deaths in the city of Mariupol have been reported (Beaumont, 2022),. At this time more than 12 million people have fled their homes and 4 million have become refugees from Ukraine (Anon, 2022b) migrated from Ukraine have been reported (Davies, 2022).

A social determinants of health perspective, on the impact of war in Europe, is current being developed in this Policy Press series (see Figure I.3).

Roadmap for exploring this book

The six parts of this book provide an insight into understanding wicked issues and approaches to responding to the complexities of a number of interrelated and wicked issues from local and national perspectives.

Part I, 'Wicked issues and relationalism', provides an introduction to the main themes of the book: **wicked issues** (Chapter 1), **relationalism** (Chapter 2), the response of the UK health and care system to COVID-19 (Chapter 3), and inequalities which have been exacerbated by the disproportionate effect of COVID-19 on Black and Asian communities (Chapter 4).

Part II, 'Regionalism and the geopolitical environment', focuses on place-based issues including the specific regional inequalities in the North East of England (Chapter 5), local authority responses to COVID-19 and the climate crisis (Chapter 6), followed by international case studies from the US (Case study 7.1 on racism and xenophobia), South Africa (Case study 7.2 on gender-based and family violence), India and Nepal (Case study 7.3 on human trafficking and modern slavery) and New Zealand (Case study 7.4 on local government and public health).

Part III, 'Public sector, COVID-19 and culture change', addresses some of the wicked issues arising from the earlier Policy Press publications, *Social Determinants of Health: Social Inequality and Wellbeing* and *Local Authorities and Social Determinants of Health*. These issues include public sector governance (Chapter 8), local authorities' financial decline (Chapter 9), climate crisis (Chapter 10), housing and homeless (Chapter 11) and the impact of COVID-19 on employment (Chapter 12).

Part IV, 'The third sector', is a heterogeneous range of organisations which, in some cases, work with the public sector for the public good. In many cases third sector organisations provide a safety net not addressed by the public sector as in the case of food banks (Chapter 13). The role of volunteering is important in community support (Chapter 14, the role of small charities), working in partnership with local authorities (Chapter 15, domestic abuse), providing a holistic faith-based approach to human need (Chapter 16)

Part V, 'The private sector', plays a significant role in supporting public services. The unregulated procurement of public services has been an

Figure I.3: Social determinants of health: Policy Press publications reflecting the impact of socioeconomic change on health and wellbeing

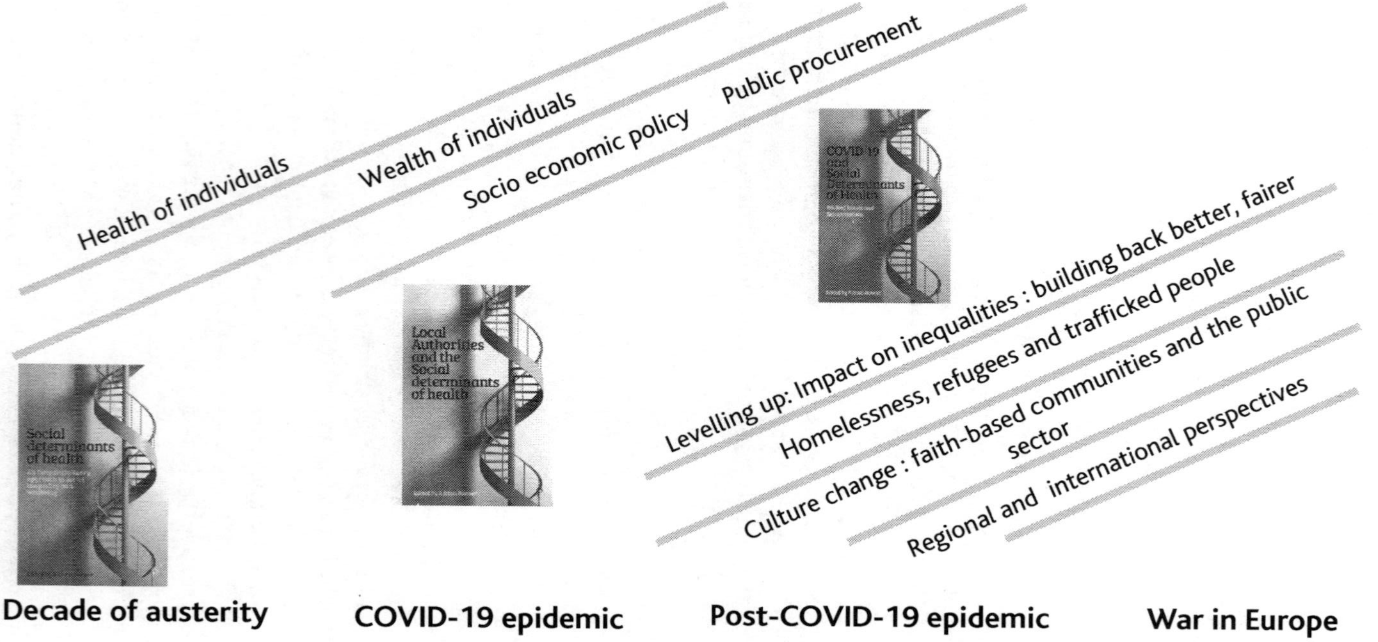

Health of individuals
Wealth of individuals
Socio economic policy
Public procurement
Social determinants of health
Local Authorities and the Social determinants of health
COVID-19 and Social Determinants of Health
Levelling up: Impact on inequalities : building back better, fairer
Homelessness, refugees and trafficked people
Culture change : faith-based communities and the public sector
Regional and international perspectives
Decade of austerity
COVID-19 epidemic
Post-COVID-19 epidemic
War in Europe

important response of the UK and other governments to COVID-19 and related **wicked issues**. In view of the wastage of public and private funds in the traditional processes of procurement, this section provides an insight into how partnerships between the public, private and third sectors contribute to **social value**, which can be amplified within the context of cultural change of relationalism. Case studies of relationalism (Case study 17.1), housing and homelessness (Case study 17.2), environmental planning (Case study 17.3), and community-based retailing (Case study 17.4) are presented with a view to introducing exemplars of public–private–third sector approaches to creating **relational dividends**.

Part VI, 'Engagement and proposed changes'. Progressing through COVID-19 and responding to the climate crisis at a time of large-scale public borrowing (following a decade of austerity budgeting relating to the global financial crash in 2008) requires new innovative planning and cultural change to promote social value and address the **social determinants of health**. These issues are presented from the perspectives of: legal protocols (Chapter 18); strategic planning of major infrastructural projects, such as the planning of housing and town centres and highways (Case study 17.1 and Chapter 19); and the socioeconomic impact of 'the lost decade', austerity and the widening inequalities gap (Chapter 20). What can be learned to enhance inter-organisational relationships and possible reforms from a transactional to a relationship-based system approach (Chapter 21)?

References

Allas, T., Canal, M. and Hunt, V. (2020) COVID-19 in the United Kingdom: Assessing jobs at risk and the impact on people and places. 11 May. Available at: https://www.mckinsey.com/industries/public-sector/our-insights/covid-19-in-the-united-kingdom-assessing-jobs-at-risk-and-the-impact-on-people-and-places#

Anon (2022a) Vaccines: Global vaccine coverage official site. Available at: https://www.google.com/search?sxsrf=ALiCzsZlYTLJt54sf_g0WiFy4JJBGml8Ag%3A1652180477773&q=vaccination%20percentage%20by%20country&ved=2ahUKEwju4e3z49T3AhXhnFwKHUNQBHkQmoICKAB6BAgCEAg&biw=1200&bih=730&dpr=1#colocmid=/m/02j71&coasync=0

Anon (2022b) How the Ukrainian refugee crisis will change Europe. *The Economist*. Available at: https://www.economist.com/europe/2022/03/25/how-the-ukrainian-refugee-crisis-will-change-europe?gclid=EAIaIQobChMIy8jWi6XV9wIVROrtCh3ZMAjWEAAYASAAEgKo6fD_BwE&gclsrc=aw.ds

Bambra, C., Lynch, J. and Smith, K. (2021) *The Unequal Pandemic: COVID-20 and Health Inequalities*. Bristol: Policy Press.

BBC (2021) COVID: How is furlough changing and when will it end? *BBC News*. Available at: https://www.bbc.co.uk/news/explainers-52135342

Beaumont, P. (2022) Ukraine civilian deaths thousands higher than official toll, wars UN. *The Guardian*. Available at: https://www.theguardian.com/world/2022/may/10/ukraine-civilian-deaths-higher-official-toll-un-warns

Bonner, A. (ed) (2018) *Social Determinants of Health: Social Inequality and Wellbeing*. Bristol: Policy Press.

Bonner, A. (ed) (2020) *Local Authorities and Social Determinants of Health*. Bristol: Policy Press.

Burstow, P. (2018) The Care Act 2014. In Bonner, A. (ed), *Social Determinants of Health: Social Inequality and Wellbeing*. Bristol: Policy Press.

Dahlgren, G. and Whitehead, M. (1991) *Policies and Strategies to Promote Social Equity in Health*. Stockholm: Institute for Future Studies.

Davies, N. (2022) The rise and fall of Mariupol. *The Spectator*, 26 June. Available at: https://www.spectator.co.uk/article/the-founding-conquering-and-destruction-of-mariupol

El-Erian, M. (2021) What can we learn from the UK's response to COVID-19? *The Guardian*, 25 January. Available at: https://www.theguardian.com/business/2021/jan/25/uk-response-covid-19-u-turns . Accessed on 29 08 2022

Fisayo, T. and Tsukagoshi, S. (2021) Three waves of the COVID-19 pandemic. *BMJ*, 97(1147).

Hale, T., Angrist, N., Goldszmidt, R., Kira, B., Petherick, A., Phillips, T., Webster, S., Cameron-Blake, E., Hallas, L., Majumdar, S., Tatlo, H. (2021) A global panel database of pandemic policies (Oxford-19 Government Response Tracker). *Nature Human Behaviour* 5: 529–538.

HMG (2022) COP: UN Climate Change Conference UK 21. Available at: https://www.gov.uk/government/topical-events/cop26

IME (2022) IHME COVID-19 insights blog. July. Available at: https://www.healthdata.org/news-events/blogs/covid-19-inIHsights-blog

KPMG (2020) COVID-19 key lessons for climate change: How can we better prepare for climate change? Available at: https://home.kpmg/uk/en/home/insights/2020/06/covid-19-and-how-can-we-use-the-lessons-learnt-from-covid-19-to-better-prepare-for-climate-change.html

LePan, N. (2020) History of pandemics: Visualising the history of pandemics. *Visual Capitalist*. Available at: https://www.visualcapitalist.com/history-of-pandemics-deadliest/

Manzanedo, R.D. and Manning, P. (2020) COVID-19: Lessons for the climate change emergency. *Science of the Total Environment* 742. Available at: https://www.sciencedirect.com/science/article/pii/S0048969720340857

Markard, J. and Rosenbloom, D. (2020) A tale of two crises: COVID-19 and climate. *Sustainability: Science, Practice and Policy* 16(1): 53–60.

Marmot, M. (2010) *Fair Society, Healthy Lives*. London: Institute of Health Equity.

Marmot, M., Allen, J., Goldblatt, P., Herd, E. and Morrison, J. (2020) *Build Back Fairer: The COVID-19 Marmot Review*. London: Institute of Health Equity.

ONS (2021) All data related to coronavirus (COVID-19). Available at: https://www.ons.gov.uk/peoplepopulationandcosmmunity/healthandsocialcare/conditionsanddiseases/datalist?lang=welsh

Rittel, H. and Webber, M. (1973) Dilemmas in a general theory of planning. *Policy Sciences* 4: 155–169.

Russell, P. (2021) COVID vaccine effectiveness 'waning over time'. *Medscape*, 26 August. Available at: https://www.medscape.com/viewarticle/957202?src=wnl_newsalrt_uk_210825_MSCPEDIT&uac=204355DN&impID=3592505&faf=1

Warren, S. and Murray, R. (2021) *Assessing England's Response to COVID-19: A Framework*. The Kings Fund, London.

WHO (2022) COVID-19 dashboard. Available at: https://covid19.who.int

PART I

Wicked issues and relationalism

Adrian Bonner

The challenges for local authorities highlighted in *Local Authorities and Social Determinants of Health* include: the problems in developing effective partnerships between health and social care services (Chapter 4); the cost of care if you do not own your home (Chapter 12); addressing inequalities in the North East of England (Chapter 7); supporting children and families (Chapter 11); and protecting future generations (Chapters 15 and 20).

Locking down populations, to reduce the spread of the virus, has involved difficult decisions by governments, often choosing between protecting the health of people or the economy. The approach using traditional management tools and leadership strategies has been found to be wanting.

Complex or **wicked issues** may be approached from multiple, sometimes competing, perspectives and may have multiple possible solutions (Conklin et al, 2017). Identifying 'a social or cultural problem that is difficult or impossible to solve due to; incomplete or contradictory knowledge, the number of people and opinions involved, the large economic burden, and the interconnected nature of these problems with other problems' (Rittel and Webber, 1977) is a first step in developing leadership in the public, private and third sectors.

Navigating wicked issues within a **social determinants of health** framework can help in managing responses to the issues. In Chapter 1, Simmons proposes that such navigation is based on the 'value that is created when the insights from different patterns of social relations are combined in the search for greater clarity about the path ahead', such that 'the impossible becomes possible when you can see it from a different point of view'. This chapter explores the nature of public services leadership using the COVID-19 crisis as a reference. Crises are true **wicked issues**; they are complex and defy routine, technical solutions. The literature reviewed in this chapter highlights the importance of the collective dimensions of leadership, how it involves a social influence process through which improvised ('clumsy') coordination and partnership emerge. The novel notion of a **relational dividend** is defined here as the sum total of benefits (or 'combined added value') that accrue from an investment in **relational work**. Chapter 1 argues that the complex and often intractable nature of wicked problems, including those relating to the social determinants of health, often means that they must be continually 'navigated' rather than 'solved'.

With reference to the interconnectivity and interdependence across the domains of the rainbow model of social determinants of health as described by Dahlgren and Whitehead, relationships matter. Relations between individuals, **relational behaviour** between people and agencies, between public, private and third sectors, relationships between national governments, are explored through the lens of **relationalism** (see Chapter 2). An application of this approach can be seen in international aid programmes where attempts are made to strengthen mutual accountability. This relational approach to **public–health ethics** is centred on three **relational values**: autonomy, social justice and solidarity (Bayliss, 2008). This **relational theory** is based on an understanding of persons as rational individuals, existing within a specific historical, economic, social and political context.

The approach to COVID-19 adopted by the UK government is reviewed from a sociopolitical perspective in Chapter 3. This exploration of the social and political contexts prevailing in a particular country can lead to a better understanding of why COVID-19 has followed a particular course.

The fundamental need to give children the best start in life was highlighted in the Marmot Reports (2010 and 2020). Chapter 4 develops this priority by reference to inequalities in the UK.

The Marmot reviews from 2010 to 2020 highlight that the top priority intervention, needed to address social and health inequalities, is to 'give children the best start'. This aspect of public policy is not only cost-effective but will also lead to improved individual and population health outcomes (Marmot, 2010; Marmot et al, 2020). Chapter 4 emphasises the urgent need for targeted and resourced plans to shield the most vulnerable while ensuring all children are supported to get over the negative effects of the pandemic. This recommendation is in line with both intergenerational and redistributive justice, prioritised in the attempts to build back better and promote a fairer society.

References

Baylis F., Kenny, N. and Sherwin, S. (2008) A relational account of public health ethics. *Public Health Ethics*, 1(3): 196–201.

Conkin, H., Ashford, J., Clark, K., Martin-Ebashesh, K., Hardy, K., Merchant, T., Ogg, R., Jeha, S., Huang, L. and Zhang, H. (2017) Long-term efficiency of computerized cognitive training among survivors of childhood cancer: A single-blind randomised controlled trial. *Journal of Pediatrics*, 41(2): 220–231.

Marmot, M. (2010) *Fair Society, Healthy Lives*. London: Institute of Health Equity.

Marmot, M., Allen, J., Goldblatt, P., Herd, E. and Morrison, J. (2020) *Build Back Fairer: The COVID-19 Marmot Review*. London: Institute of Health Equity.

Rittel, H. and Webber, M. (1973) Dilemmas in a general theory of planning. *Policy Sciences* 4: 155–169.

Using relationalism to navigate wicked issues: investing for a 'relational dividend'?

Richard Simmons

Introduction

In their seminal paper, 'Dilemmas in a general theory of planning', Rittel and Webber note that, in response to societal problems:

> [A] deep-running current of optimism seems to have been propelling diverse searches for *direction-finding* instruments [such as] ... a clarification of purposes, a redefinition of problems, a re-ordering of priorities to match stated purposes, the design of new kinds of goal-directed actions ... and a redistribution of the outputs of governmental programs among the competing publics. [However], by now we are all beginning to realize that one of the most intractable problems is that of *defining problems* (of knowing what distinguishes an observed condition from a desired condition) and of *locating problems* (finding where in the complex causal networks the trouble really lies). In turn, and equally intractable, is the problem of identifying the actions that might effectively narrow the gap between what-is and what-ought-to-be. (Rittel and Webber, 1973: 157; emphasis added)

Rittel and Webber's (1973) notion of 'direction-finding' is important. This chapter addresses the ways in which policymakers might seek to both **orientate** themselves towards policy problems and **navigate** the actions that might be taken to address them. In another seminal contribution, Lasswell's (1951) notion of the 'problem orientation' identifies 'the scientific study of problems' and 'policymaking around these problems' as the two 'poles' of policy analysis (Turnbull, 2008). Yet, as is widely recognised, phenomena such as bounded rationality (Simon, 1955) and wicked policy problems (Rittel and Webber, 1973) mean that 'policymakers must often act in the face of irreducible uncertainty – uncertainty that will not go away before a judgment has to be made about what to do, what can be done, what will be done, what ought to be done' (Hammond, 1996: 11).

The claims of evidence-based policymaking (EBPM) as a means for 'objective', technical, evidence-informed choice or 'policy selection' tend to lose traction as uncertainty and/or controversy increase (Grint, 2005; Hoppe, 2011). As Turnbull (2008: 73) observes, various objections to the EBPM approach include that it pays insufficient attention to problem framing (for example, Rein and Schon, 1977); presumes an inadequate, univocal definition of social problems (for example, Rose, 1977; Lindblom and Woodhouse, 1993); and excludes the symbolic dimension of policy meanings (for example, Yanow, 1996). In this view, sense-making thus relies on more than simply scientific analysis (Wildavsky, 1987; Hood, 1998; Rhodes, 2015).

Importantly, Lasswell (1951: 9) recognises the importance of 'values' in policymaking practice, arguing that 'practical science does involve values because the goals of policymaking should produce the type of human relations we find most desirable'. Yet it cannot be assumed that there will be agreement on such issues, or that espoused values will be universally shared. Hence, as Rhodes (2012: 15) puts it, often 'it is not a matter of solving specific problems but of managing unfolding dilemmas and their inevitable unintended consequences. There is no solution but a succession of solutions which are contested and redefined as they are "solved"'. This echoes Rittel and Webber's (1973) observation that '[social] problems are never solved. At best they are only re-solved – over and over again'. Contingent situations therefore often demand a more holistic approach, in which a wider frame of reference is taken (for example, Quinn, 1988; Simmons, 2011).

Much has been written about how problems are treated under these conditions. Navigating this terrain can be challenging, with the governance of problems often demanding different forms of response (Rittel and Webber, 1973; Grint, 2005; Hoppe, 2011). Thus policymakers must learn to 'regularly and skilfully navigate a multitude of actors and programs in the system' (McGuire and Silvia, 2010). This chapter explores how notions of orientation and navigation might contribute in practice to the governance of contemporary policymaking problems. Further, focusing in particular on the main topics for this book, it seeks to understand the role and potential of **relationalism** with regard to **wicked issues** and the **social determinants of health**. It asks: what mechanisms can be put in place to help policymakers navigate this terrain, develop clearer understandings and more effective responses?

The nature and governance of wicked problems

Policy problems vary in character. For example, Grint (2005: 1473) suggests that command-and-control approaches may be appropriate in the face of urgent and time-bound 'critical' problems. This assumes a 'formally structured' governance space, in which the question of who holds 'agenda-setting' power/authority has already been decided. This means learning not to 'question why' – accepting the legitimacy, if not always the substantive nature, of the commands of those with such power/authority. Grint also acknowledges Rittel and Webber's (1973) category of 'tame' problems: 'A tame problem may be complicated but is resolvable' (Grint, 2005: 1473). Here, policymakers occupy a 'rational', 'technical' space, in which everything from real-time data to scientific evidence can be balanced in 'problem-solving'. The prescription here is straightforward: 'simply apply science [or technical/managerial rationality] properly and the best solution will naturally emerge' (Grint, 2005: 1473). This means doing the background work to support authoritative choice between policy alternatives, perhaps via 'structured interactions in policy work' as a way to bring order to the weight of evidence and expertise (Colebatch, 2006).

In sum, each of these (critical/tame) problem-types may be encountered in relation to the social determinants of health. The prescription, which respectively assumes delegation of responsibility to either 'authority' or 'expertise', is to find the 'right' or 'best-fit' solutions in a rational-purposive process, through 'objective' informed choice or policy selection. Yet the relative claims of authority and expertise often diminish in the face of 'wicked' problems (Grint, 2005; Hoppe, 2011). For Grint (2005: 1473) 'a wicked problem is more complex, rather than just complicated. Such problems are often intractable'. In the face of this contingency, Grint (2005: 1473) observes that: 'To make any kind of progress with wicked problems, the task is to ask the right questions rather than provide the right answers.'

Asking the 'right' questions

Turnbull (2013: 124) identifies 'a key difference between the desire to reconfirm the old and *repress questions* [thereby *defending* existing policy territory], and the desire to problematize [or *explore* different options]'. In terms of 'strategic defense', the approach to wicked problems therefore may be one of **conservatism** (closing boundaries to the environment in an attempt to 'ride out change'; Mamouni-Limnios et al, 2014). This (or the more adaptive 'dynamic conservatism'/'changing to stay the same'; Pollitt et al, 1998; Ansell et al, 2015) may be appropriate for a short time or in relation to certain developments (Wildavsky, 1987), but inhibit necessary change if they are used to withstand forces that 'ought not to be resisted' (Derissen et al, 2011). In conditions of conservatism, policymakers seemingly prefer to establish and then narrow the range of possible answers than to establish and then narrow the range of possible questions.

Yet the complexity and dynamism of many policy environments place a premium on not only sound judgement, but also the ability to question, learn and adapt. Hence, in the 'complex' and 'uncertain' spaces of wicked issues a more open type of 'exploration' and policy discourse tends to be required. However, despite the very practical value of such exploration, space for this is often limited in policy work (Turnbull, 2008) – at least until 'opportunities are created by policy failure and uncertainty to put established institutions into question' (Turnbull, 2013: 125). Thus, we often lack good ways to ask questions about questions – at least, without encountering accusations of 'avoiding the problem' or 're-politicising technical concerns' (Simmons, 2018). As Turnbull (2013: 124) points out, 'despite the potential agency of individual policymakers as *questioners*, stability may occur because many choices they face are repressed or "rhetoricized" via logics of practice'. Beyond this, however, for wicked issues – where there are often more questions than answers – 'what is a good question?' is itself a good question (Rittel and Webber, 1973). Navigating this terrain is a complex and ongoing task. Yet as Sumberg (2013) points out, policymakers generally lack the 'GPS systems' of modern-day satellite navigation. Wisdom is therefore required to know when such approaches are appropriate, and when they become part of the problem rather than the solution (Grint, 2009). Relational approaches that allow such wisdom to emerge can therefore make an important contribution.

Turning 'defence' to 'offence'

In contrast to conservatism or dynamic conservatism, a third response to change – 'exploration' – implies '*strategic offense*' (Mamouni-Limnios et al, 2014). As Stirling observes, there is a contrast here between the 'opening up' or 'closing down' of policy discourses:

> If it is about 'closing down' the policy process, then the aim is to assist decision-making by cutting through the messy, intractable and conflict prone diversity of views and develop instead a clear authoritative prescriptive recommendation. ... On the other hand, if it is about 'opening up' the process, then the focus is on revealing wider policy discourses and interpretations of the available evidence. (Stirling, 2006: 101)

Exploration involves scanning the external environment for new opportunities, and engaging in strategies of experimentation, learning and repositioning (March, 1991). Rather than seeing the response to wicked policy problems through the triangulation points of authority or expertise, this approach envisages the mapping of valid information and corrective feedback through 'polyrationality' (Davy, 2016). Polyrational solutions involve 'policies and strategies that combine a variety of perspectives on what the issue at hand is, and how it should be resolved' (Verweij, 2014). Such polyrationality is derived in a plurality of **contexts**, from a plurality of **legitimate knowledges**.

In this way, research shows that the 'contexts' within which wicked problems are perceived to be located requires careful interpretation. Clarke (2013: 24) helpfully identifies a 'plurality' of contexts – spatial, political, governmental, cultural, economic, organisational, and so on that should be considered. He argues that it is only when these contexts are combined, through a lens of 'inter-contextuality', that we begin to see the particular forms of agent and types of agency that are created, which in turn create the possibility of 'imagining problems in particular ways, developing languages for naming the problem, and framing the sorts of remedial action or solution that are reasonable to pursue' (Clarke, 2013: 24). In short, it is this combination of contexts that may be seen to constitute the 'conditions of possibility' that make certain things thinkable, possible, relevant, desirable, necessary – or vice versa – and animate particular actions as solutions to a set of perceived problems (Clarke, 2013: 25).

Moreover, Table 1.1 shows how there is also a range of 'legitimate knowledges' in relation to wicked problems. Each of these has its strengths and weaknesses, and important differences may be found in actors' receptivity to others' knowledge (Argyris, 1976). An important question here lies at the 'boundary' between different forms of knowledge. In short, who is it that decides what practical action is called for – and are these the 'right' people to do so?

These perspectives give space in policy work to framing wicked problems in a relational way that seeks to resolve tensions between different constructions of values and beliefs (Colebatch, 2006), without reopening the kind of direct adversarial competition normally reserved for the realm of politics. Successful framings (which may themselves include commitments to more relational ways of working) become located within prevailing 'institutional

Table 1.1: Competing/complementary forms of knowledge

Form of knowledge	Critique
Individual (for example, consumer)	Biased
Community (for example, local community)	Anecdotal
Specialised (for example, health professional)	Inaccessible
Strategic (for example, chief executive)	Disconnected
Holistic (for example, academic professor)	Abstract

logics'. These 'focus attention on issues and solutions through a variety of mechanisms, including determining their appropriateness, legitimacy, rewarding certain forms of behaviour, and shaping the availability of alternatives' (Thornton and Ocasio, 2008: 114).

In doing so, notions of 'institutional work' are important. Institutional work has been defined as 'the purposive action of individuals and organizations aimed at creating, maintaining and disrupting institutions' (Lawrence and Suddaby, 2006: 215). Institutional work may take the form of 'mundane, day-to-day adjustments, adaptations, and compromises' (Lawrence et al, 2013: 1). It may also link with notions of cultural innovation, involving a reprioritisation or rebalancing within organisational value systems that can help reframe the conceptual or emotional view of a situation, customise new strategies and promote new behaviours (Van Ess Coeling and Simms, 1993). In turn, these values may be internalised in individuals, who become committed to them (Parsons, 1991).

In sum, at the heart of the discussion regarding wicked problems lie the key notions of **questioning**, **learning** and **adaptation**. Sanderson (2009: 713) therefore argues that 'learning is the dominant form in which rationality exhibits itself in situations of great cognitive complexity' (such as those found in relation to 'wicked' problems). For Thornton and Ocasio (2008: 117) this enables institutional change processes such as 'bricolage'; or 'the creation of new practices and institutions from different elements of existing institutions'. In turn, as Cahn (1996: 10) observes, the success of any policy lies in 'frequent reassessment and repositioning to accommodate intervening influences and maintain a course, albeit an updated course toward the predetermined policy goal'.

Policymakers often prefer to navigate this course using their own 'internal compass' (Smythe and Norton, 2007). However, in his influential management text, *Beyond Rational Management*, Quinn (1988: xv) emphasises a distinction between two institutional orientations: one that is 'purposive, static and entropic', and another that is 'holistic, dynamic and generative'. The perspective emerging in policymakers' 'purposive frame' is the equivalent of their 'internal compass', while in their 'holistic frame' they draw more widely, to also include a range of competing perspectives. Importantly, Quinn (1988) proposes that exceptional individuals do not achieve excellence by using one or other frame but by using both in conjunction.

Thus, in an environment of complexity and ambiguity, the effective navigation of wicked problems might be said to depend on such greater reflection and the 'acquisition of mastery through practical learning' (Rhodes, 2015). Sanderson (2009: 711) therefore characterises policymaking as 'a domain of *practical reason* ... not just concerned with the instrumental notion of "what works" but a broader practical notion of "*what is appropriate in the circumstances*"'. In the face of wicked problems, relationalism provides important opportunities for such questioning, reflexivity and learning.

The importance of relationalism in addressing wicked problems

Patterns of social relations are defined within social institutions and their prevailing institutional logics (Thornton and Ocasio, 2008). Thus, in an important recent contribution, Lejano (2021: 367; emphasis added) defines relationality simply as: 'The institutional logic by which established patterns of action in the public sphere emerge from *the working and reworking of relationships among policy actors.*' The evidence of this chapter so far suggests we should not pretend to be able solve wicked problems exclusively through the use of authority or rational-technical expertise, which tend towards a more narrow exploration of alternatives. Indeed, key commentators including Grint (2005) and Rittel and Webber (1973) point to the risks of treating wicked problems as critical or tame, and vice versa. Instead, there is a need to remain open and inclusive to ongoing 'exploration' (in the form of questioning, learning and adaptation) rather than discovery of a definitive 'solution'. Jessop (1997: 111) therefore identifies 'reflexive monitoring and dynamic social learning' as key processes. However, as Argyris (1976: 376) points out, often 'participants in an organization are encouraged to learn as long as the learning does not question the fundamental design, goals and activities of their organization'. Argyris (1976) calls this 'single-loop learning'. By contrast, Greenwood points out that:

> In double-loop learning the agent does not merely search for alternative actions to achieve her same ends; she also examines the appropriateness and propriety of her chosen ends. Double-loop learning therefore involves reflection on values and norms and, by implication, on the social structures which were instrumental in their development. By reflecting on the world they are instrumental in creating, human agents can learn to change it in ways that are more congruent with the values and theories they espouse. (Greenwood, 1998: 1049; emphasis added)

The search for 'progress' or 'new energy' through change (Weick and Quinn, 1999) may therefore be enabled through greater relational engagement. As Sanderson (2009: 708) observes, 'we need enhanced capacity for learning as a means of reconciling the implications of increasing social complexity with the requirement for effective public policy intervention'. Such reconciliation may well involve Greenwood's search for **greater congruence** (see also Simmons, 2016); or to put it another way, '*dissonance reduction* is an important mechanism for learning as far as selective perception and dominant interpretation is concerned' (Kemp and Weehuizen, 2005: 12; emphasis added). Patterns of social relations that can deliver greater congruence (or dissonance reduction) are therefore often valued highly.

For example, in relation to the wicked issue of climate change, Thompson (2003) identifies three competing 'stories' associated with different worldviews and patterns of social relations. In the first story, protagonists point to the profligate consumption and production patterns of the global North as the fundamental cause of global climate change. By contrast, the second story asserts that uncontrolled population growth in certain regions of the world places local and global ecosystems under pressures that quickly become dangerously uncontrollable. Meanwhile, a third story suggests that the price of natural resources is the most important factor in both controlling demand and footing the bill for environmental protection. In sum, while each story contains its own internal logic, it stands in tension with the others and holds only part of the solution to this policy problem.

Institutional pluralism ensures that the institutional blinkers are removed and appropriate attention and weight attached to each of these stories in allowing more effective policy solutions to emerge. If one story becomes dominant the system risks becoming unstable, incurring policy failure (6, 2003: 402). The lesson here is that failing to recognise other perspectives can cause considerable problems – wearing 'institutional blinkers' is not an option. For Verweij (2011; Verweij and Thompson, 2006) the policy prescription here involves constructing 'clumsy institutions' in which the voices of different worldviews, and their associated patterns of social relations, are able to be heard and responded to (as opposed to one voice being dominant and drowning out the others; Thompson, 2008). In an important recent development in defining the shape of such 'clumsy' institutions and/ or solutions, Simmons (2016, 2018) uses the Cultural Theory tradition from which such notions have emerged to provide a way to measure congruence or dissonance. Thus, in line with Rittel and Webber's (1973: 157) identification of 'the problem of identifying the actions that might effectively narrow the gap between what-is and what-ought-to-be', Simmons (2016, 2018) uses stakeholders' perceptions of how strongly represented a particular pattern of social relations *actually* is in any given context, and how strongly represented stakeholders feel it *should be* for the system to be optimally viable.

Achievements here involve the cultivation of a 'polyrational imagination' – that, through embracing more than a single perspective, takes institutional and contextual pluralism and different knowledges seriously (Verweij, 2014; Davy, 2016). In terms of institutional analysis, this involves standing back to reflect on how the weaknesses of one worldview/pattern of social relations might be compensated by the strengths of another (Hoppe, 2011), so that 'the impossible becomes possible when you see it from a different point of view' (Stewart, 1996). In this way, skilled 'reflective policymakers' can be facilitated to navigate more quickly to the 'good' questions to ask in relation to wicked issues (see also Turnbull, 2013). Notions of congruence therefore provide a way of framing more critically reflective positions on wicked issues – whether this is reflection 'in-action' (thinking carefully about the situation that is unfolding), 'on-action' (thinking retrospectively about the effects of how a situation was handled) or 'for-action' (thinking about future actions with the intention of making changes or improvements) (Schön, 1983; Killion and Todnem, 1991).

Relationalism as a 'value proposition'

In sum, value is created when different patterns of social relations are combined to consider the path ahead. In exploring the value proposition provided by relationalism as a way of navigating the terrain of wicked issues, this chapter moves on to consider several further important notions; in particular:

- a **relational imperative** (that we cannot suppose to govern wicked problems alone);
- **relational work** (where effort is invested into taking a more relational rather than more technical or transactional approach); and
- a **relational dividend** – the sum total of benefits (or 'combined added value') that accrue from this investment.

The relational imperative

In considering the importance of interactions within and between the plurality of contexts and multiplicity of knowledge contributions in exploring wicked problems, relationships take centre stage. In turn, 'relationalism' seeks to creatively combine different capacities and capabilities so that policy actors might navigate towards more adaptive policy responses. Various conceptual frameworks suggest relational approaches are particularly important in the face of wicked problems, including those related to the social determinants of health (see also Simmons, 2020).

Indeed, an absence of viable alternatives to relational approaches in the face of wicked problems provides an overarching 'relational imperative'. In part, this mirrors the moral imperative identified by Huxham and Vangen (2005: 7): that, as many crucially important public service issues simply cannot be tackled by acting alone, there is an obligation to act together. In addition, however, it addresses a related legitimate imperative: that in order to recognise the importance of information, and assimilate new knowledge (that is, learn), it is important to establish and deepen the necessary competence (ability), commitment (willingness) and culture (values, norms, beliefs) for relationalism to contribute (Simmons and Brennan, 2017). Policy systems thus require a certain level of relational capacity and capability. As Colebatch puts it:

> Relationships are important in determining the credibility of knowledge (Clavier 2010). Expert knowledge might be drawn on in some contexts, peer opinion in others (May and Winter 2009; Ritter 2009). Moreover, institutional context is likely to determine which truth claims are accepted and which rejected (Kook 2003; 6 et al 2007). (Colebatch, 2015: 212)

In this way, agreement and disagreement can each help prompt adaptation (Cameron and Freeman, 1991). This has led to increasing interest in other **relational phenomena** such as the 'spontaneity, action and "e-motion"' derived from points of connection, overlaps, interpenetrations, revisions and reformulations of knowledge (Fuchs, 2019). **Relational dynamics**, as defined in patterns of social relations, are clearly also important. If knowledge structures are rigid and their boundaries fixed, strategies to interconnect them may require greater force and be considered transgressive. If these structures are more flexible, interconnections may be permitted – or even encouraged.

Relational work

Cloutier et al (2015) develop these ideas for public administration. Taking Lawrence and Suddaby's (2006) notion of institutional work, they show how this comprises structural, conceptual, operational and relational components:

> Structural work refers to *efforts* to establish formalized roles, rule systems, organizing principles, and resource allocation models that support a new policy framework. Conceptual work refers to *efforts* to establish new belief systems, norms, and interpretive schemes consistent with the new policy. Operational work refers to *efforts* to implement concrete actions affecting the everyday behaviours of frontline professionals that are directly linked with the new policy. And finally, relational work, which underpins the other three, refers to *efforts* aimed at building linkages, trust, and collaboration between people involved in reform implementation. (Cloutier et al, 2015: 266; emphasis added)

Critically, Cloutier et al (2015: 272) identify an important 'integrative role' here for relational work, in 'gluing together' the other forms of institutional work and helping to 'navigate the pluralism and contradiction' that underpins many wicked issues. In this way, relational work functions in relation to:

- 'structural work', in enabling individuals occupying particular roles to 'establish mutually satisfactory boundaries and build trust';
- 'conceptual work', in generating 'some kind of shared understanding', connecting this to people's experience; and
- 'operational work', in locating the success of operational initiatives in 'developing personal relationships between individuals'. (Cloutier et al, 2015: 270)

In turn, the extent to which such mutually satisfactory boundaries, trust, shared understanding and personal relationships are established over time through investments in relational work, may be seen as an accumulation of **'relational capital'** (for example, Kohtamaki et al, 2012) – a point to which we will return.

It is important to note that, as defined here, all forms of institutional work require 'efforts' from policy actors. Some more rational-technical actors might be tempted to question any investment in **relational efforts** 'aimed at building linkages, trust, and collaboration' – in particular for certain critical or tame problems – as somehow non-essential, and wasteful of resources that could be better targeted on structural, conceptual or operational concerns. Arguably, however, Cloutier et al's (2015) identification of the integrative role of relational work provides an important challenge to such questions, whereby investment in relational work becomes a critical success factor in optimising actors' return on other investments of effort. The strength of this argument is multiplied in the face of the relational imperative that underpins most wicked problems (Grint, 2005). It is also worth noting at this point that while relational efforts may sound like 'hard' work, this need not be the case. Indeed, it may actually prove to be the opposite if it involves a lot of people contributing a relatively small amount to help navigate a wicked problem, as compared with alternative arrangements where a relatively small number of people (for example, policy entrepreneurs, experts, managers) seek to do a lot (see also Simmons, 2020).

Developing a more relational approach (whereby authority and expertise become more receptive to 'listening' and 'open learning') may therefore just be 'different', rather than intrinsically harder or easier. Yet as former Permanent Secretary of the Department for Education and Employment, Lord Bichard (2000: 42) has observed: 'Listening has not been one of the most precious public sector competencies, and too many senior managers are where they are because they are good at telling not listening.' Moreover, it seems that listening is not only an underdeveloped skill in the public sector, but that there are times when organisational listening devices are either underutilised or switched off (Simmons, 2011). In response, investments in 'relational work' must often seek to challenge to the prevailing culture, mindset and behaviours in established social institutions and develop the

Figure 1.1: Trust-based relationships and relational work

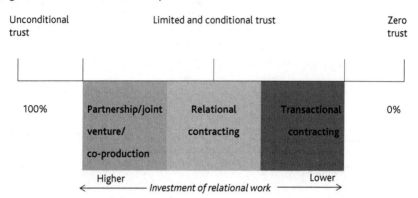

relational competence and commitment of relevant policy actors (for example, Simmons and Brennan, 2017).

In sum, it remains for policy actors themselves to decide where investments in relational work are required and how they should be made. For example, one way in which this may vary is in different forms of trust-based relationships in partnering and contracting arrangements between the public, private and third sectors. It is possible to plot these arrangements on a spectrum (see Figure 1.1). In practice, few arrangements are based at the extremes of 'unconditional' or 'zero' trust. Across the rest of this spectrum, greater investments of relational work might be anticipated to be required at the upper end and vice versa. However, this represents a first-order (or single-loop) level of analysis, which fails to question the prevailing arrangements. At the second-order (or double-loop) level, the question might instead consider whether a less relational arrangement (such as a transactional contract) has been utilised when a more relational arrangement might be more beneficial.

The evidence of this chapter suggests that these decisions should not be taken lightly, and that wherever a requirement for relational work is identified it is important that the 'appropriate' investments are made. If these are either too little (resulting in 'relational deficit', for example, Aditya, 2021, or 'moribund consensus', Simmons, 2001), or too much (resulting in 'relational overload', for example, Cross and Gray, 2013, or 'noise', Simmons, 2001), this can have deleterious effects on the 'relational dividend' that is achieved.

The relational dividend

The novel notion of a 'relational dividend' is defined here as: the sum total of benefits (or 'combined added value') that accrue from an investment in relational work. It should be noted here that the notion of relational work is important in emphasising the need for *active* attention and nurturing of the relational dividend. The dividend does *not* accrue simply from *passive* investments of relational capital – although some investment of relational capital may be critical in the start-up phase of a relational arrangement or initiative.

Thus, the relational dividend represents 'added value'. In this sense it has parallels with the notion of 'relational rents' in economics, defined as: '*a supernormal profit* jointly generated in an exchange relationship *that cannot be generated by either firm in isolation* and can only be created through the *joint idiosyncratic contributions of the specific alliance partners*' (Dyer and Singh, 1998: 662; emphasis added). Yet relational rents consider only the supernormal *financial added value within private sector contexts*. The notion of the 'relational dividend' extends this to the wider interests of different stakeholders in policy problems across the public, private and third sectors, as described in this chapter, and takes a 'combined added value' (CAV) approach that acknowledges but goes beyond financial concerns. Thus, relational attempts to navigate wicked policy issues may add 'supernormal' value in a number of important ways: from **'financial' value** (for example, cost savings); to **'functional' value** (for example, by calibrating activities to better fulfil the needs of users and citizens, and creating, sharing, transferring, adapting and embedding good practice; Hartley, 2005); to **'social' value** (for example, wider non-financial impacts of programmes, organisations and interventions, including the wellbeing of individuals and communities, social capital and the environment; Wood and Leighton, 2010) and/or **'emotional' value** (for example, through recognition, compassion, autonomy and care; Mulgan, 2007). Notably, emotional value is consistently raised as important by public service users in qualitative research into their experience (for example, Simmons et al, 2012, 2013), but is rarely considered in standard assessments of value.

The relational dividend is 'supernormal' in the extent to which it exceeds the CAV returns that could otherwise have been achieved in the absence of relational work. This takes into account both the next-best use of similar resource contributions and the opportunity costs associated with relational work. In relation to the navigation of many wicked problems, however, this may represent a low bar. Hence, where the relational imperative is strong (that is, there is a lack of viable alternatives to relational approaches), the next-best use of similar resource contributions may be as low as zero – as nothing would be done. Moreover, to the extent that relational work is able to enhance policy actors' navigation of elusive wicked problems, the opportunity costs may be heavily outweighed by the CAV returns.

Previous thinking around similar issues has often focused on the aggregation and mutual leveraging of inputs. For example, with regard to 'partnerships' Stewart (1996: 4) states that: 'There is no point in a partnership if it does not add value. It will add value by bringing in resources that are not otherwise available (financial, skills, power). In other words, partnerships depend for their value on some form of synergy.' Similarly, Bovaird et al (2015: 2) relate 'co-production' to how 'professionals and citizens make better use of each other's assets, resources and contributions to achieve better outcomes or improved efficiency'. However, while notions of 'synergy' and 'achieving better outcomes' are important and move us closer to the message of this chapter, this thinking seems to relate more to the joint investments of relational **capital** than how this is put to work in the creation and distribution of a relational **dividend**. The latter notion attempts to identify the ways in which such synergy and better outcomes might end up as the result of the former.

The 'value proposition' provided by relationalism must therefore define the manner in which stakeholders will be enticed to contribute relational work, and the mechanisms by which a relational dividend will be delivered. In turn, it must provide an account of, and account for, the ways in which the relational dividend accrues to those stakeholders for whom value is added, whether individually or collectively. Yet as Kelly et al (2002) caution, 'values and value are closely linked. Inappropriate values may lead to the destruction of value'. In response, an inclusive acknowledgment of intercontextuality, legitimate knowledges and institutional diversity can help ensure that competing and complementary values are effectively taken into account.

This author's notion of the 'relational dividend' has now been adopted by the Centre for Partnering as a key shared objective for relational policy, practice and projects, whether or not these involve the navigation of wicked problems. In further operationalising this concept, and that of CAV, it should be possible to establish a framework and methodology by which a knowledge base for relationalism might be more clearly developed and assessed.

Conclusion

This chapter has argued that the nature of wicked problems, including those relating to the social determinants of health, often means that they must be continually 'navigated' rather than 'solved'. First, this process of navigation requires the cultivation of a 'polyrational imagination' which, through embracing more than a single perspective, takes institutional and contextual pluralism and different knowledges seriously. This creates a relational imperative. Second, in order to ensure that the competing and complementary values of different stakeholders are effectively taken into account in the value proposition that is created, effort must be taken in the ongoing 'working and reworking of relationships among policy actors' (Lejano, 2021). This requires an investment in relational work. Third, this value proposition is realised where such investments of relational work result in 'supernormal' returns of functional, financial, social and/or emotional value. This constitutes the relational dividend. It should be noted that, as the scale and scope of this dividend is undermined by **relational deficits** or **relational overload**, it is important that policy actors are able to grasp the various effects of relational phenomena and relational dynamics – which requires skill. It may therefore be necessary to develop the **relational competence and commitment** of relevant policy actors, and/or to challenge the prevailing culture, mindset and behaviours in established social institutions. Investments here may find their return directly, in enhancing the scale and scope of relational dividends, but also indirectly, in the accumulation of relational capital from which future investments of relational work might be initiated.

In sum, this analysis identifies a number of possible sources of suboptimality in addressing wicked problems, including:

- underestimating the strength of the relational imperative;
- underinvesting in relational work ('deficit', 'moribund consensus');
- overinvesting in relational work ('overload', 'noise');
- failing to sufficiently consider the range of CAV in assessing the 'relational dividend';
- failing to appreciate the value of accumulating 'relational capital';
- failing to invest in relevant competences, capacities and commitment ('behaviour', 'practice');
- failing to incorporate 'relational phenomena' in key thinking ('mindset');
- failing to stabilise and/or mobilise productive 'relational dynamics' ('culture').

As the role and potential of relationalism moves to a more central position in current policy understandings of how to meet community needs and optimise outcomes (for example, Bartels and Turnbull, 2019; Lejano, 2021), it is important that these issues are given appropriate attention and consideration. In this way, policy actors need to ask both first-order and second-order questions to establish whether they have optimised their ability to:

- confront relational imperatives;
- motivate and organise relational work; and
- achieve relational dividends in line with their objectives.

Similarly, both single-loop and double-loop learning from relational initiatives, including those intended to help navigate wicked issues, will be important in continuing to understand and refine relationalism's contribution. In support, the generation of a reliable knowledge base to help people 'ask better questions' remains an important goal of the Centre for Partnering and its member universities. Through a combination of academic research and practical exemplar projects we will continue to work to operationalise the concepts of relational work, the relational dividend and CAV, and establish frameworks and methodologies by which relationalism might continually be more clearly developed and assessed, particularly in the face of wicked issues.

References

6, P. (2003) 'Institutional viability: A neo-Durkheimian theory', *Innovation*, 16(4): 395–415.

Aditya, A. (2021) 'Regime capability and relational stakes in the emerging world order', *Journal of Foreign Affairs*, 1(1): 1–36.

Ansell, C., Boin, A. and Farjoun, M. (2015) 'Dynamic conservatism: How institutions change to remain the same', in Kraatz, M. (ed) *Institutions and Ideals: Philip Selznick's Legacy for Organizational Studies*, Bingley: Emerald, pp 89–119.

Argyris, C. (1976) 'Single-loop and double-loop models in research on decision-making', *Administrative Science Quarterly*, 21(3): 363–375.

Bartels, K. and Turnbull, N. (2019) 'Relational public administration: A synthesis and heuristic classification of relational approaches', *Public Management Review*, 22(9): 1324–1346.

Bichard, M. (2000) 'The modernization and improvement of government and public services: Creativity, leadership and change', *Public Money and Management*, 20(2): 41–46.

Bovaird, T, van Ryzin, G, Loeffler, E, Parrado, S (2015) 'Activating citizens to participate in collective co-production of public services', *Journal of Social Policy*, 44(1): 1–23.

Cahn, M. (1996) Building Evaluative Models in Environmental Policy: State Innovations in Environmental Management, Working paper, Department of Political Science, California State University, Northridge.

Cameron, K. and Freeman, S. (1991) 'Cultural congruence, strength and type', *Organizational Change and Development*, 5: 23–58.

Clarke, J. (2013) 'Contexts: Forms of agency and action', in Pollitt, C. (ed) *Context in Public Policy and Management: The Missing Link?*, Cheltenham: Edward Elgar, pp 22–34.

Cloutier, C., Denis, J.-L., Langley, A. and Lamothe, L. (2015) 'Agency at the managerial interface: Public sector reform as institutional work', *Journal of Public Administration Research and Theory*, 26(2): 259–276.

Colebatch, H. (2006) 'What work makes policy?', *Policy Sciences*, 39: 309–321.

Colebatch, H. (2015) 'Knowledge, policy and the work of governing', *Journal of Comparative Policy Analysis: Research and Practice*, 17(3): 209–214.

Cross, R. and Gray, P. (2013) 'Where has the time gone? Addressing collaboration overload in a networked economy', *California Management Review*, 56(1): 50–56.

Davy, B. (2016) *Land Policy*, London: Routledge.

Derissen, S., Guaas, M. and Baumgartner, S. (2011) 'The relationship between resilience and sustainability of ecological-economic systems', *Ecological Economics*, 70(6): 1121–1128.

Dyer, J. and Singh, H. (1998) 'The relational view: Cooperative strategy and sources of interorganizational competitive advantage', *Academy of Management Review*, 23(4): 660–679.

Fuchs, T. (2019) 'Values as relational phenomena: A sketch of an enactive theory of value', in Muhling, M., Gilland, D. and Forster, Y. (eds) *Perceiving Truth and Value: Interdisciplinary Discussion on Perception as the Foundation of Ethics*, Göttingen: Vandenhoeck and Ruprecht, pp 23–42.

Greenwood, J. (1998) 'The role of reflection in single- and double-loop learning', *Journal of Advanced Nursing*, 27: 1048–1053.

Grint, K. (2005) 'Problems, problems, problems: The social construction of "leadership"', *Human Relations*, 58(11): 1467–1494.

Grint, K. (2009) 'New directions in the leadership of local public services: What has the research taught us?', Paper to ESRC public policy seminar, Leadership and Resilience: The Strategic Leadership of Local Communities and Local Services in a Time of Fragmentation, Edinburgh, 30 October.

Hammond, K. (1996) *Human Judgment and Social Policy: Irreducible Uncertainty, Inevitable Error, Unavoidable Injustice*, Oxford: Oxford University Press.

Hartley, J. (2005) 'Innovation in governance and public services: Past and present', *Public Money and Management*, 25: 27–34.

Hood, C. (1998) *The Art of the State*, Oxford: Oxford University Press.

Hoppe, R. (2011) *The Governance of Problems*, Bristol: Policy Press.

Huxham, C. and Vangen, S. (2005) *Managing to Collaborate: The Theory and Practice of Collaborative Advantage*, London: Routledge.

Jessop, B. (1997) 'The governance of complexity and the complexity of governance: Preliminary remarks on some problems and limits of economic guidance', in Amin, A. and Hauser, J. (eds) *Beyond Markets and Hierarchy: Interactive Governance and Social Complexity*, Cheltenham: Edward Elgar, pp 111–147.

Kelly, G., Mulgan, G. and Muers, S. (2002) *Creating Public Value: An Analytical Framework for Public Service Reform*, London: Strategy Unit.

Kemp, R. and Weehuizen, R. (2005) *Policy Learning: What Does It Mean and How Can We Study It?*, Oslo: Nifu.

Killion, J. and Todnem, G. (1991) 'A process for personal theory building', *Educational Leadership*, 48(6): 14–16.

Kohtamaki, M., Vsalainen, J., Henneberg, S., Naude, P. and Ventresca, J. (2012) 'Enabling relationship structures and relationship performance improvement: The moderating role of relational capital', *Industrial Marketing Management*, 41(8): 1298–1309.

Lasswell, H. (1951) 'The policy orientation', in Lerner, D. and Laswell, H. (eds) *The Policy Sciences*, Stanford: Stanford University Press, pp 3–15.

Lawrence, T. and Suddaby, R. (2006) 'Institutions and institutional work', in Clegg, S. Hardy, C. Lawrence, T. and Nord, W. (eds) *Handbook of Organizational Studies*, London: SAGE, pp 215–254.

Lawrence, T., Leca, B. and Zilber, T. (2013) 'Institutional work: Current research, new directions and overlooked issues', *Organization Studies*, 34(8): 1023–1033.

Lejano, R. (2021) 'Relationality: An alternative framework for analysing policy', *Journal of Public Policy*, 41(2): 360–383.

Lindblom, C. and Woodhouse, E. (1993) *The Policy-Making Process*, 3rd edition, Upper Saddle River: Prentice Hall.

Mamouni-Limnios, E., Mazzarol, T., Ghadouani, A. and Schilizzi, S. (2014) 'The resilience architecture framework: Four organizational archetypes', *European Management Journal*, 32(1): 104–116.

March, J. (1991) 'Exploration and exploitation in organizational learning', *Organization Science*, 2(1): 71–87.

McGuire, M. and Silvia, C. (2010) 'The effect of problem severity, managerial and organizational capacity, and agency structure on intergovernmental collaboration', *Public Administration Review*, 70(2): 279–288.

Mulgan, G. (2007) *Ready or Not? Taking Innovation in the Public Sector Seriously*, London: Nesta.

Parsons, T. (1991) 'A tentative outline of American values', in Robertson, R. and Turner, B. (eds) *Talcott Parsons: Theorist of Modernity*, London: SAGE, pp 91–105.

Pollitt, C., Birchall, J. and Putman, K. (1998) *Decentralising Public Management*, Basingstoke: Macmillan

Quinn, R. (1988) *Beyond Rational Management*, San Francisco: Jossey-Bass.

Rein, M. and Schon, D. (1977) 'Problem setting in policy research', in C. Weiss (ed) *Using Social Research in Public Policy Making*, Lanham: Lexington Books.

Rhodes, R. (2012) 'Political anthropology and public policy: Prospects and limits', Paper to Policy and Politics Conference, Forty Years of Policy and Politics, Bristol, September.

Rhodes, R. (2015) 'Recovering the "craft" of public administration in Westminster government', Paper to Political Studies Association Conference, Sheffield, March–April.

Rittel, H. and Webber, M. (1973) 'Dilemmas in a general theory of planning', *Policy Sciences*, 4: 155–169.

Rose, R. (1977) 'Disciplined research and undisciplined problems', in Weiss, C. (ed) *Using Social Research in Public Policy Making*, Lanham, MD: Lexington Books, pp 23–35.

Sanderson, I. (2009) 'Intelligent policy making for a complex world: Pragmatism, evidence and learning', *Political Studies*, 57: 699–719.

Schön, D. (1983) *The Reflective Practitioner*, London: Temple-Smith.

Simmons, R. (2001) 'Mutuality and public services', in Birchall, J. (ed) *The New Mutualism in Public Policy*, London: Routledge, pp 95–117.

Simmons, R. (2011) 'Leadership and listening in public services', *Social Policy and Administration*, 45(5): 539–568.

Simmons, R. (2016) 'Improvement and public service relationships: Cultural theory and institutional work', *Public Administration*, 94: 933–952.

Simmons, R. (2018) 'Cultural theory as a tool for policy analysis', *Policy and Politics*, 46(2): 235–253.

Simmons, R. (2020) 'Mutuality in the public, private and third sectors', in Bonner, A. (ed) *Local Authorities and the Social Determinants of Health*, Bristol: Policy Press, pp 319–342.

Simmons, R. and Brennan, C. (2017) 'User voice and complaints as drivers of innovation in public services', *Public Management Review*, 19(8): 1085–1104.

Simmons, R., Birchall, J. and Prout, A. (2012) 'User involvement in public services: "Choice about voice"', *Public Policy and Administration*, 27(1): 3–29.

Simmons, R., Brennan, C., Gill, C. and Hirst, C. (2013) *Outcomes of Complaints*, Perth: Care Inspectorate.

Simon, H. (1955) 'A behavioral model of rational choice', *Quarterly Journal of Economics*, 69(1): 99–118.

Smythe, E. and Norton, A. (2007) 'Thinking as leadership/leadership as thinking', *Leadership*, 3(1): 65–90.

Stewart, J. (1996) 'Moving partnerships forward', Paper to Policy and Performance Review Network conference, Warwick.

Stirling, A. (2006) 'Analysis, participation and power: Justification and closure in participatory multi-criteria analysis', *Land Use Policy*, 23: 95–107.

Sumberg, J. (2013) 'When evidence is thin, policy makers should learn from ancient mariners', *Future Agricultures*. Available at: https://www.future-agricultures.org/blog/entry/when-evidence-is-thin-policy-makers-should-learn-from-ancient-mariners

Thompson, M. (2003) 'Cultural theory, climate change and clumsiness', *Economic and Political Weekly*, 38(48): 5107–5112.

Thompson, M. (2008) *Organising and Disorganising*, Axminster: Triarchy Press.

Thornton, P. and Ocasio, W. (2008) 'Institutional logics', in R. Greenwood, C. Oliver, R. Suddaby and K. Sahlin-Andersson (eds), *SAGE Handbook of Organizational Institutionalism*, London: SAGE, pp 99–129.

Turnbull, N. (2008) 'Harold Lasswell's "problem orientation" for the policy sciences', *Critical Policy Studies*, 2(1): 72–91.

Turnbull, N. (2013) 'The questioning theory of policy practice', *Critical Policy Studies*, 7(2): 115–131.

Van Ess Coeling, H. and Simms, L. (1993) 'Facilitating innovation through cultural assessment', *Journal of Nursing Administration*, 23(4): 46–53.

Verweij, M. (2011) *Clumsy Solutions for a Wicked World*, Basingstoke: Palgrave Macmillan.

Verweij, M. (2014) 'Wicked problems, clumsy solutions and messy institutions in transnational governance', in Lodge, M. and Wegrich, K. (eds) *The Problem-solving Capacity of the Modern State: Governance Challenges and Administrative Capacities*, Oxford: Oxford University Press, pp 182–197.

Verweij, M. and Thompson, M. (2006) *Clumsy Solutions for a Complex World*, Basingstoke: Palgrave Macmillan.

Weick, K. and Quinn, R. (1999) 'Organizational change and development', *Annual Review of Psychology*, 50: 361–386.

Wildavsky, A. (1987) 'Choosing preferences by constructing institutions', *American Political Science Review*, 81(1): 3–21.

Wood, C. and Leighton, D. (2010) *Measuring Social Value: The Gap between Policy and Practice*, London: Demos.

Yanow, D. (1996) *How Does a Policy Mean? Interpreting Policy and Organisational Actions*, Washington, DC: Georgetown University Press.

2

Relationalism, wicked issues and social determinants of health

Adrian Bonner

Introduction

During 2020 and 2021, locking down communities, cities and countries was a public health intervention used in attempts to reduce the spread of the COVID-19 virus. Many people understood the need to reduce contact with others to reduce viral transmission, however, many objected to this threat to civil liberties either due to political reasons or the balance of risk between health and economic ruin. Sticking to the rules could mean loss of income, possibly leading to destitution or the intrinsic need to maintain social contacts with peers outweighing the need to isolate and comply with quarantine regulations. The importance of social contact to maintain mental health has become challenging during lockdown, particularly in the frail elderly at risk of dementia. The high death rate due to COVID-19 in care homes has been viewed as a moral and ethical crisis caused by government policies aimed at reducing the impact of the pandemic on acute health services, such as the National Health Service (NHS) in the UK, and ignoring the need to protect care homes from the epidemic during the first wave of COVID-19 transmission (see Case study 16.2). When this health threat to the older population in care homes was recognised they were locked down. The effects of locking down care homes, and lack of family contact for residents, particularly those with Alzheimer's disease, has been well-publicised (Anon, 2020a).

In the young, the fear of missing out changes the perception of risk such that socialising is more important than the need to adhere to guidelines and regulations designed to reduce the spread of the virus among the more vulnerable members of a family or community.

During COVID-19 there was a heightened awareness that healthy relationships are a key driver of health and wellbeing. **Social epidemics** in the 21st century were linked to stress-related depression (in pre-COVID-19 times), the second most significant health burden in the world (Parnham, 2018). Lifestyle choices contribute to modern non-communicable diseases, including cancer, heart disease, stroke, respiratory disease and liver disease

(Murray et al, 2013). The COVID-19 pandemic has refocused public health and acute health services in Western countries from non-communicative diseases to communicative diseases.

The experiences of the COVID-19 pandemic suggest that despite UK government interventions involving more than £350 billion in addressing previous underfunding of public health and social care, something other than state intervention is required. Major changes in social mixing were and are needed to reduce the spread of the virus in communities (via in families and hospitality venues), addressing a core driver, the fundamental human need for **social relationships** (Taylor, 2004). Networks of healthy personal relationships and strong social capital in communities have a profound effect on health and wellbeing (ONS, 2001). This health-psychology perspective on **relationships** is complemented by the view of sociologists, for whom an understanding of relationships in society and **relationalism** has resulted in an extensive literature contributing to our understanding of the nature of society.

Theories of relationalism

The concept of relationalism has been discussed by sociologists for many years. Marx (1990 [1876]: 932) wrote: 'Capital is not a thing but the social relation between persons which is mediated through things.' This idea is supported by Bourdieu, who regarded capital as a natural social object with an independent existence, conceptualising it in terms of relations as a social phenomena that emerges within a complex web of social factors and forces. Sociologists have drawn a distinction between relationalism and **substantialism**. Substantialism refers to agency (or freedom) commonly identified with self-action, and human will as a property or vital principle that *breathes life* into passive inert substances (individuals or groups) that would otherwise remain permanently at rest (Emirbayer, 1997). Relationalism, in contrast to substantialism, uses **agency** as part of the unfolding dynamic of situations rather like an ongoing conversation (Emirbayer, 1997). Agency can be seen as 'towards something' by means of which actors enter into a relationship with surroundings, places, meanings and events. Agency is therefore intersubjective and is never free of structure. Marx proposed that 'society does not consist of individuals, but expresses the sum of interrelations, relations within which these individuals operate' (Marx, 1997 [1939]). Bourdieu's view of **relational theory of practice**, in health promotion and public-health research, is that agency should be the focus of interventions aimed at promoting health and wellbeing. Applications of Bourdieu's theory of practice in healthcare are reviewed by Cockerham (2005, 2007), Frohlich et al (2001) and Abel and Frohlich (2012). **Health lifestyle theory** is based on the notion that structural factors such as class, age, gender, race or ethnicity, and material living and living conditions, underpin an individual's tendency to act (**habitus**) leading to choices and behaviours characteristic of healthy or unhealthy lifestyles. Relational descriptions of habitus, **doxa**, **capital** and **fields** as independent phenomena giving rise to 'coherence improvisation and innovative creative practice of actors' have been reviewed by Veenstra and Burnett (2014).

Discussions on relationalism appear in classical, modern and postmodern sociological critiques. For example, truth itself is relational and it does not signify something **absolute** or **relative**, it is 'lived in the moment and reflects an individual's connection to the whole and responding authentically to the present' (Briggs and Peat, 1999). Fuchs argues that 'things are what they are because of their location and movement in the network or system of forces; they do not assume a fixed and constant position in the network because of their essential properties'. An analogy of this can be seen in the biology of a liver cell that, in that specific way, functions differently to a brain cell, not because of its inherent nature, but because complex interactions occur between it and the selective and specific activation of its DNA (gene regulation) and the network of other cells with which it communicates. Similarly, in a social environment, people exercise and share their mental activities. Such social interactions involve an 'internal conversation [the **self–self relationship**] as well as dynamic interactions with the ever-changing social environment' (Archer, 2003). In summary, in this fast-moving, risky globalised social world everything is related to everything else, leading to the need to consider whole systems of social interaction rather than isolated phenomena. Relationalism conceives the world in terms of relationships. Network analysis is increasingly used to provide an understanding of relationalism in political science. Various approaches to this methodology are reviewed by Schneider (Schneider, 2015).

Relationalism and values

In this book a number of authors discuss the importance of **social value** which is generated by public and third sector agencies (see Chapters 8, 10 and 19). The **Centre for Partnering** is working with private sector companies to support them in their business strategies to move beyond **social responsibility** (for example, funding charitable causes) to organisational strategies which more clearly promote social value attributed to their activities (see Case studies 17.1–17.3). This ambition is increasingly observed in communication and promotional activities in the business world (see the section on 'Relationalism, culture and business development' in this chapter). Insights from theories of relationalism suggest that **values** and **objectivity** should be included in a relational approach to their activities. From a sociological perspective, value includes objects, activities, goals, careers and pursuits. However, identifying what counts as good is problematic (see Chapters 8 and 19).

The desire for an object, sensation and what situations can address the intrinsic desire for the object (value) is described by sociologists as **subjective**. This is the focus of **preference satisfaction theories**, which do not necessarily take account of moral value (Gauthier, 1986). Schmitz, 1950, proposes that there are some desires such as the desire to find something worth living for, that may change while it is being pursued. For example, choosing a career and pursuing it leads to the desire gradually dropping away as we change once the desired position is achieved. This may be viewed as a final position and is valued in itself. In this case, value has not been brought into the world. An objectivist view is that value is accrued from the desired pleasure that is independent of our affective (mental) state. This is in contrast to a subjective view that our preference has a value. '*Objectivists* argue that we have reason to pursue pleasure because it is *good* while *subjectivists* consider that *desires*, are the reasons to pursue pleasure' (Moore, 2004). In addition to considerations of objective and subjective values is the distinction between the **relational value**, that is always related to objects, persons, groups or times according to relational values defined by Mack (Mack, 1989). A relational value must be linked to a living entity which can experience different states of the world. This is contested by Moore (2004) who suggests that **goodness** exists independently of the relation to an agent, and relationalism does not require objectivity or subjectivity.

Geopolitical and regional perspectives of relationalism

A theoretical perspective of relationalism has been used in peace building (Joseph, 2018). From a territorial perspective, power and administration, social consensus and policy determination are important aspects of the analysis of **regionalism**. Prior to the development of the nation–state, local groups called tribes and clans, with attitudes and values, existed. These defined the culture of these communal and regional groupings, referred to as 'folk society' by Odom. In the 1990s an academic network emerged called the **New York School of Relational Sociology** (Mische, 2011). This sociological approach was influenced by **social network analysis**, historical studies of social structures and cultural sociology. A significant researcher in this area was Emirbayer (1997).

An application of this approach can be seen in international aid programmes where attempts are made to strengthen mutual accountability. Relationalism provides an understanding of the entities which are changeable, shaped by their position in relation to others. Messy circumstances and difficulties in measuring **quality** in aid programmes can be understood from a relational perspective. This includes analysis of processes and the complexity of the problems to be solved. Increasingly there is a recognition that effective aid may be the outcome of **relational approaches** which are rarely valued or reported. From this perspective **mutual accountability** requires the identification of powerholders and the relational power. These and an understanding of mutual responsibility, together with the effect which these factors have on each other and the wider system, contribute to measuring the effectiveness of the aid programme (Eyban, 2008).

In attempts to understand the culture in which **relational partnerships** exist social psychologists have developed methods of investigation based on relationalism (Ritzer and Gindoff, 1992). This approach has been used by both Western (or American) psychologists and also the anti-colonialism group of psychologists using an **indigenous approach**. This anthropological view is based on the idea that 'the study of human behaviour and mental processes, within cultural context, relies on *values*, concepts of *belief systems*, methodologies and all the other resources indigenous to a specific ethnic or cultural group under investigation' (Ho, 1998: 94). This approach has been criticised by cross-cultural psychologists who argue that the difference in behavioural repertoires across cultural populations should be understood against the background of the common features in these different cultures (Poortinga, 1994).

From an indigenous context, health, healing and relationalism intersect through the production of understanding and practice of health services. A cultural perspective on human activities may include religious rituals, arranging a marriage, deciding how to fight fire. An analysis of these cultural events has four factors: committee sharing, authority ranking, equality matching and market pricing (Fiske, 1991). Different combinations and arrangements of these factors are used in the social life of all cultures. In this way, sense itself, and the development of norms, motives, relationships with others and social roles, are fundamental to the establishment of institutions.

From a geopolitical standpoint, state formation, global and national policy formation and economic development, increasing inequality and civil uprising are all related to macro social change and social networks (Erikson and Occhiuto, 2017). The benefit of **collectivism** (versus **individualism**) in conflict decision-making is discussed by LeFebvre and Franke (2013).

The influence of sociological theories on international relations and relationalism has been perceived as the way in which actors interact within international relations, and the transactionalism and dynamism of those connections (Nexon, 2010; Jackson and Nexon, 2019).

Relationalism and climate change

The effects of climate change were widely recognised in 2021 as participating nations prepared for the COP26 conference that took place in Glasgow in

2021 (Anon, 2020b). The various climatic events involving floods, droughts, wildfires, and so on, provide major challenges to agricultural practice and human existence. The lives and health of many people and species of animals are at risk. This **wicked issue** involves a range of interrelated implications for populations including water and vector-borne diseases, mortality, food and water security, sanitation, shelter, settlements and the forced displacement and relocations of people (climate refugees).

There is a disproportionate contribution to the problems of climate change from the wealthy and industry-owning segments of the Western world. Doan and Sherwin promote a relational approach to **public-health ethics** centred around the idea of **relational solidarity** (Doan and Sherwin, 2016). This approach is a shift in the ethical framework from a focus on the role of individual **agents** and conversations about guilt, to issues of public-health ethics which recognises the collective nature of public health acknowledging the limitations of bioethics strategies. The primary focus of **clinical bioethics** is on individual patients and often individual providers. A **public health** approach focuses on populations not individuals, a collective understanding of ethics highlighting the activities of agents and agencies at many levels of complexity in climate change (Bayliss et al, 2008; Sherwin, 2012). This relational approach to public-health ethics is centred on three relational values: autonomy, social justice and solidarity (Bayliss, 2008). This relational theory is based on an understanding of persons as rational individuals, existing within a specific historical, economic, social and political environment, and with their interrelationships with other persons, both chosen and unchosen. **Relational autonomy** is concerned with the interests, values and commitments of those who will be affected by policy decisions and related practices. Unlike **traditional autonomy** it seeks to be sensitive to ways in which members of oppressed groups are particularly vulnerable to sacrificing their interests in favour of those with greater power. This approach acknowledges that not everyone is equally situated. An awareness of the meaningful options available for them to benefit from public-health measures should be clearly articulated (Sherwin, 2012). Relational solidarity is an important value using this relational approach, providing a more optimal approach to moral problems associated with climate change with the possibility of more meaningful responses.

A relational approach to climate change is required to raise an awareness of the interconnectedness of and interdependence of society and nature (Lehtonen, 2018).

Relationalism and the public sector

In Chapter 1 **relational leadership** has been reviewed and defined as 'a social influence process through which emergent coordination ... and change (eg, new values, attitudes, approaches, behaviours, and ideologies) are constructed and produced' (Uhl-Bien, 2006: 665). **Relational dynamics** operate within an organisation in which people live and work in relation to each other.

Relationalism and the third sector

Part IV of this book considers various forms and nature of the third sector including the role of both large and small charitable organisations, volunteering and the role of faith-based organisations (FBOs) (see Chapters 13 and 14; Case study 16.4). The various agencies working within the third sector are considered to have an understanding of the needs of service users and communities and are close to the people which the public sector (see Part III) aims to reach and finds it hard to deliver on its own. Value-driven third sector organisations are motivated by the desire to achieve social goals, for example improving the environment, or improving public welfare, and promoting social justice, rather than generating and distributing profit (NAO, 2010). The benefits of supporting and working with the third sector could be better understood by commissioners if a relationalism approach was used in determining the social value which third sector organisations bring to the community.

Third sector organisations work independently of government in line with the history and culture of the specific organisation. The values developed by these organisations have been highlighted in the Kruger Report (Kruger, 2020). This report recognises the importance of FBOs, which have a number of significant community assets including buildings/spaces, social activities, supporting vulnerable people, and the distribution of monetary and other resources including food and the provision of meals. Furthermore, FBO values contribute to the moral and ethical environment of the communities which they serve.

Working within communities, FBOs reflect a significant cultural dimension to **community organisation and development**, and are uniquely placed to work, collaboratively, with other third sector and public sector agencies.

Religions and faith-based approaches involve the promotion of relationships. Relationalism assumes that everything is connected, as noted in next section discussions on relationalism and the interplay between Marxism and Buddhism in China (Zhu, 2018). In Islam, **relational omnipotence** and collective worship might be considered to exhibit aspects of relationalism (Shah, 2020).

The theme of creation and an appreciation of beauty of creation pertains to relationships between individuals, the world and a sense of the spiritual world. A recognition of this global relationship between individuals, their activities and lifestyles increased during lockdown when people developed a greater awareness of human relationships and of nature, at a time when skies were clearer, roads were less busy, and they spent more time walking and cycling.

In summary FBOs are, or should be, grounded in their communities and add a wide range of assets, not least of which are values and an external **relational framework**. Further discussion of the third sector is presented in Part IV of this volume.

Relationalism, culture and business development

A consideration of relationalism in the private sector will be considered in Part IV of this book, with reference to a number of case studies which identify **culture**, **values** and a **relational partnering** approach which promotes trust. There is an extensive literature on systems theory, social network theory and actor networks, international relations (all influenced by sociologists), strategic alliances in the management world and **relational marketing** (for example, Kale et al, 2000; Das and Teng, 2001; Norman, 2002; Arino et al, 2010; Erikson, 2015).

From a cultural perspective, the significant economic growth in China has been directed by the dominance of the Chinese Communist Party (CCP), which has moved from the theory of class struggle to adopt a market economy and has amended its constitution to allow the protection of private properties by the state apparatus. In contrast to the Marxist approach of the past, the 21st-century CCP has attempted to open up dialogues in party schools and at regular grassroot party meetings generally supporting a community based approach in which many of the characteristics of relationalism can be identified. The invasive power of **relationalism** before and after Maoism is found within aspects of Chinese culture, across the fields of politics, sociology, psychology and diplomacy. Within this culture relationalism can be seen as the core frame of reference behind contemporary Chinese beliefs and practices. A specific example of the application of relationalism is the use of contract law in the construction industry (Cheung, 2001).

Another example of a culture which embraces relationalism is found in Japan. Hatch described Japan's techno-industrial regime as relationalism, and suggests that this approach has provided resilience for the Japanese economy during major market and political perturbations. 'A dense network of longstanding mutually reinforcing relationships between government and business, between nominally independent firms, and between labour and management' has maintained the economic strength of this country (Hatch, 2001).

From a Western viewpoint, four dimensions of a **relational environment** have been described by Young. These are: the organisational forms of marketing relationships; the governance mechanisms which exists between exchange partners; the perceived effectiveness of the organisational forms; and the expectations that the exchange relationship will continue in the future (Young et al, 1996).

Fiske (1991), from an ethnographic analysis of a West African society, proposes that the **market pricing perspective** (referring to rational self-interest) is balanced by the need to relate to one another through the medium of prices and markets. Application of these theories is seen in the relationship between marketing strategy and emergent realism in marketing channels. From a managerial perspective, managing marketing channels is critical for the successful implementation of marketing strategies (Paswan, 2011). An important aspect of marketing strategy is communication, in that individuals will interact in a way that is based on, and that is influenced by a source based on its relationalism. An individual responds socially to another social invitation even if the other is actually an inanimate object such as a computer program used in communication via digital social media (Zimmer, 2011). The extensive literature on relational marketing focuses on the manner in which companies/firms can offer the customer more than goods and services to facilitate long-term relationships and satisfy/develop long-term value relationships. An example of this would be Nissan offering after-care service (Gronroos, 1997; Porter, 2012).

In 2021, the COVID-19 pandemic and its impact on the global economy, uncertainty and concerns about the distribution of products across the world (supply chains), highlight the importance of long-term relationships between distribution channel partners. Trust and commitment between partner organisations are central to these trading arrangements. The concepts of relationalism and relational marketing (concepts that emerged in the business world in the 1950s) have become significant in the face of the threats to the global economy following the economic global crash in 2008 and the COVID-19 pandemic of 2020 (Black, 2010). Here, relational marketing has survival value.

Smith, in the previous volume in this series, *Local Authorities and Social Determinants of Health*, reviewed the 'power and value of relationships in local authorities' (Smith, 2020).

This approach is exemplified in the mid-western original equipment manufacturers, which developed an agreement with their suppliers as to how they do business by developing a trade-association-run private legal system to resolve disputes and support trade. Contracts used to consummate transactions are designed to maintain the law, with arm's-length contracting to create long-term cooperative relationships (Bernstein, 2015).

A pivotal aspect of developing a relational partnering approach is the need for **trust**. This is particularly important in inter-company relationships (Lado et al, 2008).

Relational partnering, based on **rationalism**, facilitates working across contractual boundaries, a concept developed in the US construction industry during the mid to late 1980s. Although relational partnering could be seen as increased control over the construction supply chain, a **trust-based partnering** approach encourages higher ethical standards. Trust between partners, supporting a strategic alliance, creates opportunities and the possibility of further collaborations and reduces the need for partners to continually monitor each other's behaviour, reduces the need for more controls, and reduces tensions caused by by short-term inequities (Rowlinson et al, 2002).

A critical review of relational partnering will be presented in subsequent chapters of this book (see Chapters 1, 18 and 19).

Conclusion

The COVID-19 pandemic has provided the stark reality of a world without relationships, experienced by people and communities in lockdown.

Although **relationalism** contributes to cultural changes in business practice, procurement and commissioning, it has the potential to contribute to long-standing and contemporary wicked issues. The section on 'Relationalism and climate change' gives an insight into opportunities to promote the international aims agreed in the Paris agreement (2016; see UN, 2021) and, COP26 in 2021 by shared values and trust across the developed and developing countries, as demonstrated via the need for equity in access to vaccines between developed and less well developed countries.

The third section of this chapter is a brief review of some long discussed philosophical, sociological and psychological theories which laid the foundation to the concept of relationalism. These perspectives are paralleled by the person-centred approach to health and wellbeing, a health-psychological perspective promoting relationships (relationism).

Relationism and relationalism have some common features which include trust, commitment and the development and maintenance of authentic relationships between individuals, which underpin organisational relationships in the public, private and third sectors. Relationalism provides an analytical lens to explore individualism and collectivism with respect to global issues and organisation–public relationships. The value of communication in these relationships is a core concept in relationship building (Zaharma, 2016).

The social determinants of health model, developed by Dahlgren and Whitehead in the 1990s, provides a strategic insight in to the interconnectedness and interdependence of people, their lifestyle choices, the sociopolitical environment within which public–private–third sector agencies have developed (see Bonner, 2018, 2020). Bourdieu's theory of practice in healthcare and health lifestyle theory (see the section on 'Theories of relationalism') provides a sociological perspective to the public health perspective of Dahlgren and Whitehead.

This chapter is intended to provide a translational approach, with respect to the sociological and real-world application of relationalism and relational partnering, supporting the various sections of this book, which facilitate the development of the Centre for Partnering (see Introduction of Part VI, and Footnote: CfP weblink).[1]

A key aim of this book is to review the social determinants of health framework through the lens of relationalism and relational partnering with respect to the impact and interrelationship of a number of wicked issues presented in this book.

Note

[1] Centre for Partnering Group: https://www.centreforpartnering.org

References

Abel, T. and Frohlich, K.L. (2012) Capitals and capabilities: Linking structure and agency to reduce health inequalities. *Social Science and Medicine*, 74(2): 236–244.

Anon (2020) UN climate change conference: Cop26. Glasgow, 1–12 November. Available at: https://www.ukcop26.org (accessed on 20 November 2020).

Archer M. (2003) Structure, Agency and the Internal Conversation Extract du Revue du Mauss permanent. Available at: https://asset-pdf.scinapse.io/prod/585970617/585970617.pdf (accessed on 29 August 2022).

Arino, A., Dela Torre, J. and Ring, P.S. (2010) Relational quality and interpersonal trust in strategic alliances. *European Management Review*, 2(1): 15–27.

Bayliss, F., Kenny, N. and Sherwin, S. (2008) A relational account of public health. *Public Health Ethics*, 1(3): 196–2019

Bernstein, L. (2015) Beyond relational contracts: Social capital and network governance in procurement contracts. *Journal of Legal Analysis*, 7(2): 561–621.

Black, G.S. (2010) Relationalism: A vintage but sound concept in distribution channel relationships. *Atlantic Economic Journal*, June. Available at: https://www.questia.com/library/journal/1G1-229896469/relationalism-a-vintage-but-sound-concept-in-distribution (accessed on 20 November 2020).

Bonner A. (ed) (2018) *Social Determinants of Health: Social Inequality and Wellbeing*. Bristol: Policy Press.

Bonner A. (ed) (2020) *Local Authorities and Social Determinants of Health*. Bristol: Policy Press

Briggs J., F.D. Pear (2009) *Seven Life Lessons of Chaos: Spiritual Wisdom from the Science of Change*. HarperCollins ebooks. Available at: https://silo.pub/seven-life-lessons-of-chaos-spiritual-wisdom-from-the-science-of-change.html (accessed on 29 August 2022).

Cheung, S.-O. (2001) Relationalism: Construction contracting under the People's Republic of China contract law. *Cost Engineering: Morgantown*, 43(11): 38–44.

Cockerham, W.C. (2005) Health lifestyle theory and the convergence of agency and structure. *Journal of Health and Social Behaviour*, 46(1): 51–67.

Cockerham, W.C. (2007) *Social Causes of Health and Disease*. Cambridge: Polity Press.

Das, T.K. and Teng, B.-S. (2001) Relational risk and its personal correlated in strategic alliances. *Journal of Business and Psychology*, 15(3): 449–465.

Doan, M. and Sherwin, S. (2016) Relational solidarity and climate change in Western nations. In C.C. Macpherson (ed) *Bioethical Insights into Values and Policy*. Cham: Springer.

Emirbayer, M. (1997) Manifesto for a relational sociology. *American Journal of Sociology*, 103(2): 281–317.

Erikson, E. (2015) Relationalism emergent. *Contemporary Sociology: A Journal of Reviews*. 6(January).

Erikson, E. and Occhiuto, N. (2017) Social networks and macro social change. *Annual Review of Sociology*, 43: 229–248.

Eyban, R. (2008) Power, mutual accountability and responsibility in the practice of international aid: A relational approach. Institute of Development Studies, OpenDocs. IDS working paper: 305. Available at: https://opendocs.ids.ac.uk/opendocs/handle/20.500.12413/4164 (accessed on 29 August 2022).

Fiske, A.S.P. (1991) *Structure Is a Social Life: The Four Elementary Forms of Human Relations, Communal Sharing, Authority Ranking Equality Matching, Market Pricing*. New York: Free Press.

Frohlich, K.L., Cronin, E. and Potvin, L. (2001) A theoretical proposal for the relationship between the context and disease. *Sociology of Health and Illness*, 23(6): 776–797.

Gauthier, D. (1986) *Morals by Agreement*. Oxford: Oxford University Press.

Gronroos, C. (1997) Value drive relational marketing: From products to resources and competencies. *Journal of Marketing Management*, 13(5): 407–419.

Hatch, W. (2001) Regionalizing relationalism: Japanese production networks in Asia. MIT Japan Program, Working Paper 01.07, MIT International Science and Technology Initiative. Available at: https://dspace.mit.edu/bitstream/handle/1721.1/16595/JP-WP-01-07-52125382.pdf;sequence=1 (accessed on 21 November 2020).

Ho, D.Y.F.G. (1998) Indigenous psychologies: An Asian perspective. *Journal of Cross Cultural Psychology*, 29(1): 88–103.

Jackson, P.T. and Nexon, D.H. (2019) Reclaiming the social: Relationalism in anglophone international studies. *Cambridge Review of International Affairs*. 32(5).

Joseph, J. (2018) Beyond relationalism in peace building peace: The politics of difference. *Journal of Intervention and State Building*, 12(3).

Kale, P., Singh, H. and Perlmutter, H. (2000) Learning and protecting proprietary assets in strategic alliances: Building relational capital. *Strategic Management Journal*, 21(3): 217–237.

Kenny, N.P. (2010). Re-visioning public health ethics: A relational perspective. *Canadian Journal of Public Health*, 101(1): 9–11.

Kruger, D. (2020) Levelling up our communities: Proposals for a new social covenant. A new deal with faith communities. Report commissioned by the Prime Minister. Available at: https://www.dannykruger.org.uk/files/2020-09/Levelling%20Up%20Our%20Communities-Danny%20Kruger.pdf (accessed on 14 November 2020).

Lado, A., Dant, R.V. and Tekleab, A.G. (2008) Trust-opportunism paradox, relationism, and performance in interfirm relationship: Evidence from the retail industry. *Strategic Management Journal*, 29(4): 401–423.

LeFebvre, R. and Franke, V. (2013) Culture matters: Individualism vs collectivism in conflict decision-making. *Societies*, 3: 128–146.

Lehtonen, A., Salonen, A., Cantell, H. and Riuttangen, L. (2018) A pedagogy of interconnectedness for encountering climate change as a wicked sustainability problem. *Journal of Cleaner Production*, 199: 869–867.

Mack, E. (1989) Moral individualism: Agent relativity and deontic restraints. *Social Philosophy and Policy*, 7(1): 95.

Marx, K. (1990 [1876]) *A Critique of Political Economy*, Vol 1. London: Penguin.

Marx, K. (1997 [1939]) *Grundrisse: Foundation Is of the Critique of Political Economy*. London: Penguin.

Moore, A.D. (2004) Values, objectivity and relationalism. *Journal of Value Inquiry*, 38: 75–90.

Murray, C., Richards, M. and Newton, J. (2013) UK health performance: Findings of the Global Burden of Disease Study 2010. *The Lancet*, 381(9871): 997–1020.

NAO (2010) What are third sector organisations and their benefits for commissioners? Available at: https://www.nao.org.uk/successful-commissioning/introduction/what-are-civil-society-organisations-and-their-benefits-for-commissioners/ (accessed on 29 August 2022).

Nexon, D.H. (2010) Relationalism and the new systems theory. In M. Albert, L.E. Cederman and A. Wendt (eds) *New Systems of World Politics*. Houndmills: Palgrave Macmillan.

Norman, P.M. (2002) Protecting knowledge in strategic alliances: Resources and relational characteristics. *Journal of High Technology Management Research*, 13(2): 177–202.

ONS (2001) Social capital: A review of the literature. Socio-economic Inequalities Branch, Social Analysis and Reporting Division. https://web archive.nationalarchives.gov.uk/ukgwa/20160105160709/http://www.ons.gov.uk/ons/guide-method/user-guidance/social-capital-guide/the-soc ial-capital-project/social-capital--a-review-of-the-literature.pdf (accessed on 29 August 2022).

Parnham, A. (2018) Wholistic well-being and happiness: Psychosocial-spiritual perspectives. In Bonner A. (ed) *Social Determinants of Health: Social Inequality and Wellbeing*. Bristol: Policy Press, pp 29–40.

Paswan, A., Blankson, C. and Guzman, F. (2011) Relationalism in marketing channels and marketing strategy. *European Journal of Marketing*, 45(3).

Poortinga, Y.H. (1994) Cultural bias in assessment: Historical and thematic issues. *European Journal of Psychological Assessment*, 11(3): 140–146.

Porter, M. (2012) The value chain and competitive advantage. In D. Barnes (ed) *Understanding Business Processes*. Abingdon: Routledge.

Ritzer, G. and Gindoff, P. (1992) Methodological relationalism: Lessons for and from social psychology. *Social Psychology Quarterly*, 55(2): 128–140.

Rowlinson, S., Cheung, F. (2004) A review of concepts and definitions of the various forms of relational contracting. Research programme 2A: Construction project delivery strategies. International Symposium pf the CIB W92 on Procurement Systems. Available at: http://www.construct ion-innovation.info/images/pdfs/Research_library/ResearchLibraryA/ Refereed_Conference_papers/2002-022-A/RCP_-_2002-022-A-10_A_ Review_of_the_Concepts_and_Definitions_of_the_Various_Forms_of_ Relational_Contracting.pdf (accessed on 29 August 2022).

Schneider, V. (2015) Relationalism in political theory and research: The challenge of networked politics and policy-making. *Pzeglad Politologicny*, 4: 191–206.

Shah, F. (2020) Islam and divine omnipotence a relational approach. Open Horizons. Available at: https://www.openhorizons.org/islam-and-divine-omnipotence-a-relational-approach.html# (accessed on 21 November 2020).

Smith R. (2020). The power and value of relationships in local authorities and central government funding encouraging culture change. In Bonner A. (Ed) *Local Authorities and Social Determinants of Health*. Bristol: Policy Press.

Taylor, J. (2004) Salutogenesisi as a framework for child protection: Literature review. *Journal of Advanced Nursing*, 45(6): 633–643.

Uhl-Bien, M. (2006) Relational leadership theory: Exploring the social processes of leadership and organizing. *Leadership Quarterly*, 17(6): 654–676.

UN (2021) The United Nations Framework on Climate Change: History of the Convention. Available at: www.unfccc.int/process/the-convention/history-of-the-convention#eq-1 (accessed on 21 May 2021).

Veenstra, G. and Burnett, J. (2014) The relational approach to health practices: Towards transcending the agency structure to divide. *Sociology of Health and Illness*, 36(2).

Young, J.A., Gilbert, F.W. and McIntyre, F. (1996) An investigation of relationalism across a range of marketing relationships and alliances. *Journal of Business Research*, 35(2): 139–151.

Zaharna, R.S. (2016) Beyond the individualism-collectism divide to relationalism: Explicating cultural assumptions in the concept of 'relationships'. *Communication Theory*, 26(2): 190–211.

Zhu, L. (2018) *The Power of Relationalism in China*. London: Taylor and Francis.

Zimmer, C. (2011) Information seeking behaviour: The effects of relationalism on the selection of information sources. PhD thesis, Clemson University.

3

Responding to the COVID-19 pandemic: a sociopolitical perspective

David J. Hunter

Introduction

The COVID-19 pandemic, it has been claimed, poses the gravest threat to the health and livelihoods of the British people since 1945 (Crewe, 2020). It is impossible to understand the devastating impact of the virus across the UK involving significant loss of life, and the government's much criticised response to it, without applying the lens of a sociopolitical perspective. The virus has cruelly exposed deep-seated and long-standing societal inequalities and deficiencies in the infrastructure of public services.

Following the successful vaccine rollout in the UK and growing confidence that a return to some form of normality is in sight, it is easy to overlook the incompetence of the government throughout most of 2020 and early 2021 (Calvert and Arbuthnott, 2021).

A substantial body of evidence exists to show that the virus has had a disproportionate impact on poor communities, and on care homes, reflecting widening health inequalities and the effects of deep public spending cuts since 2010 (Marmot, 2020a, 2020b; Marmot et al, 2020a). With over 200,000 deaths recorded as of 9 September 2022, the UK has suffered the highest number from the virus in Europe apart from Russia. It therefore comes as little surprise to conclude that the government's response to the virus from the outset has been found wanting and overly reliant on a public sector infrastructure that has been significantly hollowed out following a decade of austerity as part of a deliberate policy to roll back the state and reduce the size of government. This in turn has reinforced problems already evident in regard to the persistence of a dysfunctional health and social care divide, an overcentralised system of governance, a preference for uncritical outsourcing to the private sector, and a tendency to regard the National Health Service (NHS) as a special case – an institution meriting protection – while ignoring the significant public health challenges facing local government that has borne the brunt of spending cuts. Indeed, as Aileen Murphie states (Chapter 9, this volume), 'spending pressures have fallen most heavily on local authorities' adult social care, housing and public health services'. Little wonder then that local authorities are 'financially weaker than they were in 2010, with less capacity'.

None of these **wicked issues** is irrefutable or unavoidable. At their heart lie political choices about the nature of a country's governance and the priorities it seeks to pursue. Choices made by successive governments since 2010 have largely been responsible for the failure to tackle the virus in a coordinated, joined-up manner. Adopting a sociopolitical perspective, the chapter reviews the policies and systems that largely account for the UK's much criticised response to the virus and suggests lessons to be learned. Many of these are not new but have yet to be heeded.

As the Independent Panel for Pandemic Preparedness and Response (IPPPR) set up by World Health Organization (WHO) at the request of the World Assembly points out, the pandemic has challenged the assumptions that a country's wealth will secure its health. In a comment that certainly applies to the UK, the Panel is clear that 'leadership and competence have counted more than cash in pandemic responses' (IPPPR, 2021: 11).

Why adopt a sociopolitical perspective?

While much of the discourse surrounding COVID-19 has centred on its origins, aetiology and epidemiology, combined with a focus on ways of confronting and controlling the infection rate in order to limit the number of deaths and reduce pressure on hospital beds, this is insufficient as a basis for fully comprehending the trajectory of the virus or explaining why some countries have managed better than others to reduce its negative impact. Only by exploring more deeply the social and political contexts prevailing in a particular country can a better understanding emerge of why COVID-19 has followed a particular course.

A review of the data undertaken by Public Health England confirms that the impact of COVID-19 'has replicated existing health inequalities and, in some case, has increased them' (Public Health England, 2020: 4). The largest disparity found was by age, with people aged over 80 70 times more likely to die than those under 40. Risk of dying was also higher in males than females, in those living in more deprived areas, and was higher in Black, Asian and Minority Ethnic (BAME) groups. WHO's health equity status report calculated that 90 per cent of health inequalities can be explained by financial insecurity, poor quality housing, social exclusion, and lack of decent work and poor working conditions (WHO, 2019). While access to healthcare is important, it only accounts for 10 per cent of differences in health status across different socioeconomic groups. COVID-19 has shone a spotlight on all these long-standing, and worsening, weaknesses.

The UK has been especially adversely affected by the impact of COVID-19 on the social determinants of health resulting from some of the widest health inequalities in the developed world that were already well-entrenched and getting worse. As a timely reminder, shortly before the first national lockdown in mid-March 2020, a damning report appeared from Michael Marmot and his team which revisited his strategic review of health inequalities in England conducted in 2010 (Marmot et al, 2020b). The stark conclusion reached was that the UK's population is in a much poorer state of health than a decade ago and social inequalities are wider. In terms of overall health, since 2010 the rate of increase in life expectancy had slowed and, by 2018, had more or less ground to a halt. Only the US and Iceland fared worse.

When it came to health inequalities, these continued to increase with the more deprived places experiencing a higher mortality rate and shorter life expectancy. Whereas during the 2000s the gap in life expectancy between the poorest areas and the rest had narrowed, over the decade from 2010 it increased. When COVID-19 finally struck the UK after the government had played down its likely impact, Marmot noted that 'the same set of influences that led England and the UK looking unhealthy in the decade after 2010 led us to having the worst excess mortality figures in Europe' (Marmot, 2020a).

Given the deterioration in health and rise in inequalities, it is little wonder that COVID-19 has highlighted the importance of obesity as a risk factor and raised concerns over alcohol and dietary habits and mental health. As noted earlier, these behaviours tend to cluster among those social groups living in deprived places. They are also more marked in the North as another report on the North–South divide concludes (Bambra et al, 2020). Mortality rates during the first wave of the virus (March to July 2020) were higher in the Northern Powerhouse areas than the rest of England and economic outcomes, particularly unemployment rates, were hardest hit in these areas.

But if socioeconomic forces are at work, what about the political dimension? There is sometimes a reluctance to consider the political forces at work in any public policy crisis, or to do so somewhat superficially, which may serve to reveal our distaste of politics. Politics has a poor reputation (Gamble, 2019). Yet, although 'politics may be a messy, mundane, inconclusive, tangled business, far removed from the passion for certainty', it is at the heart of all that happens in public policy (Crick, 1962, p 54). In similar vein, Gamble argues that we cannot escape politics since it 'frames everything we do. It is an eradicable part of living together' (Gamble, 2019: 14).

In particular, the theories and insights offered by political science are well suited to providing a deeper understanding of the context of policymaking (De Leeuw et al, 2014; Hunter, 2015).

Political science deals with who gets what, when and how (Lasswell, 1936). It is all too easy to oversimplify social complexity by ignoring or understating the interplay of politics and power.

Complexity is not simply a case of there being many moving parts but about what happens when these parts interact in ways that cannot be predicted but will nonetheless heavily influence or shape the probabilities of later events. Political choices determine how these parts interact and to what effect. The response by government to COVID-19 has thrown these issues into stark relief.

Many of the core cleavages in health policy reflect political and ethical tensions over the balance to be struck, and negotiated, across personal and collective responsibility, across public and private interests, and between the rights of the community and personal freedoms. These are intensely political choices (Kickbusch, 2015). As will be explored further in this chapter, all these factors have been to the fore in both the UK government's efforts, and those of the governments of the devolved nations (that is, Wales, Scotland) and the jurisdiction of Northern Ireland, to confront COVID-19 in order to lower morbidity and mortality rates.

Public policy, including health, is about politics seeking to resolve (or at least attenuate) conflicts over resources, rights and morals (Marmor and Klein, 2012). All too often, however, there is a tendency to ignore, or deny, politics, regarding it as an unhelpful intrusion into the process of finding optimal solutions to complex problems. However, far from denying the place of politics, we should be seeking to repoliticise public policy in order to bring about the necessary degree of scrutiny and, where called for, change and improvement (Pfeffer, 1992).

Why has the UK government's handling of COVID-19 been found wanting?

Adopting a sociopolitical perspective allows us to identify and explore a range of factors which, taken together, help explain where the government's handling of COVID-19 has been found wanting (Horton, 2020). While most Western countries have failed to respond effectively to the challenges posed by COVID-19, the UK's overall approach has been especially lamentable as the number of excess deaths shows. Confused policy messages, dither and delay, poor communications and numerous policy reversals have seriously undermined the government's competence and exposed its inexperience and lack of preparedness.

Not surprisingly, the co-author of a highly critical analysis of UK government policymaking, *The Blunders of Our Governments* (King and Crewe, 2014), has asserted that 'the handling of the pandemic represents the most egregious failure of British governance in living memory' (Crewe, 2020: 13). Too often the government has been on the back foot, reacting too slowly to the evidence showing the virus to be out of control in some areas, and seemingly trying to steer a 'third way' between protecting the public's health on the one hand while keeping the economy afloat on the other. As a consequence, major policy and organisational failures include: the lack of a clear and coherent strategy understood and trusted by all; the delay of the first lockdown until mid–March 2020 which cost many lives combined with a further delay in introducing a second national lockdown in November 2020 followed by a third after a brief period of unlocking over Christmas; an inadequate supply of personal protective equipment (PPE) to key workers; the discharge of untested elderly hospital patients to care homes which brought havoc to that sector; and the failure to establish an efficient national system of testing, tracking, tracing and isolation.

Throughout, policies over border control and international travel have been hesitant and confused. Many of the factors giving rise to these failures have been evident for some time despite the UK having a strong and internationally recognised research base in infectious diseases and in other relevant disciplines, notably public health and epidemiology.

Public policy failures rarely have a single or common cause but COVID-19 has exposed systemic weaknesses in governance that are not new and which suggest that lessons from earlier critiques have not been heeded (Crewe, 2020). Moreover, one cause of failure stands out from all the others. The ravages of COVID-19 across the UK, with their differential impact on local communities, are a perfect illustration of what happens when government neglects and actively hollows out the public realm as successive administrations have done since 2010. In particular, the imposition of austerity has been responsible for spending cuts that have been felt most keenly in local government and in public health services, thereby rendering them incapacitated and ill-equipped to meet the challenge presented by COVID-19. Yet all the deficits that have been revealed have been the result of political choices, some having been enacted years ago but whose effects are only now being felt.

Underpinning all these failures, and the choices giving rise to them, is a UK government notably light on experience and motivated by a campaigning zeal to deliver Brexit given it was elected on such a platform accompanied by the mantra 'get Brexit done'. The government was elected in December 2019 just as the virus was hitting the headlines in China and beyond. The election resulted in an unexpected handsome majority for the new government. The continuing failure since the referendum in 2016 to strike a deal with the EU, combined with an unpopular Labour Party leader, propelled the Conservative Party into office for a further term with many of its new seats based in the North of England where it managed to breach the so-called 'Red Wall'. These seats in hitherto natural Labour territory were won on the basis of sorting out Brexit and, in so doing, 'levelling up' the North to address the widening inequalities noted earlier.

Given the nature of the 2019 general election campaign and its outcome, ministerial appointments were made largely on the basis of loyalty to the new prime minister rather than on those appointed having the necessary skill-set or experience of running a department of state. The prime minister's own decision-making and leadership skills were untested, although many who had been close to him when he was Mayor of London and in other positions remained sceptical that he was up to the job. The emerging consensus after nearly a year of living with the virus, and judging by public opinion surveys together with views expressed across the political spectrum, is that the prime minister's poor leadership has compounded the many failures already noted. Indeed, a Sunday Times investigation concluded that the prime minister was 'so fixated on Brexit and developing trade relationships that he only came to appreciate the extreme danger posed by the virus when it was too late' (Calvert and Arbuthnott, 2021: 8).

Policy failures in addressing COVID-19

Three particular policy failures, and the political choices leading up to them, are explored in this section. First, is the persistence of a command and control approach to handling the crisis which centred all decision-making in a small group of ministers and special advisers based in No 10 and the Cabinet Office, a consequence of which was to ignore the experience and expertise available locally until late in the day. Second, is the impact on the public sector, and on public health and social care in particular, of the policy of austerity introduced by the Coalition government in 2010. Third, is the heavy reliance on outsourcing activities to the private sector and management consultants to deliver on many aspects of the government's belated response to the crisis, notably the national Test and Trace system.

These three topics have been selected because of their significance in illustrating the government's overall approach to meeting (or failing to meet) the challenges presented by COVID-19. They are also all interconnected, feeding into and off each other in various ways.

Centralised approach to policy choices and decision-making

All governance systems are multilevel and involve a range of institutions and distribution of power. The UK is no exception although unlike most other European countries, and those such as the US, Canada and Australia, power predominantly resides with, and is exercised by, central government. Since 1999, the devolved administrations in Wales and Northern Ireland but especially in Scotland with its own Parliament and legal system, have exercised responsibility over many areas of policy including health. But, with exceptions in Scotland's case, control over taxation and finance remains firmly located in the UK government in London which also acts as the government for England. Local government, including more recent innovations like City Mayors and feeble gimmicks like the Northern Powerhouse, give the semblance of local responsibility but these structures resemble facades and remain very much under the control of central government despite glimmers of hope that mayors in areas like Greater Manchester and Tees Valley may be having an impact and shifting the focus from national to regional concerns.

In the government's defence, it is alleged that an advantage of a highly centralised system of governance is that it can make decisive and timely interventions, acting quickly to adapt to rapidly changing circumstances and in response to new evidence. It is also claimed to be easier to coordinate action across government departments when responsibility is located at the centre. Despite such claims, the evidence to support them is thin given the story of systemic failure (King and Crewe, 2014; Gaskell et al, 2020). The UK, and especially England, remains an outlier in Europe and beyond in maintaining such a fiction and one not borne out by the evidence. A major criticism of the government's response to managing COVID-19 has been its 'overweening and ineffectual central direction' (Gaskell et al, 2020: 524). This has been combined with a misplaced confidence in its ability to deal appropriately with the pandemic and a defensiveness when challenged. In addition, there has been a lack of trust and mutual respect between the four jurisdictions making up the UK coupled with mounting frustration in English local government at having been sidelined and ignored for much of the time.

The over-confident and ineffectual direction stems from multiple factors but permeating all of them is a campaigning style of governing that is at odds with the more technocratic style of governing that arguably the crisis warrants. To understand the precise nature of the government that was elected in December 2019, and its somewhat unorthodox style of governing, it is necessary to appreciate its ideological genesis that has been shaped by the determination to 'get Brexit done'. The unforeseen arrival of COVID-19 in early 2020 was initially viewed by the government as an inconvenient intrusion that threatened to distract it from its mission. Not only was the government unprepared for tackling the virus, as indeed any government would have been given what it had inherited in terms of a depleted and threadbare infrastructure, it was not politically prepared or equipped to rise to the challenge. A leadership style, if it can be termed as such, centred on the prime minister's unfounded, if not delusional, optimism derived from an arrogant faith in English exceptionalism, proved singularly inappropriate for the times in which we now live. The result has been dither and delay, too often being found playing catch-up instead of trying to get ahead of the game, endless policy reversals in the face of changing public opinion and revolts among the government's own MPs, and a display of control freakery that stems more from a lack of confidence in governing than in having any clear strategy.

Austerity and its impact on the public sector

Perhaps the command and control approach to the pandemic would have been less problematic had the country not been exposed to a decade of significant spending cuts aimed at freeing up the private sector to invest and to roll back the state in favour of smaller government. Such a move has always been a political choice rather than an economic necessity although the government has always denied this, maintaining it had no alternative but to cut back on public spending following the alleged profligacy of the outgoing Labour government in 2010. The result has been hollowed out public services ill-placed to rise to the challenge presented by the virus.

Local government, and the public health system for which it is responsible, have been especially hard hit by the severe spending cuts, especially those authorities in the North of the country, as noted earlier. Despite the overwhelming evidence, local authority public health teams firmly believe that their skills and somewhat depleted resources could have been harnessed sooner and more fully to assist with testing and contact tracing. Arguably, valuable time during the first lockdown from March to July was lost with central government refusing to engage fully with local government.

Partly because of the effects of austerity, the government was anxious to ensure that the NHS would not be overwhelmed by COVID-19 cases. Although the NHS had escaped the worst of the spending cuts, its budget was much reduced and it was struggling to keep pace with rising demand and costs and a failure to strengthen the workforce. But in its determination to protect the NHS, elderly people in social care or rapidly discharged from hospital to social care experienced a spike in deaths for which care homes were wholly unprepared. Austerity had effectively hollowed out those sectors − public health and social care − which, apart from the NHS, were most critical in responding to COVID-19 and its fallout. And even the NHS was in a more vulnerable state than it might have been had its funding kept pace with demand. Indeed, this reality is only now coming into focus as the full scale of the backlog of delayed NHS treatment becomes apparent (Cowper, 2021).

Outsourcing to the private sector

The third topic selected for comment has its roots in a long ideological tradition evident in both major political parties but especially present in the Conservative Party. This concerns the neoliberal love affair with outsourcing public services and activities to the private sector in the mistaken belief that it functions more efficiently and effectively. Studies have shown this belief to be a myth. For example, one study stretching back over 30 years found that as a consequence of outsourcing public services, 'far from falling, running costs rose substantially in absolute terms over thirty years, while complaints soared' (Hood and Dixon, 2015: 178). None of this experience has amounted to a lesson any recent government has been prepared to learn despite the occasional minister from time to time promising to reduce the reliance on consultants.

The sluggish response to COVID-19 and the country's lack of preparedness, combined with a threadbare public sector following a decade of austerity, made it easy for the government to claim that the only way to tackle the deficit in PPE and to set up a national Test and Trace system was to outsource such functions to the private sector. It swiftly did so to the tune of around £23 billion drawing on a two-year budget of £37 billion. In its haste, the government bypassed normal tendering and scrutiny arrangements. This proved to be convenient because it seemed to allow the government to award contracts to its donor friends in the business and to those with whom it had close connections and to make appointments to key positions involving individuals with close connections to government ministers and advisers while seemingly lacking relevant public health expertise. Led by the Good Law Project, charges of cronyism and corruption quickly gained traction which the government has unconvincingly batted away in keeping with its now customary bullish defensiveness.

In a critical report reviewing procurement activity involving 8,600 contracts related to the COVID-19 pandemic in the UK, the National Audit Office (NAO) concluded that overall the processes involved in awarding contracts 'has diminished public transparency' (National Audit Office, 2020: 11). Furthermore, the NAO stated: 'we cannot give assurance that government has adequately mitigated the increased risks arising from emergency procurement or applied appropriate commercial practices in all cases' (National Audit Office, 2020: 11). A possible casualty of such behaviour has been a loss of public trust.

The national Test and Trace has been heavily ridiculed by many in local government including public health specialists and other health professionals. As one group of former doctors put it, Test and Trace's 'privatised design by politicians is a lethal mistake' (Jones et al, 2020). Despite a widely held view in government that time should be allowed for the system to improve, critics argue that it is a victim of systemic failure and cannot improve in its present state. The system focuses too much on testing to the exclusion of the other stages in the chain of actions needed to control outbreaks, in particular tracing, isolating and supporting those who need to self-isolate. Notwithstanding such concerns, the diversion of public funds to benefit private companies, many of which, notably Serco, have on previous occasions failed to deliver on government contracts, continues. This is despite calls for the system to be brought back under the control of the NHS and local public health experts with support from general practice.

Frustrated local authorities began to operate their own test and trace arrangements so as to tap into their local knowledge of communities which is critical to the success of contact tracing and ensuring that self-isolation happens.

Going forward: an agenda for reform

With the so-called 'vaccine bounce' providing cover and a halo effect for the government's successive failures during 2020, there is a risk that the government is forgiven for its earlier errors, escapes scrutiny, is not held to proper account, and fails to learn lessons. The public inquiry now getting underway may offset that risk but we already know enough from what has happened to avoid a repeat. But for that to happen, the political stances underpinning government decision-making need to change.

From what we know of the UK government's mishandling of the crisis, the only 'world beating' feature it displays is one of 'systematic failure' (Gaskell et al, 2020). That conclusion might need to be tempered to allow for the success of the vaccine programme although that should not become an excuse for ignoring significant numbers of avoidable infections and deaths.

Numerous dysfunctional policy choices, all avoidable had lessons been learned from previous government blunders, have combined to produce a disastrous response. Little wonder the government remains in denial over its record and postponed setting up an independent inquiry until summer 2022 on the grounds that it would be a distraction from the government's single-minded pursuit of protecting the public from the ravages of the virus. The UK COVID-19 Inquiry was formally set up on 28 June 2022 with the publication of its terms of reference. The Inquiry, to be led by Baroness Hallett, has two aims: to examine the COVID-19 response and the impact of the pandemic in England, Wales, Scotland and Northern Ireland, and produce a factual narrative account; and to identify the lessons to be learned from the factual narrative account to inform preparations for future pandemics across the UK.

There are other immediate lessons to learn if a repetition of bad decision-making is to be avoided. As was suggested in the previous section, ineffectual centralisation can be seen in retrospect to have been a huge mistake. The success of the vaccine rollout via the NHS is testimony to that as well as the efforts of local government public health teams. But it is in keeping with a culture of top-down control which, if history is any guide, has not served public services or the country well. That lesson was not learned on this occasion and was compounded by a new incoming government fronted by inexperienced ministers and advisers and by a prime minister lacking the requisite leadership style. Instead of embracing complexity and displaying humility in the face of uncertainty, the government treated COVID-19 like it was akin to Brexit – an enemy to be defeated in 'whack-a-mole' style. There was an overconfidence and casualness about the virus's impact in the early months of 2020, in part the result of the prime minister's congenital optimism. The 'operational disconnect' between central and local government was especially evident with those in central government treating local authorities with contempt and choosing instead to ignore the relevant expertise and experience they possessed and which those in local government were eager to deploy. The treatment of the social care sector was perhaps the most glaring example of central government's arrogance. The term 'operational disconnect' was first employed in a study of government blunders to demonstrate the divorce between policymaking and implementation (King and Crewe, 2014). Such a divorce is unhelpful when it means those working on the frontline are ignored by those at the top of the organisation since it increases the risk of implementation failure and policies that malfunction.

Far from this lesson having been learned, evidence to the contrary shows that it continues to be ignored. The government's English Health and Care Act 2022 triggered a major NHS reorganisation (Department of Health and Social Care, 2021). In addition, and resulting in further disruption, following the sudden abolition of Public Health England in the midst of the pandemic in August 2020, two new bodies have been established to take over its responsibilities: the UK Health Security Agency and Office for Health Improvement and Disparities (Hunter et al, 2022). Apart from the wisdom of embarking on a major restructuring at a time when the NHS and its workforce remain weakened and distracted by the impact of the virus and moves are underway to clear the backlog of delayed cases, tightening the centre's grip on the NHS as the legislation envisages is unlikely to be a welcome move given the government's poor record in managing the pandemic. And while the government seeks to reform the NHS and public health, major gaps remain in regard to tackling social care and health inequalities through improved population health interventions.

In looking ahead to how things could be different with a refurbished governance system that is truly fit for purpose, there exist approaches and changes which, if adopted and enacted in the event of another pandemic, would demonstrate that we were properly prepared. Three such changes, all linked, merit urgent attention. First, is a need for reflective and consensual political leadership to replace the reactive and divisive type that has been on display in England throughout the virus and which has been counterproductive and wasteful of time, effort and resources. This would help ensure more effective joined up government at all levels, both horizontally and vertically, and a more effective and respected form of decentralised government. Second, systems need to be in place to share lessons and examples of good practice as well as to learn from mistakes – such an approach avoids apportioning blame but rather seeks to learn, as happens when adverse events occur in aviation and healthcare. Third, in place of short-term reactive and often disconnected and contradictory policy impulses, a system of anticipatory policymaking would allow governments to prepare for the unexpected before it overwhelms public services. As well as applying to the UK, these changes should also shape its global response to ensure the prevention of future pandemics.

It is difficult to single out the most egregious failure in our system of governance but perhaps what has been termed 'a deficit of deliberation' merits special attention (King and Crewe, 2014). The freedom governments have to take decisive action when they so choose can be a curse when bad decisions are facilitated. The government's management of the COVID-19 crisis is littered with poor decisions resulting in some of the highest levels of illness and death that were avoidable had there been more evidence of deliberation.

Conclusion

Hopefully any optimism arising from implementing the changes outlined in this chapter is not misplaced. However, guarding against excessive positivism is probably wise advice given the UK's current flawed, if not broken, governance system. But the problem goes wider and, in Philip Bobbitt's words, 'connects domestic politics to the global order'. As he notes, the pandemic was predictable and we knew the challenge was coming. The problem has been that 'we were politically and institutionally paralysed because the nature of the threat fit so well the vulnerabilities of the contemporary constitutional order' (Bobbitt, 2020: 68).

This leaves open the question of where the pressure for real, as opposed to the semblance of, change is going to come from. It is hard to locate with any confidence since in the past, despite what is promised in opposition by way of political and institutional change, it often mysteriously disappears from view when a new government is elected. So there is a need for realism about what can be achieved within the current constraints evident in a political system suffering from a dysfunctional state, a polarised society, a misplaced focus on tactics rather than strategy, and poor leadership. It is a toxic mix which risks leading to further failure.

Rather than expecting pressure for change to come from within the prevailing political parties embedded in Westminster, it may be that the public has to take a lead in pressing for change.

Although this will not be easy to bring about when the overwhelming temptation is to forget the litany of poor decisions in the afterglow of the successful vaccine rollout, it would be a grievous error not to try. The late historian, Tony Judt, set out the challenge facing us in his prescient book, *Ill Fares the Land* (Judt, 2011). It is 'to think the state again' and reject the misplaced faith in the market that has corrupted our politics since Thatcherism was unleashed in the 1980s. But for this to happen we urgently need a more grown-up and mature political discourse than the one currently on offer. We need, in short, to reject 'the unbearable lightness of politics' with its simplistic three-word sound-bites and silly booterish banter whatever their immediate appeal to the electorate. A first step on that journey is recognising the importance of adopting a sociopolitical perspective in understanding our present predicament, thereby appreciating why politics is important and a matter which should concern, and engage, us all. If the experience of managing COVID-19 provides the trigger, or 'burning platform', required for genuine change to occur it will have achieved what reformers have hitherto failed to do.

References

Bambra, C., Munford, L., Alexandros, A., Barr, B., Brown, H., Davies, H. et al (2020) *COVID-19 and the Northern Powerhouse: Tackling Inequalities for UK Health and Productivity*. Newcastle: Northern Health Science Alliance.

Bobbitt, P. (2020) Future scenarios. In Brands, H. and Gavin, F.J. (eds) *COVID-19 and World Order: The Future of Conflict, Competition, and Cooperation*. Baltimore: Johns Hopkins University Press.

Calvert, J. and Arbuthnott, G. (2021) *Failures of State: The Inside Story of Britain's Battle with Coronavirus*. London: Mudlark.

Cowper, A. (2021) NHS procurement: What doctors need to know about the Greensill scandal. *British Medical Journal*, 373.

Crewe, I. (2020) Points of failure, lessons for the future. In Goldin, I., Crewe, I., Hall, S., Pearce, N., Thornton, R., Cadman, D. et al (eds) *Building a Resilient State: A Collection of Essays*. London: Reform.

Crick, B. (1962) *In Defence of Politics*. Harmondsworth: Penguin.

De Leeuw, E., Clavier, C. and Breton, E. (2014) Health policy – why research it and how: health political science. *Health Research Policy and Systems*, 12: 55–65.

Department of Health and Social Care (2021) *Integration and Innovation: Working Together to Improve Health and Social Care for All*. CP 281. London: DHSC.

Gamble, A. (2019) *Politics: Why It Matters*. Cambridge: Polity.

Gaskell, J., Stoker, G., Jennings, W. and Devine, D. (2020) COVID-19 and the blunders of our governments: Long-run system failings aggravated by political choices. *The Political Quarterly*, 91(3): 523–541.

Hood, C. and Dixon, R. (2015) *A Government That Worked Better and Cost Less?* Oxford: Oxford University Press.

Horton, R. (2020) Offline: COVID-19 is not a pandemic. *The Lancet*, 396: 874.

Hunter, D.J. (2015) Analysis: Role of politics in understanding complex, messy health systems: An essay. *British Medical Journal*, 350.

Hunter, D.J., Littlejohns, P. and Weale, A. (2022) Reforming the public health system in England. *Lancet Public Health*, 7: e797–800.

IPPPR (The Independent Panel for Pandemic Preparedness and Response) (2021) *COVID-19: Make it the Last Pandemic*. Geneva: The Independent Panel.

Jones, B., Czauderna, J. and Redgrave, P. (2020) We must stop being polite about Test and Trace: There comes a point where it becomes culpable. *BMJ Blogs*, 10 November. Available at: https://blogs.bmj.com/bmj/2020/11/10/we-must-stop-being-polite-about-test-and-trace-there-comes-a-point-where-it-becomes-culpable/

Judt, T. (2011) *Ill Fares the Land*. London: Penguin Books.

Kickbusch, I. (2015) The political determinants of health: 10 years on. *British Medical Journal*, 350:h81.

King, A. and Crewe, I. (2014) *The Blunders of Our Governments*. London: Oneworld Publications.

Lasswell, H.D. (1936) *Politics: Who Gets What, When, How*. New York: McGraw-Hill.

Marmor, T. and Klein, R. (2012) *Politics, Health, Healthcare: Selected Essays*. New Haven: Yale University Press.

Marmot, M. (2020a) A decade of austerity made England easy prey for COVID-19. *The Guardian*, 11 August.

Marmot, M. (2020b) COVID exposed massive inequalities: Britain cannot return to normal. *The Guardian*, 15 December.

Marmot, M., Allen, J., Goldblatt, P., Herd, E. and Morrison, J. (2020a) *Build Back Fairer: The COVID-19 Marmot Review*. London: Institute of Health Equity.

Marmot, M., Allen, J., Boyce, T., Goldblatt, P. and Morrison, J. (2020b) *Health Equity in England: The Marmot Review 10 Years On*. London: Institute of Health Equity and The Health Foundation.

National Audit Office (2020) *Investigation into Government Procurement During the COVID-19 Pandemic*. HC959. Session 2019–2021. London: National Audit Office.

Pfeffer, J. (1992) *Managing with Power: Politics and Influence in Organisation*. Boston: Harvard Business School Press.

Public Health England (2020) *Disparities in the Risk and Outcomes of COVID-19*. London: Public Health England.

WHO (World Health Organization) (2019) *Health, Prosperous Lives for All: The European Health Equity Status Report*. Copenhagen: WHO.

4

Giving children the best start in life?

*Edward Kunonga, Victoria Cooling, Brighton Chireka and
Tsitsi Chawatama*

Introduction

It is universally accepted that giving children the best start in life should be one of the top priorities for any health and wellbeing system. A number of reports reinforce the need for evidence-based approaches to tackle health inequalities, highlighting that interventions focusing on early years are most effective, cost-effective and lead to improved individual and population health outcomes (Marmot et al, 2010; Marmot, 2020). An increasing number of reports have drawn attention to the importance of ensuring that efforts to recover from the COVID-19 pandemic not only 'build back better', but also 'build back fairer' (Marmot, 2020). For children and young people (CYP) together with their families this means addressing the significant challenges that existed before the pandemic, mitigating the negative impacts of the pandemic and also ensuring the future of our younger generation is safeguarded.

The size of the challenge before the COVID-19 pandemic

In England, over the last 15 years, social care spending on reactive services for children (including child protection and services for looked after children) has increased exponentially, with nearly two-thirds of councils reporting their 2018/2019 children's social care budget was insufficient to meet actual levels of demand and spending (LGA, 2019). In order to meet these financial pressures, many local authorities have had no option but to cut non-statutory preventative and early intervention services. This has led to massive reductions in critical infrastructure, services and programmes that support the growth and development of CYP. A few examples have been the closure of Sure Start centres, cuts to public health grants and the resultant reduction in preventative programmes, including health visitors and school nursing and the decommissioning of Family Nurse Partnerships. Even before the COVID-19 pandemic, aligning the best start in life rhetoric with the reality was a significant challenge.

Before the pandemic hit, concerns had already been raised about the health and wellbeing of CYP living in the UK. In 2020, the Royal College of Paediatrics launched their 'State of Child Health' in the UK report, raising concerns over increasing numbers of children living in poverty, the stalling of progress in infant mortality and the widening inequality in a range of health indicators (RCPCH, 2020). Of significant concern was a rise in the number of children with poor mental health, confirmed by a number of national reports calling for major improvements in mental health services for CYP (Robson et al, 2019). In 2019, the Children's Commissioner also highlighted concerns for CYP's outcomes in England (Clarke et al, 2019). Of significant concern was the rising number of CYP requiring statutory provision by local authorities, increasing numbers of families living in vulnerable circumstances and indications that growing demand was beginning to dwarf current levels of investment.

Pre-COVID-19, inequalities in economic activity and broader socioeconomic issues were blighting the lives of CYP in the UK, with CYP from different backgrounds having markedly different attainment on a broad range of social, wellbeing, physical health, mental health, education and social mobility indicators.

Progress on improving children's health and wellbeing in the UK

'The Marmot Review ten years on' highlighted failings of the UK government to progress actions to improve health, wellbeing and reduce health inequalities (Marmot, 2020). Despite local government embracing the 2010 Marmot Review recommendations, including giving children the best start in life, there was very limited national action, moreover, subsequent policies and decisions, including austerity measures, have led to widening inequalities (Marmot, 2020). 'The Marmot Review ten years on' report concluded that since 2010:

- More children and families are living in poverty, with over 4 million children affected, the highest percentage being from workless families.
- Funding for education, child/youth services has experienced significant cuts with socially deprived areas losing disproportionately more funding than affluent areas, despite increasing need.
- Socioeconomic inequalities in educational attainment have persisted with children from deprived/vulnerable environments achieving lower grades at all critical stages.
- Youth services have been cut and violent youth crime has greatly increased.

COVID-19 in the UK

Although the number of CYP dying from COVID-19 infections has been relatively small, CYP have been disproportionally affected by the social, economic, cultural and psychological consequences of the pandemic. These consequences are largely the result of the measures taken by governments and organisations to manage the disease, including the closure of educational facilities, home isolation due to national and local 'lockdowns', restrictions on business, transport restrictions and changes to the accessibility of healthcare services. While these disruptions affected everyone, those from more deprived communities have been disproportionately affected by the negative consequences.

COVID-19: direct and indirect impacts

The COVID-19 pandemic and the measures put in place to control the spread of the virus will have a lasting impact on the lives, health and wellbeing of people globally. For the most disadvantaged communities, the COVID-19 pandemic has been experienced as a 'syndemic', resulting from the intersection of pre-existing issues with the direct and indirect health, social and wellbeing effects of the pandemic creating a perfect storm for poor outcomes and widened inequalities (Bambra et al, 2020).

Summary of the evidence: direct impacts

The direct clinical impacts of COVID-19 are related to the pathophysiology of the infection, severity of disease, mortality, long COVID-19 and recovery. CYP are less likely to suffer severe disease or mortality if infected with COVID-19, with the majority having mild or asymptomatic disease (Boast et al, 2020; Viner et al, 2021). Studies indicate that unlike the situation in adults, most children are less susceptible to current strains of the virus and if they become ill are more likely to have mild disease, better prognosis and faster recovery.

However, children with pre-existing respiratory and cardiac conditions and those with complex neurodisability appear to be at increased risk of complications and poorer outcomes if infected with COVID-19. This is thought to be a similar level of risk to that seen in these groups for other respiratory viruses (Boast et al, 2020). A hyper-inflammatory syndrome (known as PIMS-TS or MIS-C) has also been identified in a small percentage of children resulting in severe disease and in some cases deaths (Bhopal et al, 2020; Boast et al, 2020).

There is consensus that the direct clinical risk of COVID-19 infection in CYP is not huge and the preventative measures for COVID-19 have predominantly focused on protecting adults among whom a larger proportion would develop severe disease, suffer complications and require hospitalisation. However, the indirect impacts of the pandemic are likely to affect children more than adults. These effects include physical, mental, social, economic, cultural and psychological damage which will have long-lasting impacts on their health, wellbeing and future opportunities/potential.

Summary of the evidence: indirect impacts

The indirect impacts of COVID-19 especially in CYP have different lag times, varying levels of impact, different durations and occur at different scales within the population (Bhopal et al, 2020; RCPCH, 2020; Save the Children UK, 2021). The indirect effects of COVID-19 on CYP are proving to be wide-ranging, complex and vary across the life-course. There are also periods during childhood when the indirect impacts of COVID-19 are thought to be particularly influential, these include during pregnancy, early years, transitions into primary and secondary school, entering the labour market and transitions into adulthood (Settersten et al, 2020).

The pandemic and its associated recession, school closures and reduced access to support services have disproportionately affected the most vulnerable and disadvantaged CYP. The indirect impacts of COVID-19 are not uniformly distributed across populations and those who were already vulnerable/disadvantaged experience the most significant and long-lasting damage from the pandemic. This is highlighted in a recent report outlining the stark differences before and during the pandemic between children in the North and South of England, with children in the North more likely to live in poverty and experience the negative indirect consequences of COVID-19 (Pickett et al, 2021).

CYP suffering the greatest impact include those: in need, in care or looked after; exposed to family violence or abuse; living in poverty; from Black Asian Minority Ethnic communities; with mental health issues or other pre-existing medical conditions; who are homeless or living in temporary accommodation; and CYP with insecure migration status (Cohen and Bosk, 2020; Douglas et al, 2020; Ghosh et al, 2020; Rosenthal et al, 2020). For these groups of CYP the pandemic has created new issues and further exacerbated existing issues they were already struggling with.

At an individual level, the impact has been poorer mental health and wellbeing, poorer physical health resulting from disruption to health services, reduced educational attainment due to interrupted education and school closures and increasing poverty and reduced employment opportunities resulting from the economic downturn. It is not easy to describe the causal pathway for most of these interconnected issues or how pre-pandemic issues have been further exacerbated by the pandemic control measures and response. This reinforces the need for a systemic and systematic approach to addressing these issues.

The following indirect impacts of COVID-19 have been identified among CYP:

- School closures resulting in reduced educational attainment and widening of the attainment gap by almost 40 per cent (Coe et al, 2020). This has affected all transitions (that is; school readiness, primary to secondary, secondary to university and other post-16 destinations). It is reported that 840 million days of in-person schooling were lost during national lockdowns, equal to around 19 weeks per pupil. While the disruption affected everyone, those from more deprived communities were disproportionately affected and are more likely to experience the long-term negative impacts of this lost education on their educational attainment, job opportunities, earning potential and social mobility. (Major et al, 2020; Save the Children, 2021). School closures also resulted in food insecurity/poverty for many families and there were significant increases in safeguarding risks (Armitage and Nellums 2020; Children's Commissioner for England, 2020b; Green, 2020; Van Lancker and Parolin, 2020).
- Over 1 million additional people in the UK, including over 200,000 children, were estimated to have been pushed into poverty as a result of the pandemic (IPPR, 2020), due to falling incomes (resulting from job losses and pay-cuts) and rising household costs. Additional vulnerability was seen in families where parents were in low-paid work, had zero-hour contracts or had a combination of self-employment/salaried work (Francis-Devine, 2021). Poverty is highly correlated with poor health, wellbeing and attainment outcomes across the life-course (Marmot et al, 2010). In addition, studies suggest that being born in a recession reduces lifespan by about 5 per cent (Banks et al, 2020).
- Reduced ability to practice healthy lifestyles with less CYP doing at least one hour a day of physical activity and increased sedentary activity, with over a million children in England not having access to a private garden, including one in three children in London (Sport England, 2020).
- A substantial impact on children's mental health and emotional wellbeing with an immediate 27 per cent increase in rates of emotional and behavioural difficulties compared to pre-pandemic levels (Pearcey et al, 2020). Pandemic-related problems included low-level concerns such as worrying, irritability, social isolation due to home confinement through to more serious concerns such as stress, self-harm, suicidal thoughts, neuropsychiatric manifestations, psychosocial stigma and deterioration of mental health (Barnado's, 2020; Ghosh et al, 2020; Jansen et al, 2020; LJMU 2020; Loades et al, 2020; Stavridou et al, 2020). It is estimated

that mental health conditions that children living in the North of England developed during the pandemic could cost £13.2 billion in lost wages over their working lives (Pickett et al, 2021).

- A rise in unemployment and numbers of young people not in education, employment or training, with disruption to most post-16 programmes, such as apprenticeships, leading to difficulties transitioning into the job market. Risks to newly employed young people of being furloughed and subsequently becoming unemployed, with under-25s most likely to be working in sectors affected by lockdown measures (that is, hospitality and retail) (Children's Commissioner for England, 2020a; Gustaffson, 2020; Joyce and Xu, 2020).
- Negative impacts from the economic recession resulting in anticipated increases in all-cause mortality over the next 50 years, for people aged 15–24 during the March 2020 lockdown, and an estimated 15,000 excess deaths equivalent to 465,000 years-of-life-lost (UK Government, 2020).
- Disruption to health, care and broader support services reduced access to treatment, rehabilitation and preventative services. This affected: continuity of treatment and care; early access to services; and access to preventative programmes including screening services, routine immunisations, and health promotion advice and support (Isba et al, 2020; Roland et al, 2020).
- An increased number of CYP were at risk of abuse due to the reduction in safeguarding arrangements, referrals (50 per cent decline) and early interventions as well as many children living in homes with increased domestic abuse, substance misuse and family violence (Baginsky and Manthorpe 2020; Bhopal et al, 2020).

Intergenerational issues and intergenerational justice

Intergenerational justice describes the duties and responsibilities that present generations have to past and future generations, and considers moral concerns when thinking through these duties and responsibilities (Baer, 2011). This is an important issue when it comes to the COVID-19 pandemic, as CYP paid a huge price in supporting the efforts to manage the pandemic. Although the necessary lockdown and social distancing measures were mainly aimed at reducing the negative clinical impact, severe disease, hospitalisations and death in adult populations, CYP are the group most likely to suffer the long-term negative impacts of the pandemic response.

It is important that the 'Covid Generation' is shielded from these harmful effects in a way that is proportionate to their level of need (Marmot, 2020; Save the Children, 2021). This will require policies and investments that strengthen universal services as well as targeted early intervention services. Shielding of the most vulnerable and high-risk individuals was a successful strategy for the clinically extremely vulnerable populations. A similar approach that identifies CYP who are vulnerable to the negative impacts of the pandemic and supports them through a wide range of measures will be important. Without this approach, many children who already had challenges before the pandemic will be severely affected and left behind.

Concerns have also been raised about the financial costs of the pandemic which could inflict a substantial economic burden on future generations, who may be subjected to increasing austerity measures and/or increasing levels of taxation. Building back approaches must take these future costs and impacts into account and ensure CYP's needs, rights and futures are prioritised and safeguarded.

Call to action

Coordinated actions are needed at a global, national and local level to ensure that efforts to respond to and recover from the pandemic do not worsen CYP's health and wellbeing. These actions need to consider the context and state of child health and wellbeing before the pandemic, how the pandemic further exacerbated these issues, as well as understand the future implications for this generation. This is not an agenda for adult-driven action without the involvement and voice of CYP and it is important that the rights of CYP and their voices are at the centre of any plans going forward. There is compelling evidence regarding rights-based approaches for improving children's health and wellbeing and this is even more important in the context of the pandemic (Peleg et al, 2021).

The actions taken so far do not provide enough evidence that children's voices and rights will be at the forefront of decision-makers' minds. Numerous examples exist where decisions that affect children have been taken without their input and contribution. For instance, the reopening of schools, the use of face coverings and lately the issue of vaccinations for CYP in the UK. These issues, despite being important for CYP, do not seem to have included their voice, considered their concerns and ensured child appropriate policy and implementation. This critical factor needs to be addressed if the best start in life is going to be more than cliché or rhetoric. CYP and their families should be engaged in approaches to measure the impacts of COVID-19, identify those at risk of the negative consequences and in developing interventions or services to address the needs of CYP.

Whole-systems, systematic and systemic approaches are required to mitigate the negative impacts of the COVID-19 pandemic and improve children's health and wellbeing. This will require action at all levels (including central and local government, local statutory and non-statutory services, local communities, families and CYP themselves). An understanding of the short-, medium- and long-term impacts of COVID-19 on CYP is vital. This will not only inform future approaches to control the virus, but will also help organisations and policymakers put in place recovery plans that will mitigate the impacts of COVID-19, help address underlying health and social inequalities and ultimately have a positive effect on the health and wellbeing of CYP.

It is important that the direct and indirect impacts of COVID-19 on CYP continue to be monitored through existing and new data collection methods and further research. This should build upon existing measures, make use of routinely collected data wherever possible, include quantitative and qualitative data and should include measures relating to: physical health, child development, mental health and wellbeing, education, training and employment, behavioural risk factors, socioeconomic factors, poverty, vulnerability and inequalities. A shift away from looking at single risk factors and indicators will help identify the intersection between risk factors as well as those CYP who might be experiencing hidden harms and risks.

Children experiencing multiple vulnerabilities and risk factors (individual, familial, community and environmental) are most likely to experience the negative indirect impacts of the COVID-19 pandemic. A population health management (PHM) approach could be adopted by local health and care systems to bring together data from different organisations to identify vulnerable children and families, better understand local needs, engage local communities and lead to improved service provision, integration and outcomes for children. In supporting efforts to give children the best start in life in a post-pandemic environment a PHM approach could be used to:

- Identify and stratify the population of CYP and families based on their risk of poor outcomes due to the COVID-19 pandemic.
- Understand the needs of these different population segments and the potential for intervention, supporting the development of a systematic and systemic approach to improving children's health and wellbeing.
- Develop and offer targeted and universal interventions that meet the needs of the population and mitigate the negative impacts of COVID-19, including targeted action for groups that are disproportionately affected, such as children living in poverty, CYP living in deprived areas, children in need/care/looked after, migrants and those who are homeless or living in temporary accommodation.
- Monitor the effects of the recovery efforts on the different groups of CYP and at different stages of childhood, to understand the short-, medium- and long-term impacts.

Conclusion

Giving children the best start in life has been embraced by many organisations, especially local authorities and local partnerships such as health and wellbeing boards. This was a priority before the pandemic and is an area in need of focused attention in the efforts to restore services. The ambition should not be about returning to the pre-pandemic environment characterised by poor outcomes for children and significant inequalities. The pandemic exposed these inequalities, further exacerbating the disadvantage and vulnerability for many children. How we respond to this crisis will either help or further confound the situation.

There is an urgent need for targeted and resourced plans to ensure all children are supported to get over the negative effects of the pandemic. Children paid a huge price in ensuring the pandemic did not result in greater numbers of deaths and even greater demands on health services. It is important, and in line with both intergenerational and redistributive justice, that the price they paid and the associated consequences are made a priority in COVID-19 recovery and future plans. Time will tell whether enough attention, effort and resources have been directed towards giving children the best start in life.

References

Armitage, R. and Nellums, L.B. (2020) Considering inequalities in the school closure response to COVID-19. *The Lancet Global Health*, 8(5): e644.

Baer, P. (2011) Intergenerational justice. In J. Dryzek, R. Norgaard and D. Schlosberg (eds) *The Oxford Handbook of Climate Change and Society*. Oxford: Oxford University Press.

Baginsky, M. and Manthorpe, J. (2020) Managing through COVID-19: The experiences of children's social care in 15 English local authorities. NIHR Policy Research Unit in Health and Social Care Workforce. The Policy Institute, King's College London.

Bambra, C., Riordan, R., Ford, J. and Matthews, F. (2020) The COVID-19 pandemic and health inequalities. *Journal of Epidemiology and Community Health*, 74(11): 964–968.

Banks, J., Karjalainen, H. and Propper, C. (2020) Recessions and health: The long-term health consequences of responses to the coronavirus. *Fiscal Studies*, 41: 337–344.

Barnado's (2020) *Mental Health and COVID-19: In Our Own Words*. London: Barnado's.

Bhopal, S.S., Bagaria, J., Olabi, B. and Bhopal, R. (2020) COVID-19 deaths in children: Comparison with all and other causes and trends in incidence of mortality. *Public Health*, 188: 32–34.

Bhopal, S., Buckland, A., McCrone, R., Villis, A.I. and Owens, S. (2021) Who has been missed? Dramatic decrease in numbers of children seen for child protection assessments during the pandemic. *Archives of Disease in Childhood*, 106(2): e6–e6.

Boast, A., Munro, A. and Goldstein, H. (2020) An evidence summary of paediatric COVID-19 literature. *Don't Forget the Bubbles*, 382: 1663–1665.

Children's Commissioner for England (2020a) *Briefing: What COVID-19 Means for Young Apprentices*. London: Children's Commissioner for England.

Children's Commissioner for England (2020b) *Childhood in the Time of COVID*. London: Children's Commissioner for England.

Clarke, T., Chowdry, H. and Gilhooly, R. (2019) *Trends in Childhood Vulnerability*. Vulnerability Technical Report 1, July. London: Children's Commissioner for England.

Coe, R., Weidmann, B., Coleman, R. and Kay, J. (2020) *Impact of School Closures on the Attainment Gap: Rapid Evidence Assessment*. London: Education Endowment Foundation.

Cohen, R.I.S. and Bosk, E.A. (2020). Vulnerable youth and the COVID-19 pandemic. *Pediatrics*, 146(1): e20201306.

Douglas, M., Katikireddi, S.V., Taulbut, M., McKee, M. and McCartney, G. (2020) Mitigating the wider health effects of COVID-19 pandemic response. *BMJ*, 369.

Francis-Devine, B. (2021) *Poverty in the UK: Statistics*. House of Commons Briefing Paper.

Ghosh, R., Dubey, M.J., Chatterjee, S. and Dubey, S. (2020) Impact of COVID-19 on children: Special focus on psychosocial aspect. *Minerva Pediatrica*, 72: 226–235.

Green, P. (2020) Risks to children and young people during COVID-19 pandemic. *BMJ*, 369.

Gustaffson, M. (2020) *Young Workers in the Coronavirus Crisis*. London: Resolution Foundation.

IPPR (Institute for Public Policy Research) (2020) Estimating the poverty impacts of coronavirus. Available at: https://www.ippr.org/research/publications/estimating-poverty-impacts-of-coronavirus#:~:text=IPPR%27s%20research%20finds%20it%20highly,the%20end%20of%20the%20year (accessed on 29 August 2022).

Isba, R., Edge, R., Jenner, R., Broughton, E., Francis, N. and Butler, J. (2020) Where have all the children gone? Decreases in paediatric emergency department attendances at the start of the COVID-19 pandemic of 2020. *Archives of Disease in Childhood*, 105(7): 704.

Jansen, D., Kosola, S., Arevalo, L.C., de Matos, M.G., Boode, K., Saxena, S. and Dratva, J. (2020) Child and adolescent health needs attention now, and in the aftermath of the COVID-19 pandemic. *International Journal of Public Health*, 65(6): 723–725.

Joyce, R. and Xu, X. (2020) *Sector Shutdowns during the Coronavirus Crisis: Which Workers are Most Exposed?* Institute for Fiscal Studies. Available on Sector shutdowns during the coronavirus crisis: which workers are most exposed? - Institute For Fiscal Studies - IFS (Accessed on 28/08/22)

LGA (Local Government Association) (2019) *Children's Social Care Budgets: A Survey of Lead Members for Children's Services.*

LJMU (2020) *Direct and Indirect Impacts of COVID-19 on Health and Wellbeing: Rapid Evidence Review.* Available at: https://www.ljmu.ac.uk/~/media/phi-reports/2020-07-direct-and-indirect-impacts-of-covid19-on-health-and-wellbeing.pdf (accessed on 29 August 2022).

Loades, M.E., Chatburn, E., Higson-Sweeney, N., Reynolds, S., Shafran, R., Brigden, A., Linney, C., McManus, M.N., Borwick, C. and Crawley, E. (2020) Rapid systematic review: The impact of social isolation and loneliness on the mental health of children and adolescents in the context of COVID-19. *Journal of the American Academy of Child and Adolescent Psychiatry*, 59(11): 1218–1239.

Major, L.E., Eyles, A. and Machin, S. (2020) *Generation COVID: Emerging Work and Education Inequalities.* London: Centre for Economic Performance, London School of Economics and Political Science.

Marmot, M. (2020) Health equity in England: The Marmot review 10 years on. *BMJ*, 368.

Marmot, M., Allen, J. and Goldblatt, P. (2010) A social movement, based on evidence, to reduce inequalities in health: Fair society, healthy lives (the Marmot Review). *Social Science and Medicine*, 71(7): 1254–1258.

Pearcey, S., Shum, A., Waite, P., Patalay, P. and Creswell, C. (2020) *Report 05: Changes in Children and Young People's Mental Health Symptoms and 'Caseness' during Lockdown and Patterns Associated with Key Demographic Factors.* CO-SPACE study. Available at: https://cospaceoxford.org/wp-content/uploads/2020/08/Co-SPACE-report-05_06-09-21-1.pdf (accessed on 29 August 2022).

Peleg, N., Lundy, L. and Stalford, H. (2021) COVID-19 and children's rights: Space for reflection, tracing the problems and facing the future. *International Journal of Children's Rights*, 29(2): 255–259.

Pickett, K., Taylor-Robinson, D., et al (2021) *The Child of the North: Building a Fairer Future after COVID-19.* The Northern Health Science Alliance and N8 Research Partnership. Project Report. Northern Health Science Alliance. Available at: https://www.thenhsa.co.uk/app/uploads/2022/01/Child-of-the-North-Report-FINAL-1.pdf (accessed on 29 August 2022).

RCPCH (Royal College of Paediatrics and Child Health) (2020) State of Child Health 2020. London: Royal College of Paediatrics and Child Health. Available at: https://stateofchildhealth.rcpch.ac.uk/ (accessed on 29 August 2022).

Robson, C., Leyera, R.U., Testoni, S., Miranda Wolpert, S.T., Ullman, R., Testoni, S., Wolper, M. and Deighton, J. (2019) *Universal Approaches to Improving Children and Young People's Mental Health and Wellbeing: Report of the Findings of a Special Interest Group.* Available at: https://assets.publishing.service.gov.uk/government/uploads/system/uploads/attachment_data/file/842176/SIG_report.pdf (accessed on 29 August 2022).

Roland, D., Harwood, R., Bishop, N., Hargreaves, D., Patel, S. and Sinha, I. (2020) Children's emergency presentations during the COVID-19 pandemic. *The Lancet: Child and Adolescent Health*, 4(8): e32–e33.

Rosenthal, D.M., Ucci, M., Heys, M., Hayward, A. and Lakhanpaul, M. (2020) Impacts of COVID-19 on vulnerable children in temporary accommodation in the UK. *The Lancet Public Health*, 5(5): e241–e242.

Save the Children 2021. *Protecting a Generation*. Available at: https://www.savethechildren.org/content/dam/usa/reports/emergency-response/protect-a-generation-report.pdf (accessed on 29 August 2022).

Settersten, Jr, R.A., Bernardi, L., Härkönen, J., Antonucci, T.C., Dykstra, P.A., Heckhausen, J., Kuh, D., Mayer, K.U., Moen, P., Mortimer, J.T. and Mulder, C.H. (2020) Understanding the effects of COVID-19 through a life course lens. *Advances in Life Course Research*, 100360.

Sport England (2020) *COVID-19 Briefing: Exploring Attitudes and Behaviours in England during the COVID-19 Pandemic*. London: Sport England.

Stavridou, A., Stergiopoulou, A.A., Panagouli, E., Mesiris, G., Thirios, A., Mougiakos, T., Troupis, T., Psaltopoulou, T., Tsolia, M., Sergentanis, T. and Tsitsika, A. (2020) Psychosocial consequences of COVID-19 in children, adolescents and young adults: A systematic review. *Psychiatry and Clinical Neurosciences*, November: 615–661.

UK Government (Department of Health and Social Care, Office for National Statistics, Government Actuary's Department and Home Office) (2020) *Direct and Indirect Impacts of COVID-19 on Excess Deaths and Morbidity*. Available at: https://assets.publishing.service.gov.uk/government/uploads/system/uploads/attachment_data/file/907616/s0650-direct-indirect-impacts-covid-19-excess-deaths-morbidity-sage-48.pdf (accessed on 29 August 2022).

Van Lancker, W. and Parolin, Z. (2020) COVID-19, school closures, and child poverty: A social crisis in the making. *The Lancet Public Health*, 5(5): e243–e244.

Viner, R.M., Mytton, O.T., Bonell, C., Melendez-Torres, G.J., Ward, J., Hudson, L., Waddington, C., Thomas, J., Russell, S., Van Der Klis, F. and Koirala, A. (2021) Susceptibility to SARS-CoV-2 infection among children and adolescents compared with adults: A systematic review and meta-analysis. *JAMA Pediatrics*, 175(2): 143–156.

PART II

Regionalism and geopolitical environments

Adrian Bonner

The communities particularly vulnerable to communicable diseases have highlighted regional variations in the UK and across the world when challenged by the transmission of the COVID-19 virus, deemed to be a pandemic by the World Health Organization in March 2020 (WHO, 2020). A complex interplay of factors has been proposed to explain these regional and geographic variations. Those include poor health status, nutritional status, cultural and ethnic practices, housing quality, and political factors related to the geopolitics of the region.

In the UK, high rates of infection have been found in the North East and North West of England and Scotland.

In the previous volume in this series, *Local Authorities and the Social Determinants of Health* (Bonner, 2020), inequalities in health and wellbeing were reviewed, from public health, cultural and geopolitical perspectives, in the North East (Kunonga et al, 2020) and the North West (Arden and Cunliffe, 2020; Dennett and Russell, 2020). In that previous publication, housing policy in Scotland (Anderson, 2020) and the needs of future generations in Wales (Farrell, 2020) provided specific geopolitically focused examples aimed at resolving identified regional needs.

In this current volume devolution to metropolitan boroughs, and the organisation of combined versus unitary local authorities, reviewed by Shutt, in Chapter 5, highlight the need for a geopolitical focus in the development of socioeconomic policy, to build back in a way that is fair for all.

A recognition of the need to address social and economic inequalities has been a key manifesto issue of the Boris Johnson government, prior to the COVID-19 pandemic. This 'levelling up' agenda has become more politically relevant during COVID-19. Although the economic consequences of the first and second lockdowns have distracted the government from its proposed 'levelling up' agenda, there is ongoing interest in Northern Powerhouse initiatives, including the high speed train line (HS2), North East infrastructure projects, Middlesbrough city centre housing initiative, 5G digital broadband and new research centres, supporting the hydrogen economy and wind farms along with new industrial strategies to support these, including the government's 'Green Deal' (see Chapter 5). This chapter will consider economic planning and consequential effects on community development and wellbeing. A major consequence of the locking down of businesses and the wider economy has resulted in emerging mass unemployment, particularly in the North of England. Employability, skills and talent management will be discussed in relation to COVID-19 and the interrelated impact of Brexit (see Chapter 12).

A significant geopolitical issue is the climate crisis. Although collaboration between the major CO_2 emitting countries (see Chapter 10) is essential, there is an important role to be played by local authorities. **Place-based** strategies were discussed in the previous volume (Dombey and Bonner, 2020). This provides a perspective on local authorities and their communities as the source of problems as well as solutions, an approach used in regeneration studies. Increasingly, local authorities are using place-based initiatives to address complex health inequalities. Since the passing of the Social Value Act (2012) and the Health and Social Care Act (2012) (see Chapter 19), public bodies have had to consider the wider social, environmental and health implications of their commissioning decisions, with local authorities required to improve health outcomes and reduce health inequalities. In building on place-based strategies in COVID-19 and post-COVID-19 planning, Abellan in Chapter 6 in this volume provides a current insight into planning, budgeting and managing a London borough. This chapter discusses the challenges of responding to urgent needs to support the local community, with respect to ensuring food supplies in lockdown and support for vulnerable people. The opportunities for behavioural change in relation to the **wicked issue** of climate change are not without public push-back, as demonstrated by Abellan.

The COVID-19 pandemic is a global threat which has elicited a range of country-wide responses, each nation having a responsibility for its own citizens, but also operating in a world community. A series of international case studies is presented in this part of the book. Brief insights into specific cultural and political approaches to interventions and outcomes from the pandemic are provided in case studies in the US, South Africa, India and Nepal. These are reflected in viral transmission rates and mortality statistics of the respective countries. These case studies highlight the more extreme consequences of COVID-19 in relation to racial disadvantage (Case study 7.1), domestic violence (Case study 7.2) and increased vulnerability to human trafficking and modern slavery (Case study 7.3). These case studies complement UK perspectives presented in Chapter 15 (domestic abuse) and Case study 16.3 (human trafficking and modern slavery).

Although there have been favourable reports regarding the containment of COVID-19 in New Zealand, the pandemic has highlighted fundamental problems in the centralised health system with limited reach into communities. McKinley and Matheson (Case study 7.4) report on the important lessons to be learnt in engaging with communities and the need for conversations with local government.

References

Anderson, I. (2020) Devolution and the health of Scottish housing policy, in Bonner A. (ed) *Local Authorities and Social Determinants of Health.* Bristol: Policy Press, pp 365–384.

Arden, K. and Cunliffe, P. (2020) Cultural change and the evolution of community governance: A north west England perspective. In Bonner, A. (ed) *Local Authorities and Social Determinants of Health.* Bristol: Policy Press.

Bonner A. (ed) (2020) *Local Authorities and Social Determinants of Health.* Bristol: Policy Press.

Dennett, P. and Russell, J. (2020) Devolution and localism: Metropolitan authorities. In Bonner, A. (ed) *Local Authorities and Social Determinants of Health.* Bristol: Policy Press.

Dombey, R. and Bonner, A. (2020) Wider determinants of health – housing, environment, economy and education more important than access to healthcare: The importance of prevention and early intervention. In Bonner, A. (ed) *Local Authorities and Social Determinants of Health.* Bristol: Policy Press.

Farrell, C. (2020) Public health and local government in Wales: every policy a health policy – a collaborative agenda, in Bonner, A. (ed) *Local Authorities and Social Determinants of Health.* Bristol: Policy Press.

Kunonga, E., Gibson, G. and Parker, C. (2020) Inequalities in health and wellbeing across the UK: A local north east perspective. In Bonner, A. (ed) *Local Authorities and Social Determinants of Health.* Bristol: Policy Press.

WHO (2020) WHO announces COVID-19 outbreak a pandemic. *WHO,* 18 March. Available at: https://www.euro.who.int/en/health-topics/hea lth-emergencies/coronavirus-covid-19/news/news/2020/3/who-announ ces-covid-19-outbreak-a-pandemic (accessed on 29 August 2022).

5

Levelling up in the North and North-East England: complex and fragmented governance and the new National Health Service and local government partnerships

John Shutt

Introduction

The 2020 book, *Local Authorities and the Social Determinants of Health* (Bonner, 2020) reported on the North East region of the United Kingdom, prior to the December 2019 UK election. The election brought Boris Johnson MP to power as British prime minister with commitments to both Brexit and to the 'levelling up' of Britain. Kunonga et al (2020) reviewed the response of the North East to austerity and reduced central government funding since 2010. They showed the scale of the North East challenge in towns and cities like Middlesbrough and Sunderland and highlighted the growing health and care gap in the North East. They argued for a more integrated approach to health and wellbeing and a whole-city and more focused place-based approach to address health inequalities, emphasising the need for long-term planning and long-term settlements to tackle health inequalities.

The 2019 general election proved cataclysmic for the Labour Party in the North East and across the North of England. Mattinson (2020) recalls: '[O]n the 12th December starting with Blyth Valley, I watched as seat after Labour seat collapsed to the Tories, challenging all conventional wisdoms about political tribalism. The Red Wall had turned Blue' (Mattinson, 2020: 5). Boris Johnson promised a levelling up process to deliver a new policy agenda for the UK and address the UK North–South divide, particularly tackling the deep-seated inequalities in regions like the North East. However, in 2021 it was still not clear what 'levelling up' means and what the geographical focus is to be. A previous Cameron and Osborne Conservative commitment to the Northern Powerhouse (HMSO, 2021a) and the three regions of the North of England appears to have now faded. A Cabinet Office Levelling Up Unit has been appointed and Neil O'Brien MP has been put in charge of bringing forward a White Paper on Levelling Up, originally for the Autumn of 2021 eventually, delayed until 2022. A recent report from the Northern Health Alliance shows the deteriorating position for the Northern Powerhouse which encompasses the three Northern regions (Bambra and Munford, 2020).

However, no sooner had the Brexit negotiations got underway in Brussels, lasting throughout 2020, when COVID-19 struck in March 2020. It brought a raging pandemic to the United Kingdom. This has increased health inequalities across the United Kingdom and brought new severe challenges to the North East in particular. At the time of writing, a year has passed, and Brexit has been done, but as Menon (2021) argues, our understanding of what this means is only now just beginning. More so, however, with the assessment of the COVID-19 pandemic, which brought three national UK lockdowns, and which is challenging English regions and the four nations to develop new partnerships and bring people together in new ways to combat the pandemic. What will be delivered to the North East through levelling up?

It is a complex picture, and this chapter summarises where we are at the end of 2021 in a fast-moving policy arena. There are many areas of public policy which are contradictory and incoherent. The ambitious plans for levelling up and a proposed new coherent approach to English devolution have not, *so far*, materialised, and over the past year central government seems to have had less faith in regional or subregional government, appearing to prefer top-down corporate private sector responses to strengthening central–local partnerships in the pandemic. This may change as the pandemic subsides, but so far there appears to be too little change and too little understanding and debate.

In February 2021, we learnt that there are to be major changes in the organisation and structure of the National Health Service (NHS), designed to recentralise control and reintroduce new integrated care systems (ICS) at local levels (HMSO, 2021b), but the detail was not finalised until 2022 and the change in health ministers in June 2021 also meant that there was also poor and negligible progress on the promised integrated Social Care Bill. The implications of policy change often remain unclear within regions, and any promised reforms may take many years to introduce and complete. How does this leave the North East, which is seeing inequalities increase?

The North East region and the North East case is interesting to international readers because it was so central to Boris Johnson's post-Brexit plan for the UK and because the UK's North–South divide is unmatched now in terms of European regional inequalities. Benyon and Hudson (2021) explore the end of the era of coal-based capitalism and argue for a new order. Boris Johnson argues that this new order in the North East will be based on sustainable and renewable energy and electric cars and battery manufacturing in the period to 2030 but appears to have little to say about health and social care and how to resolve longstanding inequalities.

Devolution and fragmentation of governance

In 2020, the Johnson era started with a commitment to devolution inherited from the 2010 Conservative/Liberal Democrat Coalition and continued by the Theresa May Conservative administration in 2016. Nine Labour Regional Development Agencies gave way in England to 39 Local Enterprise Partnerships (now 38) and to nine city- regions; new metro mayors were promoted for the new Combined Authorities and the policy momentum was with these new urban Combined Authority metro mayors (Shutt and Liddle, 2019).

In the North East, which rejected a Regional Assembly in 2004, there was a reluctance to embrace the concept of metro mayors and only in the Tees Valley had progress been made by May 2017. The proposed North East Combined Authority fell apart (Figure 5.1). Eight combined authorities were formed after 2011 and, across England, six held their first mayoral elections in May 2017. In the North East, only Tees Valley participated, and Ben Houchen was elected as the Conservative metro mayor. Eventually, the

Figure 5.1: Combined Authorities in England and the North East region

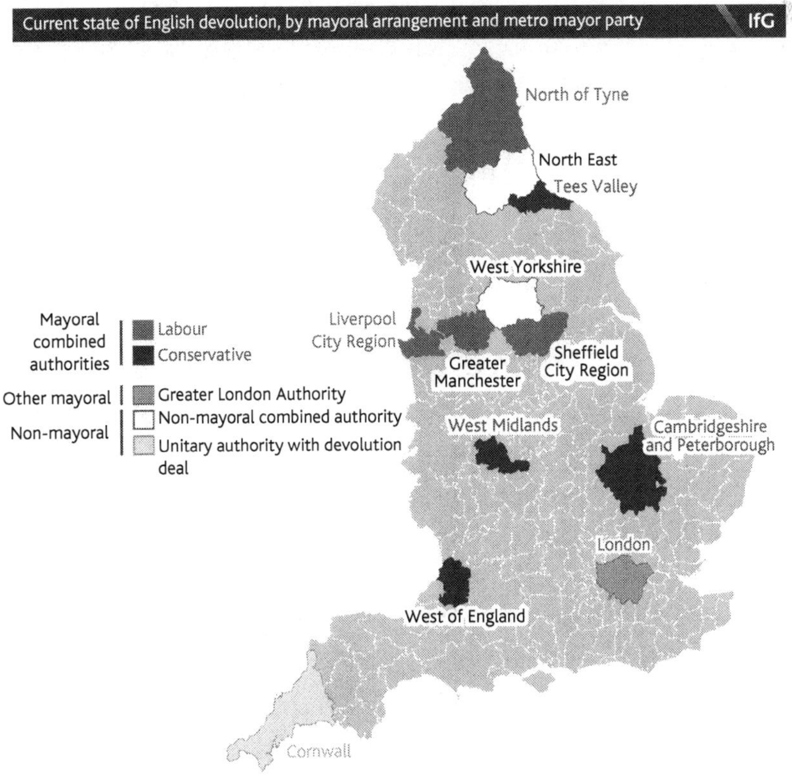

Source: Institute for Government analysis of combined authority websites, June 2019

North of Tyne Combined Authority emerged and proceeded on its own in May 2019 – a scaled down version of what was needed, and elected Labour Mayor Jamie Driscoll. This left much of the South of the Tyne without a combined authority and metro mayor and created confused and fragmented governance structures, which persisted through to 2021. This fragmented governance creates cynicism and divides: especially between Core Cities (Core Cities UK, 2021), for example Newcastle, and Key Cities (Key Cities Secretariat, 2021) and smaller towns who often feel disenfranchised and lacking in resources and policy attention. It creates public ambiguity in governance structures and resource allocations.

Quangos for recovery?

There are quangos amid the fragmentation which seek to bring more coherent policies together – on economic development it falls to the North East Local Enterprise Partnership (NELEP), continued after 2016, to seek to build a unifying role in delivering the economic and regeneration programmes of central government in the region, but it has no overarching social or authoritative planning policy remit, and it is unelected and business-led. Nexus, Transport for Tyne and Wear, and the Passenger Transport Authority continue, also, to play a larger subregional and unifying role, but transport policy too needs review, and the patchwork quilt remains.

The COVID-19 pandemic has served, however, to force the regional institutional players to work closer together throughout 2020/2021 but without resolving any of the underlying governance issues, as identified by Shutt and Liddle (Shutt and Liddle, 2019) and nationally by others (Menon, 2021), but there is a big gap between local government still suffering from austerity and seeking to rise to its pandemic roles, and the more certain centralised and directed plans for the NHS and health sector. Public health and mayors struggled to gain voice in the pandemic and yet they were crucial, forging many new partnerships to broker locally to deal with the pandemic, in the absence of clear central government direction nationally and regionally with a preference for centralised private sector contracting, which the Track and Test debacle revealed.

Health and social care: the significance of the National Health Service's long-term plan

In *The North-East after Brexit* (Liddle and Shutt, 2019), Porteous (Porteous, 2020) began the work of looking at the NHS long-term plan for the North East region and its importance to the region for the 2019–2024 period. The arrival of the Sustainability and Transformation Partnerships and ICS signalled the NHS and local government working together in new ways across the region. In June 2018 the Prime Minister announced the new five-year funding settlement for the NHS and the long-term plan and the NHS long-term plan was published on 7 January 2019 (NHS, 2019). The plan articulates the need for general practice (GP), cancer, mental health and maternity services and commits to develop new vanguard care models applied to the NHS only. It does not commit or resolve the issues with the whole health and local government social care system, but it does focus attention on the strengthening of the role of health in the life and economy of the North East. It focused attention on joined up delivery, preventative care, and the expansion of primary and community services prior to the arrival of COVID-19.

Porteous identified the significance (Porteous, 2020) of the NHS long-term plan for the region and the significant opportunities for collaboration and argued that the North East needed to build on the Due North Report (Public Health England, 2015), the Well North Report (Well North, 2019) and the work of the Northern Health Science Alliance. She drew attention to the North East and Cumbria as one of the largest ICSs in the country, serving more than 3 million people and the significance of the NHS Regional Plan for the future economy of the region.

COVID-19: impacts on the North East region 2020/2021

COVID-19 struck in March 2020 and continued for a full year, with three lockdowns: March to May 2020; October to December 2020; and the third lockdown beginning in January 2021, running through to March 2021. Vaccinations proved largely successful and unlocking took place on 19 June 2021, but in the context of a potential rise in variants, global availability and take up of vaccines, and advice for vaccinating the young, there were fears for further outbreaks and potential lockdowns in the autumn and winter of 2021.

The general picture in the North East was that the 12 local authorities, the four Integrated Health Care Services and the Trusts have been at the coalface in dealing with the big health and economic and social issues. Local authorities, as well, responded to the immediate economic concerns with supporting Treasury plans for regional business assistance programmes and bringing forward economic recovery plans for their subregions. In the first lockdown, analysis quickly showed that the North East was third in terms of the regional COVID-19 death tolls outside of London and the Midlands, and that some Health Trusts, like Sunderland and Cumbria, were bearing the brunt of the impact in the region.

Health action was initially coordinated through the three Resilience Forums in the region, bringing together all the key players. Local

Resilience Forums were developed under the Civil Contingencies Act 2004 (Government, 2004) to coordinate the actions and arrangements between responding bodies in the area – they also provide the most effective and efficient response to civil emergencies when they occur. Local Resilience Forums (LRFs) are multiagency partnerships made up of representatives from local public services, including the Emergency Services, local authorities, the NHS, the Environment Agency and others. These agencies are known as Category 1 Responders, as defined by the Civil Contingencies Act. In the North East there were three.

Around these resilience and emergency structures were grouped the leaders and key stakeholders of each local authority in the region and their joint work with the NHS Trusts and Clinical Commissioning Groups. The three groups dovetailed with their respective new Combined Authorities (CAs), so in Teesside and North of Tyne the CAs joined the groups, to play key coordinating roles and the two County Councils, Durham and Northumberland, also played critical roles. They began to coalesce around the plans for healthcare action, employment, and business support, and broadly two types of partnership have emerged in the region as the year has progressed, overlain on the ICS plans.

Health has obviously led the pandemic response and local government was in the frontline.

After the second lockdown and the introduction of the controversial regional Tier system in England the resilience arrangements began to get tightened up and the partnerships began to get stronger between the NHS and local authorities, as the three subregional case studies in Boxes 5.1, 5.2 and 5.3 illustrate.

Health and social care futures

Many people wanted the NHS long-term plan and the new place-based ICS to be developed and point the way towards the stronger local partnerships between the NHS and local government which needed to be developed at regional and local levels. It is here that the region has shown the way, but again progress is uneven and there are many obstacles to greater health devolution, not least the fact that the combined authorities in the North East do not have a health planning remit, unlike the Greater Manchester Combined Authority. Nevertheless, plans were proceeding for closer health partnerships with local government.

Some sectors are being hit harder than others, and some sectors may take longer than one year to recover. From September 2020 the group began to flesh out its second phase of work after the immediate push on employment schemes. It did so in the context of uncertainty about the future Local Enterprise Partnerships (LEPS) under levelling up plans.

Figure 5.2: Integrated care systems were being constructed and operated in the region as COVID-19 progressed

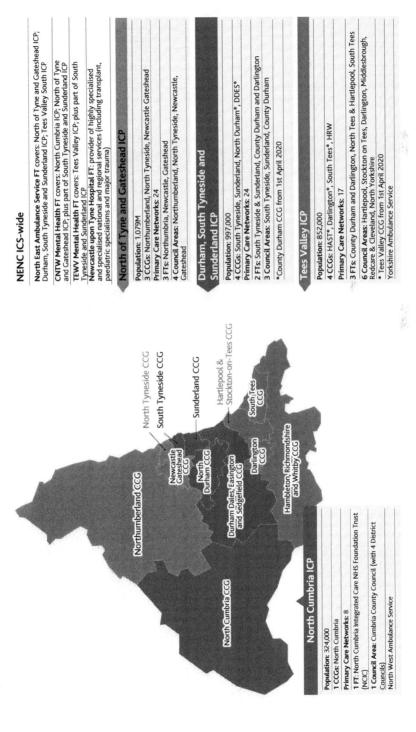

NENC ICS-wide

North East Ambulance Service FT covers: North of Tyne and Gateshead ICP; Durham, South Tyneside and Sunderland ICP; Tees Valley South ICP

CNTW Mental Health FT covers: North Cumbria ICP; North of Tyne and Gateshead ICP; plus part of South Tyneside and Sunderland ICP

TEWV Mental Health FT covers: Tees Valley ICP; plus part of South Tyneside and Sunderland ICP

Newcastle upon Tyne Hospital FT: provider of highly specialised and specialised national and regional services (including transplant, paediatric specialisms and major trauma)

North of Tyne and Gateshead ICP

Population: 1.079M

3 CCGs: Northumberland, North Tyneside, Newcastle Gateshead

Primary Care Networks: 24

3 FTs: Northumbria, Newcastle, Gateshead

4 Council Areas: Northumberland, North Tyneside, Newcastle, Gateshead

Durham, South Tyneside and Sunderland ICP

Population: 997,000

4 CCGs: South Tyneside, Sunderland, North Durham*, DDES*

Primary Care Networks: 24

2 FTs: South Tyneside & Sunderland, County Durham and Darlington

3 Council Areas: South Tyneside, Sunderland, County Durham

*County Durham CCG from 1st April 2020

Tees Valley ICP

Population: 852,000

4 CCGs: HAST*, Darlington*, South Tees*, HRW

Primary Care Networks: 17

3 FTs: County Durham and Darlington, North Tees & Hartlepool, South Tees

6 Council Areas: Hartlepool, Stockton on Tees, Darlington, Middlesbrough, Redcare & Cleveland, North Yorkshire

* Tees Valley CCG from 1st April 2020

Yorkshire Ambulance Service

North Tyneside CCG

South Tyneside CCG

Sunderland CCG

Hartlepool & Stockton-on-Tees CCG

South Tees CCG

Newcastle Gateshead CCG

North Durham CCG

Darlington CCG

Hambleton, Richmondshire and Whitby CCG

Northumberland CCG

Durham Dales, Easington and Sedgefield CCG

North Cumbria CCG

North Cumbria ICP

Population: 324,000

1 CCGs: North Cumbria

Primary Care Networks: 8

1 FT: North Cumbria Integrated Care NHS Foundation Trust (NCIC)

1 Council Area: Cumbria County Council (with 4 District Councils)

North West Ambulance Service

Note: North-East and North Cumbria Integrated Care System and Partnerships
Source: NHS Northumberland Clinical Commissioning Group (2020/2021)

Box 5.1: Durham County Council: the partnership of local government and the National Health Service

The County Durham and Darlington LRF created a Strategic Co-ordinating Group (SCG) and supporting cells and groups, under the overall strategic command of the Deputy Chief Constable for Durham and Darlington. Durham County Council strategic command was provided by the Chief Executive and corporate directors, who were key members of the SCG (see Figure 5.2). The council's Director of Public Health is a member of the LRF SCG. LRF strategic oversight transferred from the SCG to a Strategic Recovery Group at the end of June 2020, which was chaired by the Chief Executive of Durham County Council. This enabled closer oversight of testing and outbreak management arrangements and coordination with wider recovery planning. By the beginning of 2021 and the third lockdown, local authorities were beginning to play a stronger role in testing and outbreak management arrangements, after it had become clear that the centralised national arrangements were not working.

The government required all local authorities to produce a COVID-19 Local Outbreak Control Plan by mid-2020. The COVID-19 Local Outbreak Control Plans have the following key objectives:

To protect the health of local communities through:

• Provision of clear prevention messages in relation to COVID-19.
• Rapid detection of COVID-19 outbreaks.
• Controlling onward transmission.
• Provision of support to those who need to self-isolate, building on the population health management approach to the pandemic.
• Development and application of intelligence, including the knowledge and insight provided by local communities. The government has identified seven themes that were to be addressed in this plan:
  • care homes and schools
  • high risk places, locations and communities
  • local testing capacity
  • contact tracing in complex settings
  • data integration
  • vulnerable people.
• Local authority boards, which usually reported to a local Health and Wellbeing Board.

Thus, in Durham a local protection board, the Local Health Protection Assurance Board, was established. The key purpose of the Local Health Protection Assurance Board was to lead, coordinate and manage work to prevent the spread of COVID-19. As such it links with and supports wider work to help the county and its communities recover from the pandemic and restore some normality. The Board meets on a weekly basis. It has developed the County Durham COVID-19 Local Outbreak Control Plan to provide a framework for leading, coordinating and managing the outbreak prevention and control process. The key priorities of the Board are to:

- Provide a framework for leading, coordinating and managing the spread of COVID-19 including prevention and outbreak control and management.
- Establish the support mechanisms Durham County Council will provide to the Public Health England Test and Trace Service.
- Build on the established public health protection role and responsibilities of the local authority to manage outbreaks in specific settings.
- Identify further action that might be required, including considering the impact on and needs of local communities.
- Understand the local health, social and wellbeing challenges of COVID-19.
- Support the role of the Health and Wellbeing Board in engaging the public, led by Cabinet Portfolio for Adult and Health Services. The Board is chaired by the Director of Public Health and supported by a Consultant in Public Health (health protection) and Public Health Programme Manager.

Thus COVID-19 refocused attention on the NHS–local government strategic partnership arrangements at local levels, and particularly given the crisis in care homes and schools which occurred as the successive lockdowns progressed.

Box 5.2: Collaborative Newcastle

Collaborative Newcastle is an alliance between Newcastle upon Tyne Hospitals NHS Foundation Trust, Newcastle City Council, Newcastle Gateshead NHS Clinical Commissioning Group and Cumbria, Northumberland, Tyne and Wear NHS Foundation Trust, working closely with Newcastle GP Services, the GP Federation for Newcastle, Primary Care Networks and the voluntary sector.

The scope of the partnership is among the first of its kind in the country and is underpinned by a ground-breaking legal agreement between the four key health and social care organisations in the city.

The agreement, which sets out a formal co-governance structure, accelerates progress towards a fully integrated health and social care system, enabling the partners to effect significant change for residents. Their aim is to reduce the widening health inequalities, by preventing avoidable problems from arising and tackling the big things that hold people back.

In December 2020, the legal agreement was signed off by each organisation's independent Board, as well as by Newcastle City Council's Cabinet. Newcastle City Futures Board – previously the City's Wellbeing for Life Board – formally endorsed Collaborative Newcastle's ambitious plans.

Box 5.3: Teesside hospitals to continue working closer together beyond COVID-19

The strong partnership, which has played an important role in helping the two Tees Valley and North Yorkshire hospital trusts to meet the challenge of COVID-19, is to be maintained and strengthened beyond the pandemic – an unprecedented threat to health that does not respect organisational boundaries.

North Tees and Hartlepool NHS Foundation Trust and South Tees Hospitals NHS Foundation Trust are to create a new strategic board, which will bring members of the two boards together to tackle common issues that affect both trusts, while continuing as separate statutory organisations.

The two trusts are the area's largest employers, with almost 15,000 staff, and by continuing to work closely together beyond the pandemic, both organisations hope to make a bigger and lasting impact by:

• Working with local communities and partners to help improve the health and wellbeing of the populations they serve.
• Tackling the health and care inequalities that COVID-19 has exacerbated.
• Playing a leading role in helping to bring inward investment into the Tees Valley and North Yorkshire.
• Strengthening the recruitment and retention of specialist doctors and nurses.

Working more closely together will also give both trusts a stronger collective voice as they look to secure the capital investment needed to rebuild and upgrade existing hospital facilities in Teesside and North Yorkshire.

This group is very much focused on dialogue with central government and particularly the Department of Business Energy and Industry (BEIS) and Cities and Local Growth Unit in the Ministry of Housing, Communities and Local Government Unit and on the national responses from the Treasury to levelling up. Details are still not published for the UK Shared Prosperity Funds, which is to replace European funding in the regions. New infrastructure funds and the new skills programme are anticipated also. Much of the detail here awaits the results of the Chancellor's spending review, which will set the scene for the three years to the next general election in 2024 and the delayed Levelling Up White Paper.

Conclusion

Conversations with central government are largely conducted via mayors (individually and through the M9 Mayoral Network), through the LEP network nationally, the Local Government Association and the trade/ professional bodies like Confederation of British Industry, the Chambers of Commerce and the Federation of Small Businesses. The current system of North East governance is very fragmented, and the region now has limited civil service capacity since the closure of Government Offices for the Regions, and lacks one strategic, united voice for the region, but this is the framework into which new policies are being formulated and delivered.

In the North East there have been encouraging signs of new partnerships spurred on by the COVID-19 crisis in bringing both local government and the NHS closer together and producing local responses to the pandemic. However, there is a frustration that central government is too far removed from understanding both regional and local needs: frustrations have also come to the fore from the Conservative Northern Group (Rees, 2021). Beyond the day-to-day operational and delivery issues regional leaders are turning their attention to medium- and longer-term recovery planning and other plans for assessing the longer-term regional impacts of the pandemic wanting to achieve greater focus and coordination from central government. Plans for the Towns Fund, Levelling Up Fund and the UK Shared Prosperity Fund all seem too vague and uncoordinated and individual policy announcements like the £35 million Blyth Rail Fund announcement, although welcome as individual projects, pale into insignificance with the scale of the health and social care and the deprivation challenge in the North East, which is growing as the pandemic proceeds.

Alex Thomas from the Institute for Government argues that strengthening the Prime Minister's policy capacity is what is required:

> Compounding the systemic weakness at the centre of British government, the Cabinet Office and No.10 have been put under pressure during the coronavirus response, and before that by the UK leaving the EU. Both were major challenges for the state, and both responses were characterised by too much firefighting and not enough direction setting. The centre of government needs to get better at working out what is important and focusing its interventions, resources, and accountability structures accordingly. (Thomas, 2021: 10)

Others, like Gordon Brown (Brown, 2021), see the need for a more comprehensive devolution review for England and all four nations, arguing that a failing central state needs better regional representation through a second chamber, perhaps pointing the way to a more federal UK.

Changing policy directions?

Many commentators are arguing that the pandemic will provide a new opportunity for more radical long-term restructuring plans to be put in place, focused on green futures and sustainability, and reducing transport and commuting patterns, or tackling poverty and low pay, and health and social care for example. These issues will require debate and investment, but the evidence appears to suggest that regional partnerships are responding to date in a limited way and in a climate of much policy turbulence. They also suggest that we need to look at re-establishing Central Government Offices in the Regions and tackle the bigger scale restructuring and strengthening of local government and strengthen the subregional partnerships for health and social care between the health sector and local government – all of which still seem far away together with the major policy reforms which are needed.

It is not surprising that in this fragmented governance region, health inequalities are rising, even as the pandemic eases. People are still asking what levelling up means and how it will make a real difference in the period to 2030.

References

Bambra, C. and Munford, L. (2020) *COVID 19 and the Northern Powerhouse*. Manchester: Northern Health Science Alliance.

Benyon, H. and Hudson, R. (2021) *The Shadow of the Mine: Coal and the End of Industrial Britain*. London: Verso.

Bonner, A. (2020) *Local Authorities and the Social Determinants of Health*. Bristol: Bristol University Press.

Brown, G. (2021) Trust has broken down in way UK is run. *BBC News*. Available at: https://www.bbc.co.uk/news/uk-politics-55791179 (accessed 14 February 2021).

Core Cities UK (2021) About us. Available at: https://www.corecities.com/about-us (accessed 13 February 2021).

Government (2004) *Civil Contingencies Act 2004*. London: HMSO.

HMSO (2021a) *The Northern Powerhouse: One Agenda, One Economy, One North*. Available at: https://assets.publishing.service.gov.uk/government/uploads/system/uploads/attachment_data/file/427339/the-northern-powerhouse-tagged.pdf (accessed 13 February 2021).

HMSO (2021b) *Integration and Innovation: Working Together to Improve Health and Social Care for All*. London: HMSO.

Key Cities Secretariat (2021) *Key Cities Unlocking Potential: About Key Cities*. Available at: https://www.keycities.co.uk/about (accessed 13 February 2021).

Kunonga, E., Gibson, G. and Parker, C. (2020) Inequalities in health and wellbeing across the UK: A local north-east perspective. In A. Bonner (ed) *Local Authorities and the Social Determinants of Health*. Bristol: Bristol University Press, pp 121–148.

Liddle, J. and Shutt, J. (2019) *The North-East after Brexit: Impact and Policy*. Available at: http://nrl.northumbria.ac.uk/41293 (accessed 13 February 2021).

Mattinson, D. (2020) *Beyond the Red Wall*. London: Biteback Publishing.

Menon, A. (2021) *Brexit and Beyond*. London: ESRC.

NHS (2019) *The NHS Long Term Plan*. London: NHS.

Porteous, D. (2020) The NHS long-term plan and the importance to the north-east region. In J. Liddle and J. Shutt (eds) *The North-East after Brexit: Impact and Policy*. Bingley: Emerald, pp 37–54.

Public Health England (2015) *Due North: Report of the Inquiry on Health Equity for the North*. London: Public Health Publications.

Rees, T. (2021) I'm back like Gandalf to help rescue the North, says Tory MP Jake Berry. *The Telegraph*. Available at: https://www.telegraph.co.uk/business/2021/01/03/back-like-gandalf-help-rescue-north-says-tory-mp-jake-berry/ (accessed 14 February 2021).

Shutt, J. and Liddle, J. (2019) Combined authorities in England: Moving beyond devolution: Developing strategic local government for a more sustainable future? *Local Economy*, 34(2): 91–93.

Sunak, R. (2020) *Chancellor's Statement on Coronavirus (COVID 19): 26 March 2020*. Available at: https://www.gov.uk/government/speeches/chancellor-outlines-new-coronavirus-support-measures-for-the-self-employed (accessed 29 August 2022).

Thomas, A. (2021) *The Heart of The Problem: A Weak Centre Is Undermining the UK Government*. London: Institute for Government.

Well North (2019) *Inspiring Lasting Change in Our Communities*. Warrington: Well North Enterprises.

6

UK local council strategies post-COVID-19: the local economy, climate change and community wellbeing

Manuel Abellan

Introduction

Around five times a year, the 54 elected representatives of the London Borough of Sutton gather for a 'Full Council' meeting. It allows the public and backbench councillors to challenge the executive in local government's own style of Prime Minister's Questions and for political parties to trade punches on a wide range of local and national issues. These public meetings, held in mostly empty school halls, with all too often unreliable technology and without the national media spotlight, are where local democracy comes to life.

It is in this context that Sutton councillors met on a sweltering July evening in 2019. On the agenda, 'Sutton Council to declare a Climate Emergency'. A no-brainer as far as we, the Sutton Liberal Democrat administration, were concerned. To our surprise, the hall of Wallington County Grammar High School was packed. 'Extinction Rebellion Sutton' had mobilised dozens of local residents for the occasion.

As the debate progressed, it was easy to get carried away by the fervour and enthusiasm displayed by 'XR' activists. Their energy put a local face to the mass climate movement inspired by Greta Thunberg in 2018 and signalled a potential shift in public opinion. An Ipsos MORI poll in August 2019 showed that concern about climate change has reached record levels, with half now 'very concerned' and the majority thinking that the UK should bring all emissions to net zero sooner than by 2050 (Ipsos MORI, 2020). It's hard to imagine that the UK government would have single-handedly adopted a legally binding target to be carbon-neutral by 2050 and that 270 local authorities in the UK would have declared a 'Climate Emergency' had it not been for the momentum gathered by the highly mediatised climate protests in the UK and around the world.

However, as I listened to their speeches, I was also brutally aware that while on paper green initiatives are extremely popular, many of our residents are still unaware of the practical implications of these policies on their lives and the tough choices needed to achieve them.

COVID-19 has demonstrated that radical changes, both in terms of government action and people's behaviours, are possible. The shift to home working, adhering to lockdowns, wearing masks and social distancing were all implemented at pace and became socially accepted. This is encouraging as we try to preserve some of the positive changes and understand that further structural changes of this nature will be needed if we are to meet our climate targets. The experience of UK Local Council strategies post-COVID-19 has also highlighted the dangers of delivering policies at pace with minimal consultation and engagement with people. As I will explain using an example from Sutton, behaviour change risks suffering serious setbacks unless policies are well designed, set in a wider context and people are taken on a journey.

This chapter will argue that while local authorities do not have a statutory duty in relation to climate change, sustainability needs to be at the heart of their COVID-19 response. Councils have been forced to rethink their priorities. Poorer communities have been hit the hardest by COVID-19 so the focus will be on supporting the most vulnerable and addressing the growing inequalities in our society. These include environmental inequalities such as lack of access to green space, poor air quality and a higher risk of cold and damp homes.

The ambition is also to create a vibrant local economy and a pleasant place that people want to spend time in. Another focus will be to support local businesses to get back on their feet, get people back into employment and build back better and greener. The chapter will illustrate, using examples of actions from the London Borough of Sutton, how local authorities are already stepping up to the plate to reduce carbon emissions, influence behaviours and mitigate the impact of climate change in our communities (London Borough of Sutton, 2020).

Councils are ready to act but after a decade of austerity and more financial hardship to come, they will need to be better supported by the government. This means clarity over their role on this agenda, equipping them with the right powers and a credible long-term funding plan. This will enable local authorities to scale up, secure the necessary skills and influence behavioural change. It will also avoid confusion, a lack of coordination and a piecemeal approach.

Working in partnership was put to the test and crucial in our successful local COVID-19 response so I will also explain how Sutton can use established local partnerships to bring key stakeholders to the table on this agenda. In Sutton, the council is only responsible for 3 per cent of total carbon emissions in our area so it is absolutely essential that we get buy-in and concrete plans from others if we are to reach zero-carbon.

Local authorities in England

Local authorities are responsible for delivering around 800 services like social care, schools, housing, planning, waste collection, licensing and business support. In general terms, local authorities are funded by a combination of government grants (non-ring-fenced and ring-fenced), council tax (a property tax levied on residential properties), a social care precept (ring-fenced to fund adult social care services) and business rates (a property tax levied on business premises).

Since the 2008 financial crash, successive governments have pursued austerity policies aimed at reducing spending in local government. The gradual reduction in government grants combined with the requirement to hold a local referendum if council taxes are raised by more than 2 per cent annually has forced local authorities to find efficiency savings. These have ranged from commissioning services with other boroughs, reducing the number of senior managers and staff, efficiency and cutting services.

In Sutton, our core central government funding has been reduced by more than 60 per cent in real terms since 2010, meaning that for every £1 we got in 2010 we now get just 40p. In our 2020/2021 budget more than 70 per cent of the council's budget was spent on supporting the most vulnerable adults and children in Sutton (London Borough of Sutton, 2021). This perpetual search for savings has driven policy decisions at a local level and dominated our demands for more autonomy and devolution from central government.

An international comparison highlights the importance of these demands by local government over the last decade. By international standards, the UK is one of the most centralised countries in the world. According to a 2019 report by the Institute for Public Policy Research (IPPR), 95p in every £1 paid in tax is taken by central government compared to 69p in every £1 raised by Germany's central government (IPPR North, 2019). According to estimates by the Organisation for Economic Co-operation and Development, every other G7 country collected more taxes in 2014 at either a local or regional level according to estimates (IFG, 2020; see Figure 6.1).

This fiscal centralisation and policies driven by Whitehall continue to dictate the relationship between local and national government and the feeling that we are not valued as a real partner. Many experts argue that this centralised governance has played a crucial role in widening economic problems and inequalities across the UK and that longer-term funding settlements and more devolved powers would lead to economic growth and increased productivity (IPPR North, 2019). A better partnership combined with devolution and more funding will be vital if the UK is to meet its climate change targets.

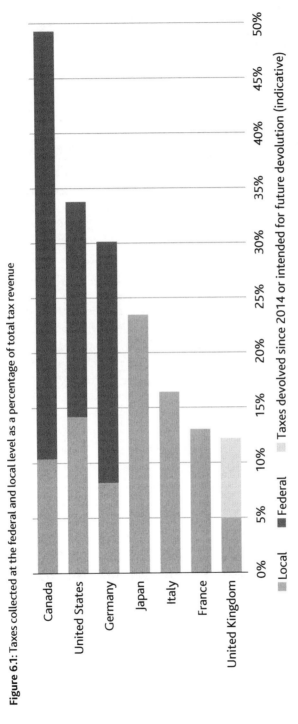

Figure 6.1: Taxes collected at the federal and local level as a percentage of total tax revenue

Source: IFG (2020); Institute for Governement analysis of OECD, Revenue Statistics; taxes by level of government, August 2016; and additional Institute for Government analysis as of March 2018

Building back better and greener

Sutton is one of the leafiest areas in London but apart from the physical amenities of the borough, our administration's actions in Sutton over the last three decades have earned us a well-established reputation for our green credentials.

For example, in the early 2000s Sutton Council helped deliver the award-winning Beddington Zero Energy Development (BedZED) taking the decision to sell land at below market value to make sustainable development economically viable. With one-third of the properties rented out to tenants nominated by the council, and designed to create zero carbon emissions, the iconic BedZED village was the first such large-scale project and continues today to be an inspiration for zero-carbon homebuilding worldwide. This proactive approach was based on the Passive-house philosophy (Passivhaus Trust, 2020).

Despite the dire financial outlook of the last decade, and the need to do more with much less, our ambition to be London's most sustainable borough has not wavered. We continue our work to embed sustainability across all teams and make sure that sustainability impact analysis of policy or decisions becomes the norm. I also still, in spite of COVID-19, detect the same sense of urgency among my Environment and Transport portfolio counterparts at a London level, as this continues to be raised at our quarterly meetings.

At the time of writing, around 75 per cent of councils and combined authorities in England have declared climate emergencies (Borrowman et al, 2020). This is quite telling especially as the Climate Change Act 2008 did not force local authorities to develop their own carbon budgets with specific targets and align them with their annual budgets (Friends of the Earth, 2019). The symbolism of these 'climate emergency' declarations locally, and the strong message it has sent to the government, should not be underestimated. It has equipped councillors with a clearer mandate for action while also empowering local residents and activist groups by providing them with a tool to hold local leaders to account. During discussions about the recovery, it has served as a helpful anchor reminding everyone of the unanimous commitment taken by all councillors and that the climate emergency has not gone away.

The consensus on climate change also reflects a recognition among local leaders that, as highlighted by the Marmot Report in 2010, 'climate change presents unprecedented and potentially catastrophic risks to health and wellbeing' (Marmot, 2010: 77). An understanding that climate change is already happening and that a failure to act urgently will lead to growing health and wealth inequalities in our communities, and put the most vulnerable at a greater disadvantage. In practice, the disruption caused by climate change would inevitably lead to much higher costs for local authorities, increase pressure on targeted services for vulnerable residents and complicate their ability to deliver some universal services.

In the summer of 2020, this consensus was solidified with the setup of the London Recovery Board, chaired by the London Mayor and the Chair of London Councils, to oversee the long-term recovery effort. The body brings together leaders from across local and regional government, together with business and civil society, as well as the health and education sectors, trade unions and the police. The Board has committed to a Green New Deal for London as one of its main missions. The deal aims to help London recover by creating new jobs and skills for Londoners, while ensuring the capital becomes a zero-carbon, zero-pollution city by 2030 and a zero-waste city by 2050.

> London is a world leader for climate action. Its growing 'low carbon and environmental goods and services' sector is worth £40bn in sales and employs nearly 250,000 people. Examples include renewable energy projects like wind and solar and other green technology and materials to make low carbon buildings and transport. London's green economy is worth more to the city than the construction and manufacturing sectors combined. Putting the environment at the centre of our recovery is a chance to reverse the looming economic downturn. It will bring new investment to London, help businesses to see long-term growth, and provide decent, skilled, local jobs. (Mayor of London, 2020)

London boroughs have so far published 24 Climate Action Plans, which set out boroughs' strategic response to climate change over the coming decade and beyond. A study by London councils shows that there is a wide variety of approaches to data sources, length and scope of activities. A majority aim to reduce emissions from the council's own estate and operations and to reduce them for the wider borough but some focus exclusively on areas within the council's direct control. As we move forward, it will be important that boroughs clarify the carbon emissions profile for the operations of the council and, in most cases, the wider area, to describe the actions the council will take to meet its net-zero target, and to clarify the extent of what the authority itself can deliver, and what it needs to work in partnership with others to achieve (London Councils, 2021).

This last point is crucial as at the moment London only has the resources to achieve 50 per cent of what is needed to become a zero-carbon city (Mayor of London, 2020). It is also clear from Sutton Council's net-zero carbon strategy that unless the government provides local authorities with much more funding and powers, it will be impossible to meet the UK's climate targets. In the next section I will illustrate some of the work that is already underway on this agenda but also touch on some of the challenges and what is needed from the government.

Energy and buildings

Homes are responsible for just over 38 per cent and workplaces for 36 per cent of London emissions (Mayor of London, 2020). On the journey to zero-carbon, one of the biggest challenges for London is to make existing buildings, 80 per cent of which will be still standing in 2050, more energy efficient and adapted to climate change (Mayor of London, 2016).

In homes, this means reducing carbon emissions with measures like better insulation, updating boilers, heating systems and windows. These actions will not only help our planet but also make homes warmer, healthier and cheaper to heat. In Sutton, this could make a real difference especially to the 10 per cent of households that are thought to be in fuel poverty, just below the national average (London Borough of Sutton, 2014: 3).

We are in the early stages, but our policy priority is to focus any funding available on these properties. This will require close partnership work with Sutton Housing Partnership and other housing associations across the borough. The good news is that we are already working closely on this agenda. In 2019, Sutton Council managed to secure significant funding from the Greater London Assembly, the Department for Business, Energy and Industrial Strategy and British Gas to trial a revolutionary low energy approach, known as EnergieSprong, in both whole house refurbishments and new builds. Sutton is the first borough in London to trial this innovative approach with a project to retrofit up to 100 council homes in the borough to a zero-carbon standard. The net-zero carbon objective is achieved by a range of measures being implemented on each property, but the overarching principle is that each property generates all the energy it uses. The retrofits are quick to complete – a complete house makeover should take less than ten days. If the 'EnergieSprong' pilot project is successful, our ambition is to roll it out across all of our social housing stock.

Just to put into perspective the scale of the challenge at hand, there are 83,700 properties in the borough (6,000 of which are council housing properties) that need to be retrofitted to a zero-carbon standard. Sutton Council estimates that this will cost between £20,000 and £100,000 per property, depending on building type and a mature supply chain. This totals between £1.7 billion and £8.3 billion for Sutton alone. It is evident that financial support will need to be offered to homeowners, landlords, housing associations and small businesses to undertake energy efficiency measures. To enable this, the government could:

> Put in place a holistic package of resourcing that enables local authorities and other registered providers to bring all public sector buildings, including as a priority social housing, up to a minimum of EPC 'C' by 2030. This should be done through whole-house

retrofits, with immediate short-term support to reduce fuel poverty rates. (ADEPT, 2020: 9)

During the pandemic, the government announced the Green Homes Grants: Local Authority Delivery Scheme (LAD) to raise the energy efficiency of low-income and low energy performance homes. These worthwhile and valuable schemes have been undermined by unrealistic delivery timetables and bureaucratic hurdles under the LAD scheme. Recent submissions to the Environmental Audit Committee revealed that the government did not consult stakeholders such as material suppliers, service providers, local authorities and trade bodies before rolling out the scheme (George, 2021). Local authorities also continued to struggle to secure the right skills, for example training apprentices, and employment benefits that the LAD should support. What is needed instead are longer-term programmes where apprentices and tradespeople can get trained into those roles to learn new skills and build the skills market.

The government should encourage and empower existing local partnerships to lead on this agenda. For example, the South London Skills and Employment Board, made up of local businesses, training providers, third sector and council representatives from the London boroughs of Sutton, Croydon, Kingston, Merton and Richmond, is an ideal forum for collaborative leadership to shape and help secure improved access to, and successful delivery of, adult skills training in our area. This will be especially important as we begin the economic recovery (South London Partnership, 2021). If we are to build a thriving and sustainable, long-term economic future for South London this work will have to include strengthening the green economy, green skills and training available and protecting jobs and organisation within the green voluntary and community sector. By working in partnership, local authorities will be able to better understand the broader green skills agenda and plan to narrow the existing green skills gap.

Active travel and air quality

Some of the most visible changes of the first COVID-19 lockdown in March 2020 were the absence of traffic on our roads, with more people enjoying walks in their neighbourhood and more families cycling to local parks. The contrast was even starker in Sutton. Our reliance on a patchy, infrequent and unattractive network of train and bus services means that our residents continue to rely on their cars for too many journeys.

The challenge to decarbonise local transport and reduce our dependence on the car is not unique to Sutton. While other sectors have made encouraging progress to decarbonise, surface transport has only seen a reduction of 3 per cent since 1990 (Department for Transport, 2020). At a time when different models estimate that the level of traffic reduction needed to reach our 2030 climate emergency targets is between 20 and 60 per cent, the UK has more cars on the road than ever before and traffic on residential roads has doubled since 2008 (*The Guardian*, 2020). This is hardly surprising. UK governments have for decades spent billions on new motorways, designed towns and villages that encourage car-dependent lifestyles and pursued transport policies that put too much emphasis on cutting car journey times. As a result, we live in a society where the car is sacrosanct. The common belief is that people have the right to drive as much, as often and wherever they want. Any intervention to manage traffic more efficiently should be discouraged especially if it risks adding to car journey times. And this is despite the fact that the rise in the emission of nitrogen dioxide (NO_2), particulates and ozone (O_3) in the last decade cause 40,000 early deaths each year and that, since 2010, the UK has broken the legal limits for NO_2 every year.

Unless we change our culture vis-à-vis cars, adopt policies to reduce car usage and shift a substantial amount of journeys to public transport and active travel, the sector will not meet its climate targets. Local authorities, with responsibilities to operate, administer and maintain public roads, are well-placed to proactively drive this transition but cannot do this alone. They need to be supported by a clear and proactive national awareness campaign and local revenue-raising powers to fund public transport infrastructure and active travel schemes.

Progress has definitely been made in the last year but, as many London boroughs have discovered with the introduction of 'low-traffic neighbourhoods', the challenge of convincing people to reduce journeys by car and cycle or walk instead is hard, often controversial and takes time. The pandemic has shown that changing human behaviours on a big scale is possible and that the application of behavioural tools and techniques are essential to this aim. In Sutton, we have successfully applied behavioural science knowledge in recent years to incentivise residents to reduce waste but this has been done sporadically across the organisation.

As we move forward, there is an opportunity to learn from these successes and for councils to increase the use of behavioural science more consistently Sutton Council (2021). This will help them sustain or change residents' behaviours especially in areas like climate change. The Local Government Association has recognised this and developed a behavioural insights programme as part of its wider support for council innovation. This programme includes a handy six-step guide for councils undertaking climate change behaviour projects with specific sections on reducing car journeys and increasing active travel (The Local Government Association, 2021).

As I reflect on the design and implementation of Sutton's five 'low-traffic neighbourhoods' pilots, it is clear that despite some encouraging schemes, these could have been significantly improved and mistakes avoided if the use of behavioural science featured more prominently. In many cases, the lack of clarity about the objectives and what was being measured, failure to understand the drivers behind certain behaviours and put together a package of relevant interventions made it harder to communicate and explain changes to residents. In addition, the requirement in the initial guidance provided by the government to local authorities, to design and implement these schemes without any public consultation, made it very difficult to build a positive relationship with communities that often felt these schemes were being imposed on them. Over the last decade, austerity and the need to find savings meant that local authorities have cut these types of non-statutory roles. In the short to medium term, councils will increasingly need to recruit and train staff with these types of skills to successfully work with residents and local partners to decarbonise local transport.

Partnership working

The previous section highlighted areas where local authorities can proactively play a role in reducing carbon emissions in their area. However, local councils only contribute a very small fraction of total carbon emissions in their boroughs. In Sutton, this amounts to only 3 per cent. This means that local authorities cannot deliver net-zero emissions in their areas on their own. Meeting our ambitious national target will require a national framework set by the government, coordination between local, regional and national government, and joint working with the rest of the public sector and private sector.

So far, the government has failed to work with councils to define the role of local authorities on climate change. Local government has indicated a will to be at the heart of our journey to carbon neutrality but without any clarity it will be difficult for councils to set the right level of ambition, plan accordingly and avoid a piecemeal approach.

It's also difficult to imagine a better partner to spearhead this agenda in every corner of the UK. Local authorities have a detailed understanding of their communities, well-established local partnerships and the ability to reach groups inaccessible to Whitehall. Councils are also democratically accountable to their communities, accepted as 'leaders' of place and experienced in community engagement. This is also reinforced by a recent public opinion survey showing that 71 per cent of residents trust their council and 75 per cent are satisfied with the way their local council runs things in their area (The Local Government Association, 2020).

Local government has the added advantage of an agile workforce that is used to delivering complex services and programmes. These strengths have been on full display during the COVID-19 pandemic as the sector has succeeded in adapting quickly and effectively to an emergency situation. In Sutton, we have been able to maintain high-quality essential services but also support the government in different ways. The council played a critical role in identifying and contacting over 7,000 vulnerable residents and then supporting with food deliveries over 1,000 residents who needed shielding. The council assisted the Department for Education by quickly distributing over 500 laptops and tablets to vulnerable children to assist them with remote learning and, in the first wave of the pandemic, was able to rapidly distribute £25.23 million in emergency funding to around 2,000 local businesses.

One of the main lessons from the COVID-19 pandemic response has been that the council could not have adapted so quickly and effectively without the well-established local partnerships. These relationships allowed us to coordinate an area-wide response and use each local partner's strengths, especially in the public and voluntary sectors. This well-coordinated response is no coincidence. As a local authority we have invested a huge amount of time and energy over the last decade to build those trusted and effective relationships with our public, private and third sector partners. These discussions, in the face of austerity, steered the council towards an outcome-based commissioning model that allowed us to think more holistically about the type of place we wanted Sutton to be and how we could work with others to build it together. Over time, this developed into a framework known as the 'Sutton Plan', bringing together over 20 public, voluntary and private sector partners in the borough. All partners have signed up to the belief that to improve the lives of our residents we should think 'Sutton first', intervene early, provide seamless coordinated services, build stronger communities and work across sectors (The Sutton Plan (2021). In practice this has meant working together on complex issues like domestic violence and health and care integration.

We are in the early stages but in the short term, I am hoping that the 'climate emergency' will become a priority under the 'Sutton Plan'. Its principles, framework and proven progress on other complex issues will form a solid foundation to start joint work with local partners on Sutton's 'climate emergency'. This forum would provide an ideal space to agree strategic objectives, raise awareness, share knowledge, identify joint opportunities and access funds. It would also empower the council to progress specific projects in partnership with individual organisations. As place-based leaders, the council would also be able to use its convening power to enable a drive to carbon emissions reductions across our whole area in ways that can also deliver better public health, reduced inequalities, a healthier environment and thriving local economies (ADEPT, 2020).

At the time of writing this chapter, the council is organising corporate leadership discussions with senior managers and delivering a carbon literacy programme across the organization Sutton Council (2021). The aim is to embed the climate emergency across the council and make sure that every team identifies areas within their work that will assist our carbon reduction efforts. This internal work is essential if the council is to reach zero-carbon and be well equipped to act as leaders of place in the borough.

Conclusion

The 270 'climate emergency' declarations to date are a powerful recognition that climate change has become a priority for local authorities in recent years. There also seems to be a consensus across all levels of government that we need to preserve some of the positive changes experienced during COVID-19 and that climate change needs to be at the heart of the economic recovery activity. At a local government level, councils recognise that unless climate change is addressed it poses a serious threat to our capacity to deliver services and build a sustainable and prosperous future for our communities.

Despite not having a statutory duty in relation to climate change, local authorities are already delivering important projects in key areas. In the short term, it is absolutely essential that the government works with the local government to define its role on the journey to carbon neutrality and, over time, equip them with the relevant powers and funding. Local government's strong understanding of their communities' needs, its well-established local partnerships, ability to reach difficult groups, experience in community engagement and ability to adapt quickly and deliver complex services makes it a unique and essential partner to move this agenda forward. As local elected representatives, we will need to balance communicating a sense of urgency and the need to be led by science with giving our community hope that they can make a difference through their own individual actions. In a post-COVID-19 world where focus might be on more immediate pressures, we will need to use our existing partnerships to assemble a broad coalition of local businesses, and other public and voluntary sector partners to get the momentum required to become carbon neutral within the legally binding target. This will enable us to extend our reach across the community, influence behaviours and ultimately reduce carbon emissions across the area.

These are many complex questions and challenges facing local and national leaders on this topic. While the risks arising from climate breakdown are much better understood in 2021, there are still many unknowns on the road ahead and the battle for hearts and minds is by no means over. The UK, as hosts of COP26 in 2021, has a unique opportunity to lead on the world stage and kick-start a green industrial revolution. Sutton will be ready to play its part.

References

AADEPT (2020) *A Blueprint for Accelerating Climate Action and a Green Recovery at the Local Level.* Association of Directors of Environment, Economy, Planning and Transport. Available at: https://www.adeptnet.org.uk/documents/blueprint-accelerating-climate-action-and-green-recovery-local-level (accessed 25 November 2020).

Abellan, M. (2021) The local economy, climate change and community wellbeing. Personal communication as Deputy Council Leader.

Borrowman, P., Singh, R. and Bulleid, R. (2020) *The Local Climate Challenge: A New Partnership Approach.* London: Green Alliance. Available at: https://www.green-alliance.org.uk/ (accessed 3 December 2020).

Department for Transport (2020) *Decarbonising Transport Setting the Challenge.* Available at: https://assets.publishing.service.gov.uk/government/uploads/system/uploads/attachment_data/file/932122/decarbonising-transport-setting-the-challenge.pdf. (accessed 26 December 2020).

Friends of the Earth (2019) *33 Actions Local Authorities Can Take On Climate Change: Policy and Insight.* Available at: https://policy.friendsoftheearth.uk/insight/33-actions-local-authorities-can-take-climate-change#:~:text=Local%20authorities%20don%27t%20have,influence%20these%20is%20very%20iportant (accessed 26 November 2020).

George, S. (2021) After green homes grant failure, government 'dodges' recommendations on energy-efficient homes. Available at: https://www.edie.net/news/11/After-Green-Homes-Grant-failure--Government--dodges--recommendations-on-energy-efficient-homes/ (accessed 3 June 2021).

The Guardian (2020) 'Rat-running' increases on residential UK streets as experts blame satnav apps. Available at: https://www.theguardian.com/world/2020/sep/25/rat-running-residential-uk-streets-satnav-apps (accessed 8 February 2021).

IFG (2020) *Tax and Devolution.* Institute for Government. Available at: https://www.instituteforgovernment.org.uk/explainers/tax-and-devolution (accessed 29 December 2021).

IPPR North (2019) *Divided and Connected: Regional Inequalities in the North, the UK and the Developed World – State of the North 2019.* Institute for Public Policy Research. Available at: https://www.ippr.org/research/publications/state-of-the-north-2019 (accessed 29 December 2021).

Ipsos MORI (2020) *Concern about Climate Change Reaches Record Levels with Half Now 'Very Concerned'.* Available at: https://www.ipsos.com/ipsos-mori/en-uk/concern-about-climate-change-reaches-record-levels-half-now-very-concerned (accessed 3 December 2020).

Local Government Association (2020) *Re-thinking Local.* Available at: https://www.local.gov.uk/about/campaigns/re-thinking-local (accessed 29 November 2020).

Local Government Association (2021) *Six Steps to Undertaking a Climate Behaviour Change Project.* Available at: https://www.local.gov.uk/six-steps-undertaking-climate-behaviour-change-project (accessed 3 June 2021).

London Borough of Sutton (2014) *Fuel Poverty Strategy 2014/15 and Beyond.* Sutton: London Borough of Sutton. Available at: https://www.sutton.gov.uk/ (accessed 2 December 2020).

London Borough of Sutton (2020) *Sutton's Environment Strategy 2019–2025 and Climate Emergency Response Plan*. Sutton: London Borough of Sutton. Available at: https://www.sutton.gov.uk/ (accessed 21 November 2020).

London Borough of Sutton (2021) *Sutton Council Approves 2021/22 Budget*. Sutton: London Borough of Sutton. Available at: https://www.sutton.gov.uk/news/article/725/sutton_council_approves_202122_budget/ (accessed 29 December 2021).

London Councils (2021) *Review of Borough Climate Action Plans*. Available at: https://www.londoncouncils.gov.uk/our-key-themes/environment/climate-change (accessed 3 June 2021).

Marmot, M. (2010) *Fair Society, Healthy Lives: The Marmot Review: Strategic Review of Health Inequalities in England post-2010.*

Mayor of London (2016) *The London Plan 2016*. London: Mayor of London. London. Available at: https://www.london.gov.uk/sites/default/files/the_london_plan_2016_jan_2017_fix.pdf (accessed 3 December 2020).

Mayor of London (2020) *A Green New Deal*. Available at: https://www.london.gov.uk/coronavirus/londons-recovery-coronavirus-crisis/recovery-context/green-new-deal#acc-i-61477 (accessed 5 June 2021).

Passivhaus Trust (2020) *What Is Passivhaus?* Available at: https://www.passivhaustrust.org.uk/what_is_passivhaus.php#2 (accessed 29 November 2020).

South London Partnership (2021) *South London Skills and Employment Board*. Available at: http://southlondonpartnership.co.uk/skills/skills-and-employment-board/ (accessed 3 June 2021).

Sutton Council (2021) *Draft Sustainable Transport Strategy*. Available at: https://www.sutton.gov.uk/info/200464/planning_policy/2232/draft_sustainable_transport_strategy (accessed 8 February 2021).

The Sutton Plan (2021) Available at: http://www.thesuttonplan.org/ (accessed 8 February 2021).

Case study: Racism and xenophobia – America's deadly pre-existing conditions during the COVID-19 pandemic's first year

Joanna Sharpless and Annie Dell

Introduction

As it rampaged through the United States during the pandemic's first year, COVID-19 exposed and exploited deep-seated racial fault-lines at a cultural and political moment particularly primed for racial conflict. The United States' long history of structural racism, permeating all aspects of life including housing, employment and healthcare, placed American minorities at disproportionate danger from COVID-19. Yet instead of fighting inequity and working to ameliorate the social determinants of health that dramatically escalated the virus's risk to America's most vulnerable citizens, the US government largely mishandled responses to the virus, and even fanned the flames of racism. The combination of American racism and COVID-19 resulted not only in spikes in hate crimes and discrimination, but also the avoidable deaths of thousands of Americans.

Structural racism's mounting death toll

Well before COVID-19's arrival, structural racism left scars on the health of the US's minority population. Heading into the pandemic, Black and Latinx Americans suffered from more medical comorbidities and poorer health outcomes compared to White Americans, and Black Americans' life expectancy was four years shorter than that of White Americans – a disparity that COVID-19 would only worsen (Bosman et al, 2021; CDC, 2021a). As the virus began to spread, minority communities were primed for a public health disaster.

From January through March 2020, the virus took root in the early hotspots of Washington and New York states, quickly exposing racial differences in infection rates, morbidity and mortality. With its high population density, New York City was a particularly ripe breeding ground for viral spread. By the end of March, the city accounted for one-third of all confirmed cases in the US (Higgins-Dunn, 2020). Heavily Black and Latinx neighbourhoods saw the city's highest infection and death rates (Schwirtz and Rogers Cook, 2020; CDC, 2021b).

These trends held true as the pandemic spread country wide. Nationally, Black, Latinx and Native American patients were more than twice as likely to be hospitalised and twice as likely to die from COVID-19 compared to White and Asian patients (CDC, 2021b). Nursing homes showed the same inequalities; facilities with more Black and Latinx residents suffered from three times as many virus-related deaths as majority-White facilities (Gorges and Konetzka, 2021).

The Navajo Nation in the American Southwest faced infection rates of 20 per cent in the early stages of the pandemic, compared to 7 per cent nationally, and its death rate exceeded that of New York, Florida and Texas. The Indian Health Service, a government-run health programme for residents of Native American tribal communities, was ill-prepared to face a surge due to insufficient funding, supplies and staffing. Tribal leaders' requests for government assistance were met with inadequate responses, such as offers of expired personal protective equipment (Walker, 2020).

These racial disparities were not surprising given the effect of centuries of structural racism on minority communities' social determinants of health. Minorities disproportionately live in neighbourhoods with more pollution and fewer healthy food and affordable housing options. These factors, among others, led to higher rates of chronic health conditions including obesity, heart disease, diabetes and chronic lung disease that put patients at greater risk of severe illness from COVID-19. In addition, minority Americans were more likely to live in overcrowded environments and rely on public transportation, and were disproportionally employed as essential workers. Consequently, they were less able to effectively quarantine or social distance to reduce infection risk (Rogers et al, 2020; Wen and Sadeghi, 2020).

Compared with White Americans, minorities also faced limited healthcare access. Data from the Kaiser Family Foundation (KFF) from 2010 to 2019 shows that Black and Latinx Americans were consistently and significantly more likely to lack health insurance compared to White Americans (Artiga et al, 2021). Moreover, because approximately half of Americans were insured through employer-sponsored health plans, millions of Americans lost their health insurance due to increased unemployment early in the pandemic (Nova, 2020: Bundorf et al, 2021). Inadequate access to COVID-19 testing was also a major issue. Minority communities had fewer testing sites and Black and Latinx patients were more likely to perceive inequities in access to testing and treatment for COVID-19 (Vann et al, 2020; Dreisbach, 2021; Grigsby-Toussaint et al, 2021).

In December 2020, the Food and Drug Administration gave emergency use authorisation for the Pfizer vaccine, shortly followed by the Moderna and Johnson & Johnson vaccines. Racial patterns in vaccination rates quickly came into focus. Data from 39 states recorded by the KFF through March 2021 showed that the vaccination rate for White people was close to twice as high as that for Black and Latinx people. In California, Latinx people made up 40 per cent of the state's population and comprised 55 per cent of COVID-19 cases and 46 per cent of COVID-19 deaths, but received only 21 per cent of vaccinations. Comparatively, vaccination rates of White Americans exceeded their corresponding infection and death rates in nearly all states reporting racial/ethnic vaccine data (Hamel et al, 2021).

The aetiology of these lower vaccination rates was likely multifactorial, inclusive of issues with vaccine access as well as vaccine hesitancy. One investigation found that vaccine sites in the Southern US were more likely to be placed in neighbourhoods that were whiter and more affluent – a problem that public health officials attempted to rectify by preferentially establishing mass vaccination sites in high-need areas (McMinn et al, 2021). Barriers to computer and internet access, a relative dearth of primary care physicians in minority communities, and other structural barriers may also have limited access to the vaccine (Njoku et al, 2021).

In addition, Black Americans had long reported lower levels of trust in the medical system. They had good reason to be mistrustful given the US's long history of systematic medical abuse of Black communities, such as the well-known 'Tuskegee Study of Untreated Syphilis in the Negro Male', in which a group of Southern Black men with syphilis was not told of or treated for their disease from the 1930s to the 1970s. In a September 2020 survey by the Robert Wood Johnson Foundation, 10.6 per cent of Black Americans reported they had been discriminated against in the healthcare system because of their race, ethnicity, disability, gender, sexual orientation or health condition – a rate twice as high as that reported by Latinx patients and three times higher than White patients reported in the same study (Gonzalez et al, 2021).

Although unclear how directly attributable it was to mistrust of the medical system, Black Americans had a much higher rate of COVID-19 vaccine hesitancy. In December 2020, 35 per cent of Black adults surveyed by the KFF stated they would probably not or definitely not get a COVID-19 vaccine, compared to 27 per cent of the US population at large. Half of Black adults surveyed reported they were reluctant to get vaccinated because they didn't trust vaccines in general or because they worried the vaccine would give them COVID-19. Many told researchers that they were not confident that the needs of Black Americans were taken into account during vaccine development. However, as more evidence emerged supporting vaccine safety and efficacy and as more Americans received the vaccine, vaccine hesitancy began to decrease. The percentage of Black adults who said they had gotten or would get the vaccine as soon as possible rose 14 per cent between February and March of 2021 (Hamel et al, 2020, 2021).

Notably, there were other Americans with even higher rates of vaccine hesitancy: Republicans and white Evangelical Christians (Hamel et al, 2021). Like Black Americans, their reluctance was related at least in part to mistrust of the government and the public health system, though this mistrust was rooted in a very different type of cultural conflict.

Culture wars and clashes: the US political landscape during COVID-19

COVID-19 arrived at an inopportune time for President Donald Trump, who was in the final year of his first four-year term and facing re-election in November 2020. The booming economy had been one of his strongest campaign issues, so as the financial ramifications of the virus and associated shutdowns became clear, President Trump and other conservative leaders sought to minimise the virus' threat, stating that it was 'under control' and would 'disappear' with the arrival of warmer weather (Bump, 2021; NPR, 2020). President Trump later told journalist Bob Woodward that he intentionally sought to 'play it down' to avoid triggering a 'panic' (NPR, 2020).

Perhaps to deflect blame for the pandemic's effects, President Trump also sought to portray COVID-19 as a foreign invader from Asia, reigniting xenophobic sentiments reminiscent of 19th-century portrayals of Asians as a 'Yellow Peril'. In multiple public appearances, President Trump referred to COVID-19 as the 'Chinese virus' and 'kung flu', language echoed by other conservative politicians and pundits (Nakamura, 2020). A study showed that within the two days after politicians used the terms 'Chinese virus' and 'Wuhan virus' in the media, there was an 800 per cent increase in online news articles using stigmatising language to refer to the virus (Darling-Hammond et al, 2020).

In tandem with this rhetoric, hate crimes against Asian Americans spiked precipitously. Data from the Federal Bureau of Investigation showed a 73 per cent increase in anti-Asian hate crimes in 2020, compared to a 13 per cent rise in total hate crimes (Venkatraman, 2021). The non-profit organisation Stop AAPI Hate reported 6,603 hate incidents between March 2020 and March 2021, 12.6 per cent of which were violent in nature (Jeung et al, 2021). Yet while governmental agencies had made efforts to respond to increases in hate crimes during 9/11 and the 2003 SARS outbreak (which comparatively infected only eight people in the US), the Trump administration did not direct the Department of Justice or the Centers for Disease Control and Prevention to intervene in early spring of 2020 (Fernández Campbell et al, 2020).

Despite imposing aggressive measures aimed at restricting travel and immigration to the US, President Trump and other leaders in his administration were hesitant to endorse equally aggressive public health policy measures such as mask wearing, social distancing and lockdowns. As the spring surge escalated, President Trump implied that mask wearing should be optional and encouraged state governors to begin to reopen their states (Victor et al, 2020). He also spread virus-related misinformation, suggesting that COVID-19 could be killed by injecting or ingesting disinfectants, or prevented by taking the drug hydroxychloroquine, which was later shown to be false (Clark, 2020; Saag, 2020).

President Trump also consistently disregarded public health recommendations in service of his re-election campaign. He continued to hold large in-person rallies with many maskless attendees, which were later linked to spikes in infections (Lovelace, 2020). In October 2020, President Trump and the First Lady were diagnosed with COVID-19 after attending a large White House event, at which tens of others also became infected (Schoenfield Walker and Conlon, 2020). President Trump was admitted to Walter Reed Medical Center for three days – a dramatic turn of events so close to the election. Yet despite his personal brush with the illness, Trump continued to resist mask wearing and social distancing measures (Noack, 2020). Under his guidance, mask wearing and social distancing rapidly became partisan issues, the effect of which was reflected in disproportionate increases in infection and death rates in Republican-led states through the summer and fall of 2020 (Gregorian, 2021).

Parallel to the virus's spread throughout the spring and summer of 2020, news reports began to circulate about several Black Americans, including Rayshard Brooks, George Floyd and Breonna Taylor, who were killed in encounters with police. Public outrage over their unjustified deaths, which occurred on a backdrop of a long history of police violence against Black Americans, grew and reignited the Black Lives Matter movement, inspiring the largest mass protest movement in the nation's history. An estimated 15–26 million protestors filled streets across the nation to demand action on police brutality and racial injustice in the criminal justice system, among other issues (Buchanan et al, 2020). Though public health officials raised concerns that these mass gatherings might trigger COVID-19 outbreaks, this did not occur, perhaps in part because many protestors wore masks and most protests occurred outside (Beer, 2020).

President Trump opposed the Black Lives Matter movement, labelling protestors 'THUGS' and threatening a violent response to protests (Madani, 2020). He also suggested that the protests were linked to rising COVID-19 cases, despite evidence to the contrary (Smith, 2020). Encouraged by President Trump, millions of his supporters developed a shared ideology that linked opposition to the Black Lives Matter movement, mandatory masking and lockdowns.

Despite mishandling the pandemic response and actively fanning the flames of racial unrest, President Trump received over 74 million votes in the November election, or 46.9 per cent of the voting population. Yet Joseph Biden was ultimately declared the winner, with 51.3 per cent of the vote and 306 electoral votes (CNN, 2020). The new administration quickly moved to accelerate the country's response to COVID-19, which had killed 400,000 Americans by the time of the inauguration in January 2021 (Smith-Schoenwalder, 2021).

On his first day in office, President Biden implemented a federal mask mandate and issued executive orders targeted at increasing COVID-19 testing and addressing the economic impacts of the virus. His first executive order, titled 'Advancing Racial Equity and Support for Underserved Communities Through the Federal Government', identified combating the impacts of systemic racism as one of his administration's top priorities (Executive Office of the President, 2021). In March 2021, Congress passed a $1.9 trillion American Rescue Plan, which included billions of dollars aimed at combating the pandemic and accelerating vaccination efforts, particularly in underserved communities (Collins and Sullivan, 2021).

As the pandemic stretched into its second year, glimmers of hope emerged as more and more Americans got vaccinated. However, new variants of the virus continued to emerge, triggering recurrent surges and ongoing high infection and death rates. With the public's growing pandemic fatigue, many political leaders from both political parties were hesitant to resume widespread or intensive lockdowns. These factors, combined with persistent vaccine hesitancy in large portions of the population, meant that Americans continued to perish at alarming rates. The end of the pandemic appeared tantalisingly close, yet remained frustratingly out of reach.

Conclusion

While no American remained untouched by the devastating effects of COVID-19, the US's minority communities bore the brunt of its fury. Strategies to fight the pandemic effectively demanded action against prejudice and racism, yet on this front, the Trump administration was inactive at best and divisive at worst. While some individuals and non-governmental organisations moved to fill voids left by government inaction on racism and xenophobia, others actively sought to escalate racial tensions. The structural racism and social determinants of health that set the stage for the harm American minority communities endured in the pandemic's first year and beyond remain deeply ingrained in the American cultural, political and social systems. As the pandemic extended into its second and third years, it nevertheless remained clear that its end would likely come much sooner than the systemic change needed to safeguard American minorities from similar public health catastrophes in the future.

References

Artiga, S., Hill, L., Orgera, K. and Damico, A. (2021) Health coverage by race and ethnicity, 2010–2019. Kaiser Family Foundation, 16 July. Available at: https://www.kff.org/racial-equity-and-health-policy/issue-brief/health-coverage-by-race-and-ethnicity/

Beer, T. (2020) Research determines protests did not cause spike in coronavirus cases. Forbes, 1 July. Available at: https://www.forbes.com/sites/tommybeer/2020/07/01/research-determines-protests-did-not-cause-spike-in-coronavirus-cases/?sh=27c199307dac

Bosman, K., Kasakove, S. and Victor, D. (2021) US life expectancy plunged in 2020, especially for Black and Hispanic Americans. The New York Times, 21 July. Available at: https://www.nytimes.com/2021/07/21/us/american-life-expectancy-report.html

Buchanan, L., Bui, Q. and Patel, J. (2020) Black Lives Matter may be the largest movement in U.S. history. The New York Times, 3 July. Available at: https://www.nytimes.com/interactive/2020/07/03/us/george-floyd-protests-crowd-size.html

Bump, P. (2021) A year after Trump said coronavirus was 'under control,' a look back at the first news stories. The Washington Post, 24 February. Available at: https://www.washingtonpost.com/politics/2021/02/24/year-after-trump-said-coronavirus-was-under-control-look-back-first-news-stories/

Bundorf, M.K., Gupta, S. and Kim, C. (2021) Trends in US health insurance coverage during the COVID-19 pandemic. JAMA Health Forum, 2(9): e212487.

CDC (2021a) Impact of racism on our nation's health. CDC. Available at: https://www.cdc.gov/healthequity/racism-disparities/impact-of-racism.html

CDC (2021b) Risk for COVID-19 infection, hospitalization, and death by race/ethnicity. CDC. Available at: https://www.cdc.gov/coronavirus/2019-ncov/covid-data/investigations-discovery/hospitalization-death-by-race-ethnicity.html

Clark, D. (2020) Trump suggests 'injection' of disinfectant to beat coronavirus and 'clean' the lungs. NBC News, 23 April. Available at: https://www.nbcnews.com/politics/donald-trump/trump-suggests-injection-disinfectant-beat-coronavirus-clean-lungs-n1191216

CNN (2020) Presidential results. CNN. Available at: https://www.cnn.com/election/2020/results/president

Collins, K. and Sullivan, K. (2021) Biden administration to provide $150 million to boost COVID response in underserved and vulnerable areas. *CNN*, 19 April. Available at: https://www.cnn.com/2021/04/19/polit ics/american-rescue-plan-funding-vulnerable-communities/index.html

Darling-Hammond, S., Michaels, E., Allen, A., Chae, D., Thomas, M., Nguyen, T., Mujahid, M. and Johnson, R. (2020) After 'the China virus' went viral: Racially charged coronavirus coverage and trends in bias against Asian Americans. *Health Education and Behavior*, 47(6): 870–879.

Dreisbach, E. (2021) Black, Hispanic or Latinx adults twice as likely to report worse COVID-19 access. *Healio: Infectious Diseases*, 28 January. Available at: https://www.healio.com/news/infectious-disease/20210128/black-hispanic-or-latinx-adults-twice-as-likely-to-report-worse-covid19-access

Executive Office of the President (2021) Advancing racial equity and support for underserved communities through the Federal Government. Executive Order 13985, 20 January. Available at: https://www.federalregister.gov/documents/2021/01/25/2021-01753/advancing-racial-equity-and-supp ort-for-underserved-communities-through-the-federal-government

Fernández Campbell, A. and Ellerbeck, A. (2020) Federal agencies are doing little about the rise in anti-Asian hate. *NBC News*, 16 April. Available at: https://www.nbcnews.com/news/asian-america/federal-agencies-are-doing-little-about-rise-anti-asian-hate-n1184766

Gonzalez, D., Skopec, L., McDaniel, M. and Kenney, G. (2021) Perceptions of discrimination and unfair judgement while seeking health care: Findings from the September 11–28 coronavirus tracking survey. Robert Wood Johnson Foundation Urban Institute, April. Available at: https://www.urban.org/sites/default/files/publication/103953/perceptions-of-discrim ination-and-unfair-judgment-while-seeking-health-care.pdf

Gorges, R. and Konetzka, R.T. (2021) Factors associated with racial differences in deaths among nursing home residents with COVID-19 infection in the US. *JAMA Network Open*, 4(2): e2037431.

Gregorian, D. (2021) States with Republican governors had highest COVID incidence and death rates, study finds. *NBC News*, 11 March. Available at: https://www.nbcnews.com/politics/politics-news/states-republican-governors-had-highest-covid-incidence-death-rates-study-n1260700

Grigsby-Toussaint, D., Shin, J.C. and Jones, A. (2021) Disparities in the distribution of COVID-19 testing sites in Black and Latino areas in New York City. *Preventive Medicine*, June. Available at: https://www.scienc edirect.com/science/article/pii/S0091743521000475?via%3Dihub

Hamel, L., Kirzinger, A., Muñana, C. and Brodie, M. (2020) KFF COVID-19 vaccine monitor: December 2020. Kaiser Family Foundation, 15 December. Available at: https://www.kff.org/coronavirus-covid-19/rep ort/kff-covid-19-vaccine-monitor-december-2020/

Hamel, L., Lopes, L., Kearney, A. and Brodie, M. (2021) KFF COVID-19 vaccine monitor: March 2021. Kaiser Family Foundation, 30 March. Available at: https://www.kff.org/coronavirus-covid-19/poll-finding/kff-covid-19-vaccine-monitor-march-2021/

Higgins-Dunn, N. (2020) New York City is the new coronavirus epicentre with one-third of all US cases, Mayor de Blasio says. *CNBC*, 20 March. Available at: https://www.cnbc.com/2020/03/20/new-york-city-is-the-new-coronavirus-epicenter-with-one-third-of-all-us-cases-mayor-de-blasio-says.html

Jeung, R., Yellow Horse, A. and Cayanan, C. (2021) Stop AAPI Hate national report. Stop AAPI Hate, 31 March. Available at: https://stopaapihate.org/wp-content/uploads/2021/05/Stop-AAPI-Hate-Report-National-210506.pdf

Lovelace, B. (2020) Trump campaign rallies led to more than 30,000 coronavirus cases, Stanford researchers say. *CNBC*, 31 October. Available at: https://www.cnbc.com/2020/10/31/coronavirus-trump-campaign-rallies-led-to-30000-cases-stanford-researchers-say.html

Madani, D. (2020) Trump's warning as Minneapolis burns over George Floyd's death: 'When the looting starts, the shooting starts'. *NBC News*, 28 May. Available at: https://www.nbcnews.com/politics/donald-trump/trump-s-warning-minneapolis-burns-over-george-floyd-s-death-n1217571

McMinn, S., Chatlani, S., Lopez, A., Whitehead, S., Talbot, R. and Fast, A. (2021) Across the South, COVID-19 vaccine sites missing from Black and Hispanic neighbourhoods. *NPR*, 5 February. Available at: https://www.npr.org/2021/02/05/962946721/across-the-south-covid-19-vaccine-sites-missing-from-black-and-hispanic-neighbor

Nakamura, D. (2020) With 'kung flu,' Trump sparks backlash over racist language – and a rallying cry for supporters. *The Washington Post*, 24 June. Available at: https://www.washingtonpost.com/politics/with-kung-flu-trump-sparks-backlash-over-racist-language--and-a-rallying-cry-for-supporters/2020/06/24/485d151e-b620-11ea-aca5-ebb63d27e1ff_story.html

Njoku, A., Joseph, M. and Felix, R. (2021) Changing the narrative: Structural barriers and racial and ethnic inequities in COVID-19 vaccination. *International Journal of Environmental Research and Public Health*, 18(18): 9904. Available at: https://www.ncbi.nlm.nih.gov/pmc/articles/PMC8470519/

Noack, R. (2020) Trump's resistance to face masks, even while he is infected with coronavirus, sets him apart from other world leaders. *The Washington Post*, 7 October. Available at: https://www.washingtonpost.com/health/2020/10/07/trump-coronavirus-face-masks-world-leaders/

Nova, A. (2020) Millions of Americans have lost health insurance in this pandemic-driven recession. Here are their options. *CNBC*, 28 August. Available at: https://www.cnbc.com/2020/08/28/millions-of-americans-lost-health-insurance-amid-pandemic-here-are-options.html

NPR (2020) Trump tells Woodward he deliberately downplayed coronavirus threat. *NPR*, 10 September. Available at: https://www.npr.org/2020/09/10/911368698/trump-tells-woodward-he-deliberately-downplayed-coronavirus-threat

Rogers, T., Rogers, C., VanSant-Webb, E., Gu, L., Yan, B. and Qeadan, F. (2020) Racial disparities in COVID-19 mortality among essential workers in the United States. *World Medical and Health Policy*, 5 August. Available at: http://europepmc.org/article/MED/32837779

Saag, M. (2020) Misguided use of hydroxychloroquine for COVID-19: The infusion of politics into science. *JAMA*, 324(21): 2161–2162. Available at: https://jamanetwork.com/journals/jama/fullarticle/2772921

Schoenfeld Walker, A. and Conlen, M. (2020) Tracking coronavirus infections in the White House and Trump's inner circle. *The New York Times*, 8 December. Available at: https://www.nytimes.com/interactive/2020/11/11/us/politics/white-house-covid-outbreak.html

Schwirtz, M. and Rogers Cook, L. (2020) These N.Y.C. neighbourhoods have the highest rates of virus deaths. *The New York Times*, 18 May. Available at: https://www.nytimes.com/2020/05/18/nyregion/coronavirus-deaths-nyc.html

Smith, D. (2020) Trump falsely ties climbing COVID-19 cases to Black Lives Matter protests. *The Guardian*, 22 July. Available at: https://www.theguardian.com/us-news/2020/jul/22/trump-coronavirus-briefing-black-lives-matter-protests

Smith-Schoenwalder, C. (2021) U.S. coronavirus death toll tops 400,000 day before Bidens's inauguration. US News and World Report, 19 January. Available at: https://www.usnews.com/news/national-news/articles/2021-01-19/us-coronavirus-death-toll-tops-400-000-day-before-bidens-inauguration

Vann, W., Kim, S.R. and Bronner, L. (2020) White neighbourhoods have more access to COVID-19 testing sites: Analysis. *ABC News*, 22 July. Available at: https://abcnews.go.com/Politics/white-neighborhoods-access-covid-19-testing-sites-analysis/story?id=71884719

Venkatraman, S. (2021) Anti-Asian hate crimes rose 73% last year, updated FBI data says. *NBC News*, 25 October. Available at: https://www.nbcnews.com/news/asian-america/anti-asian-hate-crimes-rose-73-last-year-updated-fbi-data-says-rcna3741

Victor, D., Serviss, L. and Paybarah, A. (2020) In his own words, Trump on the coronavirus and masks. *The New York Times*, 2 October. Available at: https://www.nytimes.com/2020/10/02/us/politics/donald-trump-masks.html

Walker, M. (2020) Pandemic highlights deep-rooted problems in Indian Health Service. *The New York Times*, 29 September. Available at: https://www.nytimes.com/2020/09/29/us/politics/coronavirus-indian-health-service.html

Case study: Safe at home? Exploring intersecting vulnerabilities under COVID-19 and the role of faith actors in the South African context

Selina Palm

Introduction

In the early stages of the COVID-19 pandemic, South Africa recorded the fifth largest number of COVID-19 infections globally. By March 2021, it had over 1.5 million cases recorded with an estimated 50,000 COVID-19-related deaths (Reuters, 2020). Yet at the same time, it received early commendation from the WHO for its swift response (Ryan, 2020). An integral part of this was an early, strict national lockdown from March 2020 declared by President Ramaphosa (Relief Web, 2020). This helped flatten the curve and enabled health systems to prepare. A unique, but contested, aspect of South Africa's lockdown was a total ban on the sale of alcohol over three periods,[1] strongly influenced by third sector voices, in order to mitigate lockdown's impact on women and children (Harrison, 2020).

Globally COVID-19 is seen to be escalating pre-existing, intersecting inequalities especially between rich and poor and between genders (Peterman and O'Donnell, 2020). South Africa remains highly unequal with a structural legacy of colonialism and apartheid. Public health and education systems are fragile, and thousands of families remain food insecure (May et al, 2020). COVID-19 has further entrenched inequalities with women and children bearing the brunt of increased household stresses and lockdown (Dartnell and Gevers, 2020). South Africa also has a toxic relationship with alcohol, partly shaped by its socio-structural history. Heavy drinking patterns by some have serious social costs (Matzopoulos et al, 2014; Trangenstein et al, 2018). This reality and its impact on violence against women and children (VAW/C) has drawn increased policy attention under COVID-19.

South Africa also has some of the highest rates of gender-based violence and femicide in the world (WHO, 2018). President Ramaphosa has focused on this issue with a 2018 presidential summit, a 2019 inter-ministerial task team and a National Plan of Action focused on violence against women and children (National Strategic Plan on Gender-based Violence and Femicide, 2020). However, a significant gap remains between legal and policy provisions and lived realities. COVID-19 and VAW/C are **wicked issues** characterised by social complexity, multiple actors and disagreement on how to respond appropriately. They also intersect. South African scholars reinforce global evidence that COVID-19 is a gendered pandemic (Lefafa, 2020). Some responses to COVID-19, especially strict lockdowns, may put vulnerable women and children at greater risk (Dartnell and Gevers, 2020). Gender-based violence has been termed COVID-19's shadow pandemic (Majumdar and Wood, 2020) and has been highlighted within South Africa (Adebayo, 2020). President Ramaphosa has insisted that these links have to be taken seriously, stating in his 17 June 2020 speech that, '[A]s a country, we find ourselves in the midst of not one, but two, devastating epidemics. Although very different in their nature and cause, they can both be overcome – if we work together' (Ramaphosa, 2020). This reinforces the need for an intersectional lens on COVID-19 that pays attention to the compounding risks of violence and requires collaboration with the third sector. Women's organisations have played important roles in moving VAW/C up the policy agenda. At the same time faith institutions also need engagement if entrenched patriarchal social norms and hierarchical power relations within households are to change (Palm and Le Roux, 2018).

COVID-19 and violence against women and children

COVID-19 is seen to be compounding pre-existing vulnerabilities globally (Spiranovic et al, 2020) and making visible a broader landscape of inequalities which interact in new ways. Scholars showcase studies that connect COVID-19 with increased risks of VAW/C, including crisis-related unrest, social isolation, poverty-related stress and an inability to escape abusive partners (Peterman and O'Donnell, 2020; Peterman et al, 2020). At the same time, COVID-19 responses can further invisibilise violence within homes which often flourishes in social isolation (Majumdar and Wood, 2020). Responses protective for COVID-19, such as lockdowns or school closures, may escalate risks of violence for women and children, creating a 'perfect storm' of isolation, online abuse, hunger, economic and psychological stress (Nombembe, 2020; Spiranovic et al, 2020). Concern exists regarding reduced protections and increased barriers to access VAW/C prevention services, including suspension of services, less access to justice, a culture of impunity for perpetrators, and lack of privacy to report violence (Dartnell and Gevers, 2020). At the same time, opportunities exist to develop new social innovations to prevent VAW/C by refusing to 'return to normal' post-pandemic (Majumdar and Wood, 2020). This places a responsibility on everyone to work towards a post-COVID-19 future which tackles root causes, avoids reversing policy gains and transforms unjust household power relations that fuel VAW/C.

The most dangerous place for both women and children in South Africa is within the home, and from those they know (Palm and Le Roux, 2018). Women in South Africa also face additional gendered pressures under COVID-19. Many have lost significant household income, reducing their financial ability to leave abusive situations (Harrison, 2020). At the same time, a sense of helplessness and failure by more men to provide financially can increase their risk of perpetrating family VAW/C.

South Africa's policy decision to ban the sale of all alcohol over successive COVID-19 lockdowns was influenced by these twin pandemics, and by the coordinated grassroots lobbying of civil society groups. While rigorous evidence is still needed, and a perceived reduction in reporting VAW/C does not automatically mean a reduction in experiencing VAW/C (Dartnell and Gevers, 2020), anecdotal figures suggest that this ban may have tempered the rise in violence against women and children in South Africa (Gould, 2020; Harrison, 2020) in ways apparently not observed in other countries. Harrison claims that while in many other countries, reporting of domestic violence cases increased during lockdown, in South Africa, one of a few countries to implement a total ban on alcohol sales, the reverse happened, with a significant drop in reported cases of the number of women seeking assistance at Thuthuzela Centres (Harrison, 2020). This insight, if verified longer term, may provide opportunities to address South Africa's toxic relationship with alcohol (Mkise, 2020; Trangenstein et al, 2020).

Collaboration within the third sector including faith actors

South Africa's civil society organisational network forms an important asset in relation to the twin pandemics. A history of collaboration under apartheid and HIV/AIDS provides resources on which to draw, especially in the light of state systems mired in corruption and inefficiency. Civil society offers important resources for COVID-19, such as communicating information, providing food support and holding the government to account on social issues, such as VAW/C. They are seen as playing critical roles in: identifying who is 'left at the back of the queue' in COVID-19 responses; giving a voice to ordinary people; and developing social innovations by working together (Harrison, 2020).

VAW/C is one area where political rhetoric needs to be matched with social responses to tackle root causes in the risk environment of COVID-19. The banning of alcohol sales under lockdown offers one example of effective collaboration between civil society organisations concerned with VAW/C and government policy (Harrison, 2020). However, some gender activists have expressed concerns that blaming alcohol can be misused to enable perpetrator impunity or to blame the victims of violence. While social patterns around alcohol abuse play a role in VAW/C, tackling the patriarchal social norms and toxic masculinity which underpin male entitlement and superiority here must also be addressed (Dartnell and Gevers, 2020; Palm, 2020). A successful June 2020 petition to the South African government to reinstate the alcohol ban was signed by over 166 academics, researchers and civil society partners. It noted that while gender-based violence is driven by gender inequality, it is made worse by social and economic marginalisation, failures of policing and justice, and the abuse of drugs and alcohol as a contributing factor, and requires interventions which tackle these factors simultaneously (Petition, 2020).

Gender activists, government and civil society can collaborate on these issues to develop synergies and avoid fragmented polarisation. Alcohol abuse can be recognised as an important trigger around the severity and frequency of violent patterns of domestic violence while also engaging underlying drivers. The role that alcohol also plays in constructing toxic masculinities (Mkise, 2020) must be engaged alongside tackling other patriarchal social norms that underpin forms of VAW/C.

Faith-based organisations and local church programmes form a significant part of civil society here where over 80 per cent of South Africans indicate strong Christian affiliation. Mobilising their constructive engagement under COVID-19 has been essential for adherence to public health measures including the long-term closure of faith meetings as well as strict limits or bans on important religious events such as weddings and funerals. Getting religious leader support was critical for a coordinated response to COVID-19 that reached people with consistent messaging (Palm and Melane, 2020).

Local faith actors can also play important roles around the prevention of VAW/C if they are appropriately capacitated (Palm, 2020). This offers opportunities and risks. Faith leaders played important roles in the HIV pandemic only once they had been capacitated to rethink harmful theologies, such as seeing HIV as a punishment from God. Likewise, faith leaders need to ensure that their theologies do no harm in relation to the pandemics of COVID-19 and VAW/C. Faith leaders were recognised early as critical partners in the lockdown especially as religious events were identified as super-spreaders and a decision was taken to close all religious gatherings, even over key religious festivals. While most faith leaders were supportive, a vocal minority resisted these restrictions and some mounted legal challenges.

Faith leaders' action on VAW/C however has been less active and more ambiguous. However, positive collaboration with faith actors is critical for a comprehensive multisectoral response in South Africa especially where social behaviours play such a strong role both under COVID-19 and in relation to VAW/C. Promising collaborations between VAW/C prevention researchers, faith leaders and faith-based organisations have emerged. Four promising examples are briefly noted in what follows.

The Unit for Religion and Development Research at Stellenbosch University has engaged with the roles of faith actors under COVID-19 to prevent VAW/C. A webinar series on *Healthy Households* equipped local faith leaders to help to prevent VAW/C (Palm, 2020). It drew attention to patriarchal social norms used to justify VAW/C.

The South African Council of Churches also ran a series of seminars on ending gender-based violence over 2020, drawing attention to how COVID-19 is a gendered pandemic and the risks of lockdown for VAW/C. It interrogated patterns of power within households that legitimate violence and invited faith leaders to engage with their traditions differently (SACC, 2020).

Third, the Circle of Concerned African Women Theologians captured lived experiences of many South African women under COVID-19 and the challenges they face, putting together a compendium of voices entitled *A Time Like No Other: COVID19 in Women's Voices* (Hadebe et al, 2020) which was driven by local women faith leaders offering prophetic voices for change on gender-based violence (Gennrich, 2021).

Finally, lobbying the government around practical longer-term restrictions on alcohol and support for those seeking to overcome addiction can be an issue where faith-based entities collaborate with other civil society organisations. The South African Catholic Parliamentary Liaison Office ran a webinar in 2021 on alcohol and the lockdown, related to the safety needs of children (CPLO, 2021).

Conclusion

South Africa can make important contributions to the wicked intersections between COVID-19 and VAW/C within a structural context of pre-existing inequalities. Its policy decisions around alcohol under lockdown offer insights that need further analysis to influence long-term policy gains that centre women and children. However, protectionist responses to complex social issues must be avoided. New policies on alcohol need support from the third sector to build back differently. However, religious leaders moralising about the evils of drinking must not use alcohol to avoid looking at how harmful gendered beliefs underpin social norms which justify male entitlement, gendered household roles, female inferiority, silence and submission, and child violence. Faith actors must also transform entrenched harmful social norms if women and children in South Africa are to live in houses of freedom. COVID-19 responses must engage with these gendered power relations if women and children are not to be placed further at risk. Promising signs of collaboration are seen between women's organisations, feminist academics and local faith leaders which can contribute to global conversations on involving faith leaders in preventing VAW/C.

Note

1   The sale of alcohol ban began in mid-March 2020, was lifted in mid-June and then reimposed from 12 July until 7 September 2020 and again over the second lockdown (28 December 2020 until 7 February 2021). This covered a total period of over five months.

References

Adebayo, B. (2020) 'South Africa has the continent's highest COVID-19 cases: Now it has another pandemic on its hands', *CNN*, 19 June. Available at: https://edition.cnn.com/2020/06/19/africa/south-africa-gender-violence-pandemic-intl/index.html (accessed 12 March 2021).

CPLO (Catholic Parliamentary Liaison Office) (2021) 'Alcohol and the lockdown', Webinar, 21 March. South Africa.

Dartnell, E. and Gevers, A. (2020) 'Domestic violence during COVID-19: Are we asking the right questions?', 3 July. Blog. Available at: https://www.svri.org/blog/domestic-violence-during-covid-19-are-we-asking-right-questions (accessed 15 December 2020).

Gennrich, D. (2021) 'Gender-based violence and the church: A church gender activist's reflections', in N. Hadebe, S. Rakoczy and N. Tom (eds) *A Time Like No Other: COVID19 in Women's Voices*. South Africa: Circle of Concerned Women Theologians, pp 15–32.

Gould, C. (2020) 'Why is South Africa not showing the rise in domestic violence cases reported elsewhere in the world?', Institute for Security Studies, 11 May. Available at: https://issafrica.org/iss-today/gender-based-violence-duringlockdown-looking-for-answers (accessed 5 September 2020).

Hadebe, N., Gennrich, D., Rakoczy, S. and Tom, N. (2020) 'A time like this: COVID-19 in Women's Voices'. Available at: https://www.partner-religion-development.org/fileadmin/user_upload/PaRD_GAM_South_Africa_2021_A_time_like_no_other_Women_and_Covid-19_e-book.pdf (accesed 22 August 2022).

Harrison, D. (2020) *Harnessing the Thunder: Civil Society's Care and Creativity in South Africa's COVID Storm*. Johannesburg: Porcupine Press.

Lefafa, N. (2020) 'COVID-19 lockdown provides "perfect storm" for SA's GBV crisis', 29 April. Available at: https://health-e.org.za/2020/04/29/covid-19-lockdown-provides-perfect-storm-for-sas-gbv-crisis/ (accessed 20 March 2020).

Majumdar, S. and Wood, G. (2020) *UNTF EVAW Briefing Note on the Impact of COVID-19 on Violence against Women through the Lens of Civil Society and Women's Rights Organizations*. New York: UN Trust Fund to End Violence Against Women.

Matzopoulos, R., Truen, S., Bowman, B. and Corrigall, J. (2014) 'The cost of harmful alcohol use in South Africa', *South African Medical Journal*, 104(2): 127–132.

May, J., Witten, C. and Lake, L. (eds) (2020) *South African Child Gauge 2020*. Cape Town: Children's Institute, University of Cape Town.

Mkise, V. (2020) 'South Africa's toxic relationship with alcohol', *BBC News*, 11 August. Available at: https://www.bbc.co.uk/news/world-africa-53699 712 (accessed 22 August 2022).

National Strategic Plan on Gender-based Violence and Femicide (2020) Pretoria: South African Government. Available at: https://justice.gov.za/vg/gbv/NSP-GBVF-FINAL-DOC-04-05.pdf (accessed 20 March 2021).

Nombembe, P. (2020) 'Hunger, poverty and lockdown adds up to domestic violence crisis', *The Times*, 6 April. Available at: https://www.timeslive.co.za/news/south-africa/2020-04-06-hunger-poverty-and-lockdown-adds-up-to-domestic-violence-crisis/ (accessed 20 March 2021).

Palm, S. (2020) 'Homes of bondage or households of freedom? The role of faith in underlying harmful social norms', Webinar, 7 July. Available at: http://blogs.sun.ac.za/urdr/files/2020/07/Palm_7-July-webinar-slides.pdf (accessed 20 March 2021).

Palm, S. and Le Roux, E. (2018) 'Households of freedom? Faith's role in challenging gendered geographies of violence in our cities', in S. De Beer (ed) *Just Faith: Global Responses to Planetary Urbanization*. Pretoria: AOSIS Online, pp 135–164.

Palm, S. and Melane, A. (2020) 'The role of FBOs during a pandemic', *Cape Talk*. Available at: https://omny.fm/shows/weekend-breakfast-with-afr ica-melane/the-role-of-faith-based-organisations-during-a-pan (accessed 5 September 2020).

Peterman, A. and O'Donnell, M. (2020) *COVID-19 and Violence against Women and Children: A Third Research Round Up for the 16 Days of Activism*. Centre for Global Development. Available at: https://www.cgdev.org/sites/default/files/covid-and-violence-against-women-and-children-three.pdf (accessed 10 March 2021).

Peterman, A., Potts, A., O'Donnell, M., Thompson, K., Shah, N., Oertelt-Prigione, S. and van Gelder, N. (2020) *Pandemics and Violence against Women and Children*. Centre for Global Development Working Paper 528. Available at: https://www.cgdev.org/publication/pandemics-and-violence-against-women-and-children (accessed 15 December 2021).

Petition (2020) 'Abuse of alcohol linked to GBV: Put the rights of women and children first'. Available at: https://awethu.amandla.mobi/petitions/five-urgent-and-effective-measures-needed-now-to-curb-the-abuse-of-alcohol (accessed 22 August 2022).

Ramaphosa, C. (2020) 'Address on South Africa's response to the coronavirus pandemic', 17 June. Available at: https://www.gov.za/speeches/president-cyril-ramaphosa-south-africa%E2%80%99s-response-covid-19-coronavirus-pandemic-17-jun-2020# (accessed 15 February 2021).

Relief Web (2020) 'WHO encouraged by South Africa's declining COVID-19 trend', press release, 17 September. Available at: https://reliefweb.int/report/south-africa/who-encouraged-south-africa-s-declining-covid-19-trend (accessed 15 December 2020).

Reuters (2020) *COVID-19 Global Tracker.* Available at: https://graphics.reuters.com/world-coronavirus-tracker-and-maps/ (accessed 11 March 2021).

Ryan, M. (2020) 'WHO commends South Africa's response to COVID-19 as one of the best in the world', 23 April. Available at: https://youtu.be/qn05I9ihuWQ (accessed 12 March 2021).

SACC (South African Council of Churches) (2020) 'GBV and churches', Webinar, 26 August. Available at: https://www.facebook.com/302306103119496/videos/1207910869548223 (accessed 15 December 2020).

Spiranovic, C., Hudson, N., Winter, R., Stanford, S., Norris, K., Bartkowiak-Theron, I. and Cashman, K. (2020) 'Navigating risk and protective factors for family violence during and after the COVID-19 "perfect storm"', *Current Issues in Criminal Justice*, 33(1): 5–18.

Trangenstein P.J., Morojele, N.K., Lombard, C.L.O. Jerniigan, D.H. and Parry, C.H. (2018) 'Heavy drinking and contextual risk factors among adults in South Africa: Findings from the International Alcohol Control study'. *Substance Abuse Treatment, Prevention, and Policy*, 13(43).

Case study: COVID-19 and increased vulnerabilities to human trafficking and modern slavery – perspectives from India and Nepal

Tribeni Gurung, Nishan Lo, Lallian Kunga and Vijaya Lama

Introduction

This case study is an accumulation of our own personal reflections of what we have experienced and observed during the COVID-19 pandemic in our country contexts. We include stories we have gathered from our partners, personal contacts and community members and grey literature (including academic, media reports and journal articles) found through online searches. Responding to modern slavery and human trafficking during this time has never been so difficult. Despite lockdowns implemented in our respective contexts, we have continued responding to modern slavery and human trafficking, as we recognise the urgency and severity it brings in an emergency.

We outline the COVID-19 situation in our countries, followed by some of the consequences of COVID-19 that have made people vulnerable to modern slavery and human trafficking. We describe some new forms of vulnerabilities that are emerging as well as how different organisations are working together to not only tackle the virus but also to reduce vulnerabilities. Finally, we conclude with some key recommendations of responding to modern slavery and human trafficking during a time of crisis.

COVID-19 situation in Nepal and India

There has been much attention on Asia since the COVID-19 virus was discovered in late 2019 in Wuhan City, China (WHO, 2020). Unsurprisingly, the virus spread to neighbouring countries causing a domino effect and eventually a surge in COVID-19 cases globally, establishing a pandemic new to our generation. The first known cases of COVID-19 in South Asia were detected in Nepal on 25 January 2020 and later in India on 30 January 2020, both students, carrying the virus, returning from China to their respective home countries (Andrews et al, 2020; Behal and Mukherjee, 2020). As with the rest of the world, India and Nepal imposed a nationwide lockdown in March 2020 in order to retain the virus and in fear that the health system could collapse if there was a sharp rise in cases. Nepal and India share a 'long, porous border' (Aljazeera, 2021a) whereby the government on either side chose to close their doors to both domestic and international visitors. At a local level transport was banned, masks were to be worn and social distance to be maintained. A violation of the rules or anyone breaking the standard operating procedures (Sarma, 2021) laid out by the government resulted in fines and penalties. With a high proportion of the population adhering to the guidelines due to an uncertainty around COVID-19, combined with both the Nepali and Indian governments' efforts to contain the virus, infection rates were kept low and hospitalisation to a minimum.

The second wave of COVID-19 in early 2021 exposed the rigid healthcare system in both Nepal and India. The 'Delta' variant, a much more dangerous form of the COVID-19 virus that has dominated the world's headlines since the spring of 2021, was first discovered in India, pushing health services to the brink of collapse (Chauraisa and Ellis-Petersen, 2021). Resources such as ventilators, hospital beds and oxygen cylinders have been in short supply, leading to thousands of deaths per day: the highest at 4,200 deaths on a single day in May 2021 (*The Guardian*, 2021). Nepal faced a similar fate with many patients unable to access COVID-19 treatment and the disparity can be observed among disadvantaged communities who cannot afford medical expenses, therefore avoiding health support altogether. The vaccination programme in both Nepal and India had a successful start although both countries faced barriers in completing their programme. In Nepal, the vaccination programme set out by the government initially targeted key workers followed by the general population, but since the discovery of the Delta variant, vaccine supplies from India have been halted and Nepal has faced a vaccine shortage with only 2 per cent of the population fully vaccinated at the end of May 2021 (Rankin and Citrin, 2021). Health experts have predicted that it will take approximately three years to vaccinate the entire Nepali population. In North East India, the landscape is slightly different. Vaccines are available free of charge in public hospitals while private hospitals require a vaccine fee. However with a higher proportion of the population opting for a free vaccine, access is a challenge for some members of the population. There are also mixed feelings towards the vaccine with many hesitating to take their dose, convinced that it is a conspiracy.

With no formal test and trace system in both Nepal and India, COVID-19 is being spread unknowingly among communities. Multigenerational living arrangements are common in Nepalese and Indian cultures and this has exacerbated transmission of the virus to family members. It is acknowledged that attitudes towards the virus have largely been dictated by societal norms whereby illnesses and diseases are often associated with the weak, poorly and marginalised groups. The same can be said for COVID-19. In North East India, our culture tends to discourage the sharing of problems in fear of shame or loss of face; similarly in Nepal, stigma is associated with matters that deviate from societal norms and values. Given the damaging impact of COVID-19 on health and wellbeing, negative connotations have been associated with the virus – people are hesitant to admit to having, or testing for, COVID-19 if they have symptoms in fear that they and their families would be stigmatised and discriminated against (Sethy, 2020). There is a culture of denial when it comes to COVID-19 with those who may have symptoms similar to a common cold and resorting to home-made herbal remedies for treatment. In the national fight against COVID-19 this sense of denial can hamper the collection of accurate figures of COVID-19 cases and the prevalence of the virus in communities, leading to further infections and deaths. Feelings of fear, anxiety and apprehension have been common emotions throughout the pandemic, especially due to the uncertainty around employment, health and life in general. Lockdowns have also affected mental health with reports of increase in depression and ultimately suicide (Pathare et al, 2020; Shrestha et al, 2021).

Increased vulnerabilities to modern slavery and human trafficking

The effects of the pandemic were not only prevalent in the health sector; COVID-19 has promoted criminal activity and exploitation of the vulnerable. Modern slavery and human trafficking, a **wicked issue** prevalent long before COVID-19, has been exacerbated as a result of the pandemic, pushing the trade further underground (UNODC, 2021).

When nationwide lockdowns were enforced in Nepal and India it activated a total shutdown of the economy. Businesses were forced to close, creating a ripple effect of financial insecurity for employers and their workers. In Nepal, the Central Bank reported that industries such as tourism, hospitality, forestry and agriculture were particularly affected by the pandemic with workers facing an average salary cut of 18 per cent or more, and 61 per cent of businesses forced to close (Sharma, 2020). A very similar picture is illustrated in North East India, with workers being laid off, particularly those from a younger age group (Deori and Konwar, 2020). With a lack of jobs and employment opportunities available, thousands of workers are desperate for survival, placing them at greater risk of accepting false opportunities offered by human traffickers.

As economies across the world also faced closures, the COVID-19 pandemic has resulted in movement of people both domestically and internationally, forcing many to return to their home communities.

Migrant workers in particular have been severely impacted by the pandemic with thousands of Nepali and Indian workers returning home, from countries such as Saudi Arabia and Qatar (IOM, 2020; Foley and Piper, 2021), to limited employment opportunities in their home country, leading to a rise of unemployed workers. For instance in Mizoram, North East India, there are very few industries that are appropriate for the specialised skills that migrant workers bring, thus hindering their chances of finding employment after returning home. Domestically there has been an influx of migrant workers escaping the city and returning to their villages to avoid being stranded in jobless cities (Aljazeera, 2021b); in North East India, we have witnessed 10,000 migrant workers returning home and isolating in some of our church premises, used as isolation centres. At the Nepal–India border, we have also heard accounts of labourers and workers crossing the border – on returning to their home communities, they are being blamed for bringing the COVID-19 virus with them.

For others, international travel restrictions have posed a prevailing challenge with many migrant workers trapped in their host countries, jobless, homeless and penniless (Srivastava and Nagaraj, 2020). Their foreign status in the host country positions migrant workers as a minority population where accessing benefits or services during the COVID-19 pandemic can be difficult. Many are constrained in accommodation for migrant workers, often which are poorly maintained and crowded, creating a base for the virus to spread. Some are bound to their employers and compelled to pay off any debt or costs of being offered employment pre-COVID-19, indicating high levels of desperation of sustaining some form of employment and putting them at enhanced risk of forced labour (GoodWeave International, 2020).

During the lockdown, educational institutions were also forced to temporarily close in Nepal and North East India (Dawadi et al, 2020; UNICEF, 2021a). Educational institutions have had to adapt and undertake alternative teaching approaches, mainly moving from face-to-face classes to online platforms. This has placed children at greater risk of online exploitation such as sexual exploitation, since human traffickers have also intensified their recruitment methods on the Internet, in particular social media sites and online gaming platforms (Equality Now, 2020).

UNICEF (2021a) reports that school closures can in fact threaten the future of millions of children and students since Internet access is not always readily available and for the most disadvantaged communities, educational institutions are not only a learning hub, but also a means to access food, health services and refuge from 'abuse, neglect and dysfunctional parenting' (Gough, 2020). A lack of digital access to education during the COVID-19 pandemic raises fears of a literacy gap among children and students that are either disadvantaged or marginalised, and the exclusion is felt greater in rural communities, thus widening the life chances gap between rural and urban communities. With schools closed and families facing financial hardships, children are having to help in supporting the family by undertaking paid work, raising concerns of an increase in child trafficking and child labour (Ellis-Petersen and Chaurasia, 2020; Human Rights Watch, 2021).

In larger cities such as Delhi and Kathmandu, accessing medical treatment for COVID-19 has brought about challenges due to a lack of an effective healthcare system and no health insurance. Patients are expected to pay for hospitalisation, which is often expensive and based on a 'first come, first served' basis. High expenses associated with healthcare, combined with loss of employment and school closures, have led to some families resorting to marrying off their daughters at a young age (UNICEF, 2021b) in anticipation of receiving a dowry (which is a tradition of receiving a monetary gift in a marriage, practised in communities in Nepal and India), thereby reducing the financial burden on a household. Early child marriage violates girls' rights, health and education (Girls Not Brides, nd) and many married girls may experience long-term suffering such as physical and emotional abuse, coercion and control – acts which are commonly associated to slave-like conditions (Anti-Slavery International, nd) – or trafficked for various forms of exploitation.

New forms of vulnerabilities

Despite the Nepal–India border being sealed at the start of the pandemic, the border has in fact become a point of more perverse activities with traffickers finding new routes or new reasons to target vulnerable populations (Betteridge-Moes, 2020). For instance, Neupane (2020) reported the interception of a group of Nepalese women transiting through the state of Manipur in North East India – a less common route for trafficking victims before heading to central India and countries in the Middle East. Our government partners have also shared with us that in North East India, women are putting themselves at risk of falling into the hands of human traffickers. Since lockdown has restricted the freedom of movement, women who are reliant on drugs and women in prostitution are travelling with lorry drivers in order to source income and obtain drugs and clients. During lockdown, lorry drivers have had the freedom to cross between borders to channel essential commodities, but some have recognised this as an opportunity to escape the harsh consequences of COVID-19. Furthermore, in Nepal, we are also aware that social media has been vital during lockdowns, firstly as a source of information and secondly as a form of escapism when lockdown was beginning to place strain on families. Quarrels between family members have increased and, to avoid these, people resorted to the Internet and social media. Many people felt lonely and thought that their family members were unable to understand them and so befriending strangers became common practice, although this can also result in people unknowingly exposing themselves to potential traffickers, posing as someone in a similar situation.

Working together

The COVID-19 crisis has brought people together to tackle the issue, collaboratively. In both Nepal and North East India, we witnessed various levels of government, non-governmental organisations, civil society organisations and community groups coming together to help families and communities get through the lockdown. The governments in Nepal and India introduced similar initiatives to support the COVID-19 response, which became a national priority while other issues took a back seat, including responding to modern slavery and human trafficking. The Nepalese government introduced a partnership policy where non-governmental organisations, clubs and community groups were invited to support the national response to COVID-19. As part of this, efforts were made by several organisations to provide items such as face masks, hand sanitisers and oxygen cylinders. Non-governmental organisations and faith-based organisations also set up isolation wards to support those who had contracted COVID-19. Similarly in North East India, a Chief Minister's COVID-19 relief fund was set up to contribute towards tackling the pandemic. The government also requested church premises to be used as isolation centres. Although this provided assistance in tackling the health crisis, the vulnerabilities created by COVID-19 were still to be addressed. As such, local task forces were created in pockets of communities within North East India. These task forces consisted of representatives from non-governmental organisations, local government, faith-based organisations, civil society organisations, community groups and women's groups and they were responsible for ascertaining vulnerabilities throughout the communities. Dry goods and essential necessities were distributed to firstly ensure people had the basic means for survival and secondly to prevent them from making any risky decisions such as accepting false job opportunities presented by human traffickers. In Nepal, vulnerable communities were identified where different organisations and groups selected a community to work with and provide relief aid and support. We express the value of working together as we have been able to share learning and resources to address vulnerabilities to modern slavery and human trafficking, despite challenges presented to us as a result of COVID-19 such as lack of funding opportunities, restriction on movement to carry out activities and staff shortages as a result of contracting the virus.

Conclusion

Our case study has highlighted the volatile situation in Nepal and North East India, as a result of the COVID-19 pandemic. While fighting the virus, our governments should not overlook the real and concrete risks that this unprecedented situation presents for vulnerable individuals and groups, who are not always visible in our societies. A much-needed focus on alleviating the economic impact of the COVID-19 pandemic should not exclude disadvantaged and marginalised groups. Recovering from the pandemic offers a unique opportunity to look at our economic development model that can explore marginalisation, gender-based violence, exploitation and human trafficking. Based on our experiences of responding to both COVID-19 and modern slavery and human trafficking, we recommend the following in reducing vulnerabilities:

- integrating a response to trafficking in persons within the COVID-19 response and recovery plans;
- maintain the identification and protection of victims/survivors of trafficking during the crisis;
- ensure trafficked survivors have access to essential protection services and provision of care;
- prioritise flexible and long-term funding for prevention of modern slavery and human trafficking and not diverted elsewhere during a time of crisis.

The Salvation Army is a significant partner in these collaborative efforts to address COVID-19 (see Case study 16.3).

References

Aljazeera (2021a) 'Nepal COVID infections surge, fuelled by India's mutant strains'. *Aljazeera*, 26 April. Available at: https://www.aljazeera.com/news/2021/4/26/nepal-covid-infections-surge-fuelled-by-indias-mutant-strains

Aljazeera (2021b) 'Life is precious: India's migrant workers flee COVID-hit cities'. *Aljazeera*, 29 April. Available at: https://www.aljazeera.com/news/2021/4/29/life-is-precious-indias-migrant-workers-flee-covid-hit-cities

Andrews, M.A., Areekal, B., Rajesh, K.R., Krishnan, J., Suryakala, R., Krishnan, B. et al (2020) 'First confirmed case of COVID-19 infection in India: A case report', *Indian Journal of Medical Research*, 151(5): 490–492.

Anti-Slavery International (nd) 'Out of the shadows: Child marriage and slavery'. Available at: https://www.ohchr.org/Documents/Issues/Women/WRGS/ForcedMarriage/NGO/AntiSlaveryInternational2.pdf

Behal, S. and Mukherjee, D. (2020) 'COVID-19: A South Asia update', *Observer Research Foundation*.20 March. Available at: https://www.orfonline.org/expert-speak/covid-19-a-south-asia-update-63529/

Betteridge-Moes, M. (2020) 'Human trafficking persists during COVID at Indo-Nepal border'. Available at: https://study.soas.ac.uk/indo-nepal-border-human-trafficking-persists-amid-pandemic/

Chauraisa, M. and Ellis-Petersen, H. (2021) 'COVID rips through rural India's threadbare healthcare system', *The Guardian*, 7 March. Available at: https://www.theguardian.com/world/2021/may/07/covid-rips-through-rural-indias-threadbare-healthcare-system

Dawadi, S., Giri, R.A. and Simkhada, P. (2020) 'Impact of COVID-19 on the education sector in Nepal: Challenges and coping strategies', *Sage Submissions*. https://doi.org/10.31124/advance.12344336.v1

Deori, U. and Konwar, G. (2020) 'Impact of COVID-19 in north eastern states of India', *International Journal of Health Sciences and Research*, 10(6): 213–217.

Ellis-Petersen, H. and Chaurasia, M. (2020) 'COVID-19 prompts "enormous rise" in demand for cheap child labour in India', *The Guardian*. 13 Oct Available at: https://www.theguardian.com/world/2020/oct/13/covid-19-prompts-enormous-rise-in-demand-for-cheap-child-labour-in-india

Equality Now (2020) 'COVID-19 conversations: The crisis of online child sexual exploitation'. Equality Now, 8 May. Available at: https://www.equalitynow.org/news_and_insights/covid_19_online_exploitation/

Foley, L. and Piper, N. (2021) 'Returning home empty handed: Examining how COVID-19 exacerbates the non-payment of temporary migrant workers' wages', *Global Social Policy*, 7 May. https://doi.org/10.1177/14680181211012958

Girls Not Brides (nd) 'About child marriage'. Available at: https://www.girlsnotbrides.org/about-child-marriage/

GoodWeave International (2020) 'Hidden and vulnerable: The impact of COVID-19 on child, forced and bonded labour'. Available at: https://goodweave.org/wp-content/uploads/2020/11/GoodWeave-Hidden-and-Vulnerable-Report-Final.pdf

Gough, J. (2020) 'Urgent action is required to protect the learning of all South Asian children'. UNICEF, 23 November. Available at: https://www.unicef.org/rosa/stories/urgent-action-required-protect-learning-all-south-asian-children

The Guardian (2021) 'India records almost 4,200 COVID deaths in a day'. The Guardian, 8 May. Available at: https://www.theguardian.com/world/2021/may/08/india-records-almost-4200-covid-deaths-in-a-day

Human Rights Watch (2021) 'I must work to eat'. Human Rights Watch, 26 May. Available at: https://www.hrw.org/report/2021/05/26/i-must-work-eat/covid-19-poverty-and-child-labor-ghana-nepal-and-uganda

IOM (2020) 'Status of Nepali migrant workers in relation to COVID-19'. IOM, 17 December. Available at: https://publications.iom.int/es/node/2576 https://publications.iom.int/es/node/2576

Pathare S., Vijayakumar, L., Fernandes, T., SZhastri, M., Kapoor, A., Pandit, D., Lohumi, I., Ray, S., Kulkarnari, A. and Korde, P. (2020) 'Analysis of new media reports of suicides and attempted suicide during the COVID-19 lockdown in India'. *International Journal of Mental Health Systems*, 14(88).

Rankin, K. and Citrin, D. (2021) 'Nepal was inoculating its people with great success – until India stopped sending it vaccines'. Scroll, 28 May. Available at: https://scroll.in/article/996040/nepal-was-inoculating-its-peo ple-with-great-success-until-india-stopped-sending-it-vaccines

Sarma, J. (2021) 'As COVID-19 virus marches east, India's north east states float new SOPs, restrictions'. HealthSite.com, 15 May. Available at: https:// www.thehealthsite.com/news/as-covid-19-virus-marches-east-indias- north-east-states-float-new-sops-restrictions-813851/

Sethy, P. (2020) 'The myth of South Asian exceptionalism'. *Think Global Health*, 1 October. Available at: https://www.thinkglobalhealth.org/arti cle/myth-south-asian-exceptionalism

Sharma, G. (2020) 'Nearly a quarter of Nepal's workers lose jobs due to coronavirus – central bank'. Reuters, 13 August. Available at: https:// www.reuters.com/article/health-coronavirus-nepal/nearly-a-quarter-of- nepals-workers-lose-jobs-due-to-coronavirus-central-bank-idINKCN259 1A8?edition-redirect=uk

Shrestha, R., Siwakoti, S., Singh, S. and Shrestha, A.P. (2021) 'Impact of the COVID-19 pandemic on suicide and self-harm among patients presenting to the emergency department of a teaching hospital in Nepal', *PLoS One*, 16(4). https://doi.org/10.1371/journal.pone.0250706

Srivastava, R. and Nagaraj, A. (2020) 'No way back: Indian workers shun city jobs after lockdown ordeal', *Thomson Reuters Foundation*, 28 May. Available at: https://longreads.trust.org/item/india-coronavirus-migrant- workers-reluctant-return

Neupane, S.R. (2020) '21 trafficked Nepali women coming home after nine months'. *The Katmandu Post*, 1 September. Available at: https://kathma ndupost.com/national/2020/07/13/21-trafficked-nepali-women-com ing-home-after-nine-months

UNICEF (2021a) 'COVID-19: Schools for more than 168 million children globally have been completely closed for almost a full year, says UNICEF'. UNICEF, 10 March. Available at: https://www.unicef.org/india/press- releases/covid-19-schools-more-168-million-children-globally-have-been- completely-closed

UNICEF (2021b) '10 million additional girls at risk of child marriage due to COVID-19'. UNICEF, 8 March. Available at: https://www.unicef.org/rosa/ press-releases/10-million-additional-girls-risk-child-marriage-due-covid-19

UNODC (2021) 'The effects of the COVID-19 pandemic on trafficking in persons and responses to the challenges'. UNODC, Available at: https://www.unodc.org/documents/human-trafficking/2021/The_effects_of_the_COVID-19_pandemic_on_trafficking_in_persons.pdf

WHO (2020) 'COVID-19 China'. World Health Organization, 5 January. Available at: https://www.who.int/emergencies/disease-outbreak-news/item/2020-DON229

Case study: COVID-19 and governing for health and wellbeing in New Zealand – putting communities at the centre

Peter McKinlay and Anna Matheson

Introduction

We have learned tough lessons from the COVID-19 pandemic about trust in government and that when our systems are disrupted, many communities are immediately vulnerable to hardship (Henrickson, 2020). With the government poised to make significant changes to the health system there is an opportunity in New Zealand (NZ) to revisit our social infrastructure and put communities at the centre of decision-making. An important part of this infrastructure is the untapped potential of local government and local *iwi* (Māori tribes) to strengthen the ability for communities to act on their own needs. Understanding the history, legislative context and current challenges and opportunities for local governance, provides direction for how community and public health action could be more impactful and sustainable.

For decades, public health has had community health and empowerment at its theoretical core. The 1986 Ottawa Charter for Health Promotion is a widely used framework for action to improve health (World Health Organization, 1986). Two central elements are a greater focus on community action on health and to reorient health services towards patients and communities. This built on the 1978 Alma Ata declaration on primary healthcare which also called for communities to be central actors within the health system (World Health Organization, 1978).

In 2008 the World Health Organization convened a Commission on the Social Determinants of Health which found, while the health system itself is one determinant, most of health and illness results from interactions with, and within, the places in which we are born, live, work, play and age (Commission on the Social Determinants of Health, 2008). And this is no different in NZ. We have a rising burden of non-communicable diseases (NCDs; heart diseases, cancers, mental health disorders) which are linked to shared risk factors found in our surrounding social and physical environments (Ministry of Health, 2013). NCDs are also the biggest drivers of health inequality, but as COVID-19 has shown, infectious diseases will also follow patterns of existing inequality if given the opportunity to spread.

For 50 years we have known in NZ of significant health inequities by ethnic group – in particular Māori and Pacific people (Blakely et al, 2005). And we have a substantial socioeconomic gradient in health outcomes where people who are poorer have worse health outcomes than people who are richer (Crampton et al, 2004). On income, an influential determinant of health, we are not doing well. A recent national Household Economic Survey finds that our already high income inequality has become higher, and globally – the United Nations has reported – wealth inequality is on a runaway trajectory (United Nations, 2020).

Despite all this evidence – and attempts at different times to devolve health decision-making and resources to local areas – the reach of public health and the health sector into communities has been limited. In NZ this has become increasingly evident in the lack of improvement in our big health trends. Recent health system reviews have all found we have made limited progress over the past few decades despite both intention and investment (Health Quality and Safety Commission, 2019; Health and Disability System Review, 2020).

These findings make clear that a big challenge has been our approach to communities. The way devolution has been implemented through services and decision-making compounded the already low value placed on community, rather than led to a strengthening of control and voice. A recent review of our health system confirmed its fragmentation and challenges in connecting locally to diverse communities (Health and Disability System Review, 2020). This is despite whole-of-government and intersectoral action having been goals of the public sector for a long time.

Our initial success in NZ at controlling COVID-19 was not because we were prepared. We did have a plan but this was predicated on a well-connected public health sector – which we did not have immediately. But as the pandemic has unfolded it has become apparent that we did have latent strength in our systems with collaboration and responsiveness between levels of government and communities swinging into action to provide resources, information and support. Although the recent vaccine rollout has made clear that there are significant barriers still for communities.

In both limiting the spread of the virus and ensuring timely vaccination uptake responding with speed, and across sectors, has been critical, showing the importance of system strengthening beyond centralised decision-making.

In NZ we already have some policy initiatives doing this. Initiatives that are showing we can break our attachment to top-down solutions, silos and single issues and instead focus on multiple outcomes and government, sector and community relationships. Whānau Ora has been a leading example. Launched in 2010, this is a Māori-led initiative aimed at joining up health and social services for individuals and their *whānau* (extended families) (Boulton et al, 2013). Similarly, and introduced in 2015, Healthy Families NZ is a multi-community health and wellbeing initiative led from community priorities. It aims to foster collective impact and strengthen community prevention systems (Matheson et al, 2019).

NZ currently has an expressed commitment to wellbeing as the principal objective of public policy. In 2019 the government committed to a wellbeing budget with the Treasury taking a lead role in the development of wellbeing indicators and assessing both departmental expenditure bids, and performance, against those indicators. This approach differs from wellbeing practice in some other countries which have a more explicit focus on involving communities – such as in Wales (public service boards), and Scotland and Northern Ireland (community planning partnerships). In these places there are legislative requirements for local authorities to work with communities.

Local governance and communities in New Zealand

There has been limited experience in NZ of working with communities as a natural part of formal or informal governance. One important exception is *te ao Māori* – a Māori worldview. NZ's indigenous Māori population have a very long history of collective decision-making within a tradition which is significantly different from the more functional approach typical of European governance even at the lowest levels.

In NZ, local authorities' legal existence and powers depend on legislation – currently the Local Government Act 2002. And, as a result it has become common to think of councils as creatures of statute, dependent on and deriving all their authority from central government. This view exists throughout the government sector despite the early history of local government in NZ which was community driven and bottom-up. Government responding to representations for statutory enablement rather than acting as initiator (Cardow, 2007).

NZ's Productivity Commission has recently observed that local authorities are sometimes characterised as agents of central government, required to implement national priorities and directions, and accountable to central government (New Zealand Productivity Commission, 2020). This view persists despite the Local Government Act 2002. The Act states the purpose and role of local government is to enable local democratic decision-making and action by and on behalf of communities and to promote community wellbeing – described broadly as economic, social, cultural and environmental (sections 10 and 11, Local Government Act 2002).

Rethinking the place of community

Recent innovations in central government policy thinking, influenced by the 2019 adoption of a wellbeing budget, has emphasised the place of community. For example, Section 13 of the Public Service Act 2020 states that 'the fundamental characteristic of the public service is acting with a spirit of service to the community'. While a recent briefing to the Minister of Local Government by the responsible department states: 'Local authorities know their communities and are best placed to lead, represent and respond to the needs and interests of those communities' (Department of Internal Affairs, 2020: 3).

The report (Health and Disability System Review, 2020) which has led to the current health reforms states that '[i]mproving population health outcomes and equity requires the system to truly focus on communities and what they need', and proposes a community led system.

At the same time as this increasing rhetoric on the importance of communities, central government is paradoxically acting to reduce significantly the role of local government in major aspects of infrastructure and regulation. The principal group of NZ councils, Territorial Local Authorities (TLAs), have traditionally been responsible for the ownership and management of water, wastewater and stormwater services. A current central government initiative will remove this responsibility and transfer it to four standalone entities.

TLAs have also been largely responsible for land-use planning, preparing district plans and handling consents for developments which are not predominant uses (something which applies to the majority of significant developments). Current reforms of resource management legislation will remove this function from TLAs. Although there is merit in more robust national standards and more effective stewardship, these two reforms will significantly reduce the role of TLAs in shaping important infrastructure, service and regulatory functions to reflect the preferences of their communities.

For all TLAs the impact on their scope of activity and influence within their communities will be significant. In the case of most rural and provincial councils, it could see them lose the core part of their activity. As a result, many TLAs are rethinking their roles and are pivoting towards strengthening relationships with their communities, emphasising community voice on needs and preferences, especially in relation to health and social services.

What are some possibilities for the future of local governance in New Zealand?

There is opportunity in NZ to learn from international experience. One commonly taken option is to focus on working with and empowering existing community organisations. Another is to enable place-based entities which are representative of, and engage all of, the people within a community.

An important factor in making this choice in NZ is the relationship between place-based communities and *mana whenua* – the indigenous people who have historic and territorial rights over the land. But at the heart of this choice is how to put communities at the centre of decision-making. How to create an environment in which communities will have both the interest and the capability needed to participate and lead.

Lessons from the UK on working with communities show if this is to be done effectively it needs to be firmly based within place-based localities, and facilitated by people and organisations who have fostered understanding and trust within those communities (Locality, 2018). In NZ this is clearly an area where local government can play a role.

Lines on a map may satisfy an electoral commission, but they do not create attachment to place and a sense of belonging. In the UK, working with communities often means working with community or voluntary sector organisations, themselves anchored in place. It can mean working through different forms of community level governance such as parish, town and neighbourhood councils. A recent development is the emergence of community-based groups in response to initiatives such as participatory budgeting or Crowdfund London. Also promising, and which would feed directly into rethinking NZ's health and disability system, is to adopt an anchor institutions strategy. This commits major local institutions to undertake their activities in ways which optimise positive economic and social impacts within the local economy especially for marginalised communities (Centre for Local Economic Strategies, 2020).

NZ can also learn from experience in the United States. Portland, Oregon supports a network of 95 residents' associations under a policy adopted to recognise and support communities of place. Any group seeking to be recognised was required to demonstrate it had: an agreed boundary and broad support for its role as the community's representative organisation; a constitution which ensured open and democratic governance; and a reasonable level of demonstrated capability. Residents' associations are grouped into seven district coalitions which in turn appoint a citywide body to represent the entire network. The city provides governance training and capability development, and funds each of seven district offices to employ staff who can work full-time on policy development, research and other activities to support individual associations (Alarcon de Morris and Leistner, 2009).

The UK and US examples illustrate a tension between working through established structures and finding ways of working with the entire community (whether of place or of interest) including those with voices seldom heard. The emphasis within NZ's looming health reforms on equity of access is to adopt ways of engaging with communities which provide user-friendly means for communities to be engaged on matters which are important for them. Options which could be considered include Portland's approach to enabling self-identifying communities, alongside participatory budgeting and civic crowdfunding.

NZ has some important choices ahead. With so much government policy potentially reorienting around community, key will be peoples' voice, choice and control over decisions affecting their place – and services available to them (Locality, 2018). There is a powerful role that local government can play in enabling empowered communities because of proximity to need and relationships, as well as connecting to central government.

Conclusion

Two alternative futures lie ahead for NZ local government. Either it declines into insignificance or asserts its role as the enabler of empowered communities, taking a lead in supporting community engagement. Enabling community-led health systems provides an important opportunity for local government to demonstrate its capability. The evidence suggests ensuring communities have voice, choice and control over decisions which affect their place (or interest) is central for achieving wellbeing for all.

References

Alarcon de Morris, A. and Leistner, P. (2009) From neighborhood association system to participatory democracy: Broadening and deepening public involvement in Portland, Oregon. Available at: https://www.portlandore gon.gov/civic/article/440644

Blakely, T., Fawcett, J., Atkinson, J., Tobias, M. and Cheung, J. (2005) *Decades of Disparity II: Socio-economic Mortality Trends in New Zealand, 1981–1999.* Wellington: Ministry of Health.

Boulton, A., Tamehana, J. and Brannelly, T. (2013) Whanau-centred health and social service delivery in New Zealand. *Mai Journal: A New Zealand Journal of Indigenous Scholarship*, 2: 18–31.

Cardow, A. (2007) The foundation and development of New Zealand local government: An administrative work in progress. *Transylvanian Review of Administrative Sciences*, 21: 18–27.

Centre for Local Economic Strategies (2020) *Own the Future: A Guide for New Local Economies*. Available at: https://cles.org.uk/blog/own-the-fut ure-a-guide-for-new-local-economies/

Commission on the Social Determinants of Health (2008) *Closing the Gap in a Generation: Health Equity through Action on the Social Determinants of Health*. Geneva: World Health Organization.

Crampton, P., Salmond, C. and Kirkpatrick, R. (2004) *Degrees of Deprivation in New Zealand: An Atlas of Socioeconomic Difference*. Auckland: David Bateman.

Department of Internal Affairs (2020) Briefing to the incoming Minister of Local Government. Available at: https://www.dia.govt.nz/diawebsite. nsf/Files/Brieifngs-to-incoming-ministers-2020/$file/Local-Governm ent-BIM-Oct-2020.pdf

Health and Disability System Review (2020) *Health and Disability System Review: Final Report – Pūrongo Whakamutunga*. Wellington: HDSR. Available at: www.systemreview.health.govt.nz/final-report

Health Quality and Safety Commission (2019) *A Window on the Quality of Aotearoa New Zealand's Health Care 2019*. Available at: www.hqsc.govt.nz

Henrickson, M. (2020) Kiwis and COVID-19: The Aotearoa New Zealand response to the global pandemic. *The International Journal of Community and Social Development*, 2: 121–133.

Locality (2018) *People Power: Findings from the Commission on the Future of Localism*. Available at: https://locality.org.uk/about/key-publications/findi ngs-from-the-commission-on-the-future-of-localism/

Matheson, A., Walton, M., Gray, R., Wehipeihana, N. and Wistow, J. (2019) Strengthening prevention in communities through systems change: Lessons from the evaluation of Healthy Families NZ. *Health Promotion International*, 35(5): 947–957.

Ministry of Health (2013) *Health Loss in New Zealand: A Report from the New Zealand Burden of Diseases, Injuries and Risk Factors Study, 2006–2016*. Wellington: Ministry of Health.

New Zealand Productivity Commission (2020) *Local Government Insights*. Available at: https://www.productivity.govt.nz/research/local-governm ent-insights/

United Nations (2020) *World Social Report 2020: Inequality in a Rapidly Changing World*. Washington: United Nations, Department of Social and Economic Affairs.

World Health Organization (1978) *The Alma Ata Declaration*. Geneva: World Health Organization.

World Health Organization (1986) *The Ottawa Charter for Health Promotion*. Ottawa: World Health Organization.

PART III

Public sector, COVID-19 and culture change

Michael Bennett

One way of understanding the idea of a **wicked issue** is as an issue that escapes the grasp of standard, professional knowledge (Rittel and Webber, 1973). While tame problems can be grappled with within the confines of organised disciplines, a wicked problem may be unresolvable and any conceivable solution will be unique and temporary. It follows that where we face wicked problems, because we do not understand them, we are likely to fail when we first try to solve them.

Thus while professional knowledge is adept at searching for ever more in-depth scientific knowledge about the disciplines that exist, there is both an epistemological and organisational problem when experience, the outside world, presents a problem that does not fall within the boundaries of these established disciplines and knowledge.

This part of the book addresses some of the **wicked issues** arising from the earlier Policy Press publications, *Social Determinants of Health: Social Inequality and Wellbeing* and *Local Authorities and Social Determinants of Health*. These issues include public sector governance, local authorities' financial decline, climate crisis, housing and homeless, and economic challenges to families which include loss of employment (particularly affecting young people).

One way in which wicked issues map on to organisational endeavour and resource allocation and leadership in the public sector is through innovation and partnering. Local authorities, in particular, have developed new ways of governing and working with others in the realisation that they alone do not have the resources, the knowledge, the capacity or the capability to deliver the outcomes they believe are required – and wanted – in their areas.

As Liddle argues in Chapter 8, this has led public managers and leaders to collaborate and create relationships with a wide range of stakeholders to innovate and develop novel ways of meeting citizens' needs. Governance form has flexed to follow the novel and complex functions.

The availability of funding is pivotal to implementing public sector activities. This is addressed in Chapter 9, in which Aileen Murphie reviews the effect of COVID-19 on the sustainability of local government. The challenging conclusion is that the scale of the current crisis could mean systemic financial failure across the sector. As Murphie points out, this would not just be an existential crisis for local governments. It would also be a profound failure by the Ministry of Housing, Communities and Local Government in its role as steward of the local government finance system and its policy aim to create 'sustainable communities'.

It is difficult to disagree with Murphie's analysis of the structural inadequacies of a finance system – which pays for a wide range of essential, statutory services – that it is implausible that local government's future can be founded securely on a council tax system rooted in 1992 property values; a business rates system increasingly divorced from actual business activity hard hit by the pandemic; a diminishing and reactive grants programme and locally generated income dependent on the business cycle. These arrangements are the result of short-term deals, plastering over the cracks. This is inconsistent with and clearly not a sufficient basis for the delivery of a long-term, joined-up and holistic approach necessary to address the wicked issues outlined in this volume.

The following three chapters provide case studies of the deeply insolvable challenges that defy professional knowledge and traditional approaches and that require such a holistic and long-term approach.

In Chapter 10, Rob Whiteman and his colleagues from the Chartered Institute of Public Finance and Accountancy analyse the problem of the climate crisis for the public sector, linking the concept of **social value** with Sustainable Development Goals within the framework of the **social determinants of health**. They argue that only if a more collaborative relationship can be built between central and local government can we collectively tackle the wicked issue of climate change in this country.

The provision of housing and shelter is another wicked problem that from a social determinants of health perspective, is a key factor underpinning health and wellbeing. The promotion of inclusive, safe, resilient and sustainable cities and human settlements is enshrined in the 11th Sustainable Development Goal of the United Nations. Housing policy has singularly failed to deliver adequate homes for all over recent decades. The overriding reliance on the market to provide new houses has led to social housing being reduced to residual provision for the very poorest in society on an emergency basis. This is far from the municipal dream of social housing as part of shared and sustainable communities which adequately accommodate all citizens, and where housing makes a positive, rather than a negative, contribution to a healthy and prosperous society.

For Peter Murphy in Chapter 11, the UK's purely economic approach continues to fail even in its own terms and he calls for the focus to return to a 'social policy perspective' that takes a more holistic approach to the enduring problem of housing policy by understanding the interrelationships between the complex multidimensional influences that housing has on the health and wellbeing of citizens.

Chapter 12 introduces the role of employment policy and employment support. In light of the COVID-19 pandemic and those lessons that come from it, this intersection between public health and employment support will require further examination by researchers. The role of local authorities in both of these areas, and others, is crucial. This role is explored in this chapter after a first section that provides a historical mapping of employment support policy and provision.

The emerging theme from the chapters in Part III is that the public sector faces challenges without resolution if the systemic and structural underpinnings of its strategic environment are left as they are. The current system treats public sector bodies as atomised components, in competition for capacity and resources. It is only by building new relationships between these different components that the structural weaknesses can be overcome.

Relational partnering may offer a new way of conceiving of the necessary holistic approach to public sector governance that delivers additional value, greater than the sum of the individual parts.

References

Rittel, H. and Webber, M. (1973) 'Dilemmas in a general theory of planning', *Policy Sciences*, 4: 155–169.

8

The changing context of public governance and the need for innovation and creating public value

Joyce Liddle

Introduction

In the UK's HM Treasury Spending Review (November 2020), the Chancellor of the Exchequer confirmed a major reform to **value for money** assessments of large infrastructure spending which has been biased against Northern cities for too long. HMT Green Book (the rules used to determine value generated by government intervention schemes) and planned investments of £600 billion on transport, energy, schools or hospital investment were widened beyond a narrow definition of benefit compared to cost. Those calculations had inherently favoured the government investing continuously in the South East of England and London. Values of economic return are influenced by existing high property prices in those regions. Additionally, the UK National Infrastructure Commission updated its assessment framework on infrastructure interventions. The novelty lies in the government's declared commitment to a broader definition of 'value', and 'levelling up' as a central plank of the UK government's spending plans for COVID-19 recovery and post-Brexit to address **wicked issues** and inequalities (HM Treasury, 2020). There is an acknowledgement that measuring the success of multibillion-pound infrastructure projects alone ignores the wider causes of regional imbalances as traditional indicators of gross value added and gross domestic product (GDP) are inadequate (economic activity and productivity – see Figure 8.1 for regional imbalances). Significantly, and probably for the first time, this is an attempt to achieve a balanced portfolio of policy interventions, a broader impact assessment to capture intraregional disparities, within and between clusters of cities, towns and other settlements, for the achievement of wider social outcomes. Not since the creation of the Index of Multiple Deprivation has there been any comprehensive attempt to measure the impact of policies on inequality and deprivation.

Figure 8.1: Share of UK gross domestic product at current prices

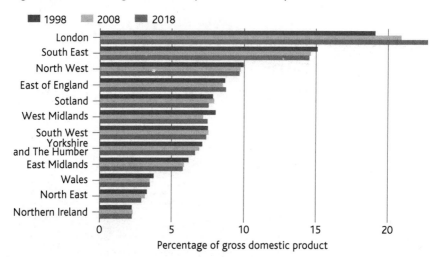

Source: Office for National Statistics (2018)

New forms of assessment aim to identify and remove constraints to growth, and show how lagging localities can be transformed. Earlier in 2020, the Royal Town Planning Institute had called for a reform of local and strategic planning of utilities and infrastructure to drive economic recovery across London. They advocate place leadership to drive growth, which can only be achieved by engaging a range of civic stakeholders in **assessing needs** for transforming quality of life and wellbeing. What these reports have in common is the need to achieve wider societal value from policy interventions, and an acceptance that factors affecting social determinants of health and wellbeing must be included in 'levelling up' and equalising all areas of England. The Prime Minister convinced traditional Labour voters to switch allegiance at the 2019 general election, creating the fall of the political 'Red Wall' across the North of England, allowing a much larger majority in the House of Commons. Global uncertainty, threats posed by COVID-19 and Brexit heightened the imperative to reward voters in Northern regions with more policy interventions to improve localities. Assessing 'wicked' problems in deprived localities must be set within debates surrounding the changing context of public sector reform; the significance of innovative and experimental solutions; and a fundamental examination of what constitutes 'public and social value'.

The pressure for reform of public services globally

Increased performance requirements, rising citizen demands and a need to relate to broader stakeholders (see Figure 8.2) has led many public service organisations to develop innovative service delivery mechanisms in response to wicked issues, by creating and adding value to service delivery.

Figure 8.2: Social and public value

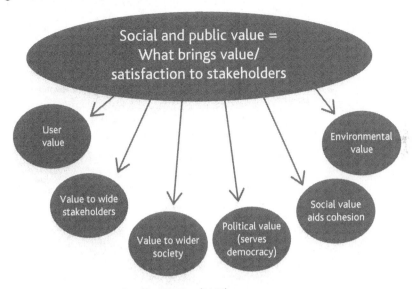

Source: Adapted from Moore (1995) and Talbot (2008)

'One size fits all' universal solutions to complex social problems no longer suffice, and it is generally agreed that no one public agency can satisfy all citizen demands for tailoring services to personal needs. Pressures for reform in all public agencies have forced public managers and leaders to collaborate in partnership with other stakeholders to develop novel methods of delivery, evaluation and measurement of services. Creating **public and social value** is an essential part of a comprehensive approach to transforming and continuous improvement of modern governance and effective public services delivery for wider society. Public services have changed cultures and behaviours more akin to commercial sectors and citizens are no longer passive consumers but empowered individuals who expect state (and non-state) agencies to provide more personalised services and choice increasingly through a wider range of providers.

Historically the 'reinventing government' literature stimulated discussions and debates on downsizing and reducing the size of government, and brought management processes closer to business methods. Total quality management and continuous improvement led (in the UK, at least) to initiatives such as market testing, contracting out, Best Value, Better Government, Total Place, to raise service quality standards and bottom-up stakeholder engagement. Reinventing, re-engineering and reimagining the state led to empowered public employees and innovative and enterprising solutions to customer needs. Privatisation led to enhanced entrepreneurial engagement with the commercial and private sector, either to leverage resources or capacities, or wholly reconfigure service delivery.

Nowadays governance is exemplified by a plurality of inter-relational connections between state, market and civic institutions as a focal point for co-production on service delivery and creation of public and social value. New **relational** forms of governance[1] are not only a challenge to the role of traditional hierarchical forms of government in advanced democracies in the 21st century, but raise questions on type of institutions, organisational and capacities to synergise the state's own resources, capacities and knowledge with those of market and civic institutions (Liddle, 2016a). **Traditional Public Administration** was supplanted over a 40-year period by successive ideas exemplifying as **New Public Management** (NPM). In essence, NPM was a hotchpotch of academic, policy and practice ideas, then overtaken by New Public Governance (NPG). NPG at core illustrates public service delivery through multiple, interdependent agencies and inter-organisational negotiated, relational contracts governing processes to achieve 'public value' (Liddle, 2016a). Public value emanated from a long debate started in the early 1990s by Mark Moore (1995), and continued until the present day, but in the last five years attention has been focused more on how social value can be created.

The changing context of public governance

Contemporary public sector reform initiated in the 1980s was a response to public sector expansion after the Second World War to assess how well various programmes were operating (Liddle, 2016a). Focused on improving performance and reshaping structural configuration of states, radical NPM reform programmes in advanced democracies such as the UK, New Zealand and Australia emphasised deregulation, privatisation and marketisation, and structural devolution, disaggregation and single-purpose organisations became the bywords for continued reform. All governments need to balance resources and investment with results and outcomes at local, regional, federal or national levels, and public leaders came under greater public scrutiny as many citizens expected efficiency, accountability, productivity and responsiveness. Public managers embraced reform, but the scale of reform and the tools and techniques adopted, differed considerably between states. NPM only partly addressed concerns on efficiency, because it did not address larger challenges such as declining government resources, the growing size of government agencies, and the complex, developing linkages between state, non-state and civic institutions to deliver public goods and services and create public value. Scholars and practitioners then began to seek novel ways of redefining the role of the state, its purpose and ways of functioning, operating and managing (O'Flynn, 2007). The post-bureaucratic and post-competitive public value approach of Moore (1995) gathered apace as others have added ideas, to explain decision-making gaps between formalised, hierarchical 'tiers' of regulatory government jurisdictions and informal, unregulated inter-relationships between a plurality of actors (O'Flynn, 2007).

The public value literature acted as a stimulus for entrepreneurial public managers working with plural actors across organisational boundaries for the common good, but in the intervening years a much broader definition has emerged as public service delivery within society is no longer limited to public managers and state officials. This approach had some resonance and utility, but quickly became outdated as all types of non-governmental and private organisations seek to address a multitude of wicked issues, create public and social value, and satisfy broader societal aims (Meynhardt, 2019). As there is no longer 'one' best solution to addressing wicked issues, combining public and social value for societal enhancement and reform means that characteristics, doctrines and components within the public value paradigm served as a good basis to explore other ways that organisations take the lead in seeking solutions to some of the more urgent dilemmas of the 21st century.

Defining public and social value, and assessing historical antecedents

The way in which public value is created is highly contested territory. One definition is '[a] new paradigm including a set of doctrines and approaches aimed at promoting "common good" by incorporating "public values" across the political system'. The concept facilitates an understanding of interconnections, interdependencies, interactions between complex issues and across multiple boundaries, to reach agreement between diverse stakeholders influencing what constitutes 'public value' (Liddle, 2020). Moore's original formulation of public value (Moore, 1995) associated with NPM used a **Strategic Value Triangle** (SVT) to understand what citizens expect from public managers and how virtue was incorporated into executive activities. His diagnostic framework satisfied three key tests: (i) it identified publicly valuable outcomes; (ii) it mobilised authorisation and political sustainability for ongoing support; and (iii) it was operationally and administratively feasible (Moore, 2006). Prominent scholars challenged Moore's definitions for normative and empirical reasoning; loose definition of public management; inability to understand regulatory state activity, power relationships between state officials and others; how entrepreneurial managers shape policies; deference to private sector management models free of accountability and democratic politics. Stoker extended Moore's SVT with a **Collective Preferences** model, to include **value conflict resolution**, because although strategic implementation was important, it failed to deal with how public managers reflect on intervention choices and actions, or build vital networks for delivery (Stoker, 2006). Osborne (2010) extended

Moore and Stoker's ideas on public value creation by drawing from several other strands of research on reform.

Limited research exists on the key dimensions of social and public value; importance stakeholders place on changes needed; enhancing service quality to benefit communities and address wicked issues. Moreover, which stakeholders' view should prevail in relational encounters; or how value is, or can be, co-created, designed, delivered and measured? These limitations demonstrate that 'value' creation is very complex, operates at multiple levels, and attempts at quantifying/monetising produce partial success. New metrics can capture social and public value, but digital and social media in complex encounters complicate things further. We need more nuanced approaches to redefining the state, its purpose and functions, operations and management, in relation to non-state agencies and actors. New relational forms of engagement challenge the role of 21st century government in advanced democracies because of questions on type of institutions, organisational and leadership capacities needed to synergise the state's own resources, capacities and knowledge with those of market and civic institutions.

Social value quantifies the relative importance that people place on changes they experience in their lives, and capacity to capture broader influences on wellbeing. It can be captured in market prices, but social value must be viewed from the perspective of those affected by an organisation's work. Examples could be value placed on increased confidence, living next to a community park, good neighbours, or anything that materially enhances general wellbeing. Things of importance to people, but rarely expressed or measured, like financial value, social value has huge potential to help individuals and groups make appropriate decisions on where resources should be invested. It can also be utilised to explain assets and resources locked into public agencies or how public services can be privatised or taken over by local communities.

There have been many attempts to quantify 'value' in public and private sectors, for example, by using a mixture of accounting and economic measures developed by bodies such as the Chartered Institute of Public Finance and Accountancy (CIPFA) and Deloitte (drawn from international standards and accounting bodies) but driven increasingly by social values embodied in UN Sustainability Goals. Many commercial companies are developing 'social value' mechanisms developed to measure corporate social responsibility. The World Bank, International Monetary Fund and EU have created 'wellbeing indices' to capture and measure economic, social and environmental vulnerability and a National Well-being Index was introduced by the Coalition government of 2010–2014. Local authorities, police, social service departments and health trusts developed their own definitions to classify disadvantaged groups with metrics to capture how 'value' was added within neighbourhoods and communities. Business associations and individual companies produced Vulnerability Assessment Tools (for example, VSAT, Birmingham Resilience) and the Confederation of British Industry developed its own 'Well-being and Vulnerability Index'. Meynhardt (2019) created a public value scorecard to show how business and public sectors work together to create 'social value'.

Interpretation of the concept differs at community levels as it is difficult to standardise public and social value, due to a variety of actors with their own individual or organisational perspective on 'value'. Public value involves public managers working in collaboration with citizens to co-create 'value', but the impact that service delivery has on overall personal wellbeing and broader physical infrastructures also affect the 'common good' varies. Each group has a different perspective on what constitutes 'the common good'. If you were to ask a local business person the response might be 'to create more employment', a local community group 'to have a local park', health agencies would suggest 'more hospitals' whereas a local authority chief executive officer would argue for educational spending on schools. Identifying or creating 'value' is multidimensional, meaning different things to different groups.

The need for novel solutions to 'wicked issues': global, national and local 'experimental and innovative governance'

Wicked problems are cross-cutting and require enterprising solutions. Such enterprise is embodied in leaders who drive change as well as in resources and capabilities found in constellations of public/private and other organisations acting to address them. Public sector innovation and entrepreneurship, or any new ideas that create value for society, are not new, and there are many conscious and systematic approaches to creating innovative solutions for effectively addressing some of the most pressing societal challenges. Managers of public services, and increasingly managers from third sector, voluntary and charitable sectors, continually seek innovative ways of adapting structures, processes and operations. We still lack understanding on how to identify opportunities for transformation, who are the key actors, what are the rules of the game, constraints on public and social entrepreneurship, novel approaches to use resources creatively are evident, and how the linkages and relationships between public and other forms of entrepreneurship can be harnessed to achieve greater overall added value. Internationally, since 2000, governments have introduced numerous experiments on citizen engagement, innovation and enterprise (OECD Report on Partnerships, 2013). All were aimed at adding social and public value, but some governments also felt the need to nudge citizens into behavioural change and enable them to make better choices about health, wellbeing and happiness. The following list provides a selection of innovation initiatives:

- NESTA – body for innovation, UK
- LA27E Region – laboratory for innovation on policy, France
- UK Cabinet Office, Office for Civil Society and Social Investment Office, UK
- New Age to New Edge, San Francisco, US
- School of Design Konding, Denmark
- DesgnGOV, Australia
- MultiMedia Design, Rotterdam University, the Netherlands
- OECD Digital Government
- Government at a Glance Observatory for Public Innovation, US
- Gov Innovator, podcast, US
- Public Innovation, Chile
- MindLab, Denmark
- South African Centre for Public Innovation, South Africa
- Harvard Kennedy School, Ash Center for Democratic Governance and Innovation, US
- Behavioural Insights Team, UK
- The Young Foundation, UK
- OECD Red Tape Reduction Commission
- Australian Government Review of Government Services, Australia
- Office for Implementation and PA Reform, Spain
- Committee on Evaluating National Programmes, Korea. (Office for National Statistics, 2018)

David Cameron's idea of creating a **Big Society** was meant to enable local communities to develop thousands of social and community enterprises and non-profit organisations to engage 'third', 'voluntary' and 'charitable' sectors into local service delivery. To add public and social value, government attempted to nudge citizens into behavioural change, and innovative programmes created by the Behavioural Insights Team and Office for Civil Society, both located in UK Cabinet Office, produced numerous reports and established a Centre for Social Impact Bonds, Centre for Social Action and Commissioning Academy. Programmes such as the Social Outcomes Fund, Innovation Fund and Public Service Mutuals Fund allowed local communities to run enterprises and grow the social investment market. The recently created Centre for Public Impact has further developed thinking on such social value creation. Continued privatisation and outsourcing through Private Finance Initiatives and Public Private Partnerships enabled government to continue the performance management regime but develop an evidence base of 'public and social value' and more citizen self-regulation, local service provision and comprehensive strategic commissioning and procurement. Commissioning and procurement moved from outputs (activities) to outcomes (results) to the end value created by services and interventions. Outcomes based performance measures not only encouraged managerial entrepreneurialism but shifted the focus to creating customer and societal value within multisector partnerships for delivery. During 2020, mid-COVID-19, a controversial, CIPFA-inspired 'COVID OneView' profiling system was developed by Xantura, to identify vulnerable individuals and households considered 'at risk'. Then a 'Levelling Up' Index was developed to identify localities that are in need of support.[2]

Innovation in local governance to create 'public and social value'

Big Society had piloted devolution and 'localism' by allowing communities to challenge local government and establish their own services. A 2010 Total Place initiative had enabled local authority areas to develop a 'whole systems' approach to service delivery, including co-designing approaches to reducing worklessness, building transport plans to get people back to work and build infrastructure for growth (and inclusion). Other experimental and innovative ways of configuring the structural forms and delivery mechanisms of local government were suggested, that is, as commissioning bodies; co-operatives and co-production models; enterprising, or trading companies. The need for innovation was accelerated by fiscal austerity and the need for smarter interventions. Moreover, innovative and experimental architectures and financing models to build up community capacities and assets included Community Asset Funds, Community Innovation Funds, Asset Buy Outs, Asset Transfer Partnerships, Social Impact Bonds, Social Enterprises, Mutuals, Co-operatives, and Community and Development Trusts, Community Interest Companies, Participative budgeting, Co-financing, and co-procurement and commissioning, income-generating subsidiaries of charities, independent social enterprises, social firms, Companies Limited by Guarantee, Industrial and Provident Societies. These were experiments at the time, and each met with varying success.

The Community Right to Bid (Localism Act, 2011) led to discussions about how to make the most of assets to meet community needs in ongoing and challenging economic climates. A centrally created 'Advancing Assets Programme' worked with 88 councils on their strategic approach to community asset transfer and supported numerous pilot projects. Over 154 councils in England developed community asset transfer strategies and policies, and 1,500 individual community asset transfer initiatives were taken over, and run by local community groups. At the time there were fears that there would not be much left within public ownership, but there was a huge effort to facilitate community empowerment and quantify social value.

Quantification of social value

Many states and non-state organisations are increasingly required to have formal standards and measures of performance in place (Local Government Association, 2019, 2020). They are being called upon to assess the outcomes of their activity in order to demonstrate their social, economic and environmental value. Indeed, decision-making on local service delivery was affected by how social and public value and performance were measured, so in order to ensure that all people involved in procuring and commissioning public service contracts should have an awareness of securing benefits for all stakeholders in a particular locality (with wider social, economic and environmental benefits), the UK government introduced the Public Services (Social Value) Act, to appreciate the gaps between citizens' and users' expectations.[3] By changing the way that value is accounted for, it was claimed that society would become more equal and sustainable.[4]

A review of extant literature reveals that there is no one preferred method used to evaluate and demonstrate social impact. All organisations drew on a burgeoning set of methodologies, toolkits and consultancy reports to identify, measure/evaluate and demonstrate the value and impact of social return on investment. Organisations were urged to understand, manage and report on the social, environmental and economic value created by an organisation and price became a proxy for value. New Economics Foundation (NEF) led the field in the UK but other methods include: Social Return on Investment, The Balanced Scorecard, Well Being Portfolio Evaluation Review, Social Accounting and Audit, Local Multiplier 3, AA1000 Assurance Standard (Social accounting), Global Reporting Initiative Framework (sustainability), Business in the Community and a Corporate Responsibility Index. All had differing strengths and weaknesses, and many were adopted but, regardless of their utility, it is important to examine how valuable these concepts are in a real-world situation of social determinants of health and inequality.

'Public and social value' in the context of social determinants of health and inequality?

Societal development and improving people's lives lie at the heart of public and social value. A growing body of literature suggests that the social element has become embedded in the principles and practice of public value due to the need to effect social change for the common good, generating social benefits, evoking social impacts and socially valued outcomes. One simple way of articulating social and public value is to argue that different stakeholders articulate their own social values and then public agencies deliver on these values because, it is argued, in a complex and changing environment, policymakers, public managers, private, voluntary sector organisations and informal community actors interact dynamically to create public and social value that numerous recipients perceive as valuable. It is very important to understand what is meant by social and public value in that health and wellbeing and quality of life of vulnerable and disadvantaged individual groups in society encompasses all aspects of life as represented in the rainbow model of Dahlgren and Whitehouse (Bonner, 2018). Moreover, wicked issues or the most challenging and complex problems of our time, many with undefined causes, and to which there are no ready solutions, can be affected by social, psychological and biological factors as well as much broader economic, political and environmental influences (Dahlgren and Whitehead, 1991, adapted in Bonner, 2018: xxi).

For Moore, the value that an organisation contributes to society is equivalent to shareholder value (Moore, 1995). Though originally limited to specific public management settings to assess economic, political and social costs and desirable actions and impacts on individual and collective life of citizens, it is now more broadly used by all types of organisations to enable managers to juggle multiple goals beyond performance targets (Meynhardt, 2019). They steer networks of service providers in the quest for creating public value, maintaining trust and responding to collective voices. It is also a stimulus to allow managers to be entrepreneurial for the common good and general wellbeing of citizens, though undoubtedly public value emerged as contested democratic practices. Given the different stakeholder interpretations of what constitutes 'value' and incorporated debates around rights, duties and the restructuring of government agendas across Europe, globally and cross-culturally has focused relationships between state, non-state/private, para-state agencies and civic society to attain public and social value. Many governments have experimented with citizen engagement, innovation and enterprise to create value added services. However, very different approaches to value creation are evident in states with very different models of governance, leadership, visions, objectives and strategies, due to their differing administrative cultures, legal systems and political traditions. Current analyses of public and social value creation differ hugely across international jurisdictions, and no one model prevails, but relational partnering to such creation offers some hope.

Conclusion

Is **relational partnering** the key to achieving public and social value and reform of public services? This chapter has demonstrated how state architectures were transformed to achieve overall strategic objectives, with central and local states providing leadership and direction (more steering than rowing) within new governance arrangements based on a series of complex, overlapping jurisdictions and formal/informal collaborative arrangements, rather than traditional, hierarchical control mechanisms.

Over the coming decades, key challenges face public sector agencies worldwide, not least the need to provide high quality services with diminishing resources, and success will depend on how well public services are delivered and types of support and resources leveraged from non-state partners. Global public sectors have a poor record on productivity despite dramatic investment, so the ongoing global pandemic (and any potential fall-out from Brexit) will continue to adversely impact 'left behind' areas of the UK. They also highlight the need for a focus on an 'innovation and enterprise imperative' (Brown and Osborne, 2013; my italics) of how we create social and public value to aid commissioning and procurement of services for the poorest and most disadvantaged groups and individuals in the country.

To consider value creation represents a way of thinking which is post-bureaucratic and post-competitive, and moves beyond the narrow market versus government failure approaches so dominant in earlier analyses of NPM. It is, therefore, a new paradigm for thinking about government activity, policymaking and service delivery, and has implications for public managers (O'Flynn, 2007). In seeking to create 'social and public value', public services can be delivered by multiple, interdependent agencies, with inter-organisational relational commissioning and procurement of contracts governing the processes across boundaries and between diverse stakeholders. Resource allocation and decision-making are negotiated between actors who share values, meanings and relationships, and power inequalities between stakeholders identified and meaningful policy and service outcomes agreed.

The wider determinants of health and inequalities have been further exposed during the COVID-19 pandemic as the crisis has brought into sharp focus the need for enhancing the quality of life and wellbeing for many more vulnerable groups and individuals (Anon, 2020. In the UK and many Western nations, wealth, if measured in purely material and physical aspects such as GDP and the economy. However considerations of mental, emotional, relational and social dimensions lead to re-evaluation of the concept of 'wealth' (Parnham, 2018). Half of the UK population reported having at least one adverse childhood experience and many vulnerable families continue to face acute and ongoing economic pressures that lead to stress and mental health issues (Fallaize and Lovegrove, 2018, chapter 4, in Bonner, 2018), regardless of multiple past health policy interventions.

It is clear that Dahlgren and Whitehead's **social determinants of health** rainbow model (1991) and Moore's original definition of public value (1995) were classic, ground-breaking analyses with social and public value embedded therein. However, in the intervening period, other scholars have contributed further components and merged/blended different perspectives on how to define, capture and measure social, public and collective values. Globally, at the same time as wellbeing and social and public values moved up political agendas, many governments placed citizen engagement at the centre of policymaking, in theory at least, by creating bodies to either nudge or change citizen behaviour. At core, these initiatives represent experimental, innovative and enterprising government for transformation.

Relational partnerships are the latest manifestation of innovation and enterprising governance, because, as described by Smith (2020: 205–206), they have potential for building up long-term relationships between public and private organisations (and more latterly, voluntary, third sector and other organisations) for enhanced local government procurement, contracting and commissioning services. Previous attempts to establish relational partnerships in local areas ultimately failed to gather momentum due to the incapacity to develop robust models incorporating the ways in which resources are captured effectively in commissioning and procurement processes for the long term.

Many local government and health chief executive officers in the UK have argued that COVID-19 may stimulate a rethink of public finances, reshape services in line with what local citizens and other stakeholders believe to be of 'value', tackle inequalities, and shine a light on the wider social problems. Other local leaders have seen COVID-19 as a catalyst and major anchor to the transformative power of local action, adding social and public value to the outcomes of entire supply chains of services (Municipal Journal event, 25 September 2020). For many place leaders inequalities in deprived communities can only be addressed by developing integrated and targeted commissioning of local authority services in partnership in response to budget cuts and escalation of vulnerable groups with complex needs (Kunonga et al, 2020: 121–148). Indeed, the Mayor of Tees Valley, Ben Houchen, giving evidence to the Select Committee on 'Levelling Up and Devolution' (October 2020), called for integrated policies to tackle 'left behind places'. Smith (2020: 197–214) also advocated new longer-term relational partnering as an alternative to traditional local authority commissioning services to build up trust and transparency and deliver successful community outcomes as well as profits. However, it is recognised that to unlock value different forms of resources from both sets of partners need to be reconfigured because a past focus on resources and financial returns had missed out on value to be gained from the socioeconomic benefits of partnering over the medium to long term.

Notes

[1]   The concept of relational partnerships is drawn from a wider body of contested theoretical and multidisciplinary research in fields such as international relations, sociology, strategy, management, leadership and theatre direction, among others.

[2]   https://wpi-strategy.com/levellingupmap

[3]   https://www.gov.uk/government/publications/social-value-act-information-and-resour ces/social-value-act-information-and-resources

[4]   https://www.socialvalueuk.org

References

Anon (2020a) Municipal Journal, Future Forum webinar, 25 September 2020.

Anon (2020b) Municipal Journal event, The Future of Local Government, virtual webinar, 25 September 2020.

Bonner, A. (2018) The individual growing into society. In Bonner, A. (ed) *Social Determinants of Health: An Interdisciplinary Approach to Social Inequality and Well-being*, Bristol: Policy Press, pp 1–16.

Brown, K. and Osborne, S.P. (2013) *Managing Change and Innovation in Public Service Organisations*, London: Routledge.

Dahlgren, G. and Whitehead, M. (1991) *Policies and Strategies to Promote Social Equity in Health*. Stockholm: Institute for Future Studies.

Fallaize, R. and Lovegrove, J. (2018) Nutrition in marginalised groups. In Bonner, A. (ed) *Social Determinants of Health: An Interdisciplinary Approach to Social Inequality and Well-being*, Bristol: Policy Press, pp 41–54.

HM Treasury (2020) Spending Review, 25 November. Available at: https://www.bbc.co.uk/news/business-55022162 (accessed 2 November 2020).

Kunonga, E., Gibson, G. and Parker, C. (2020) Inequalities in health and well-being across the UK: A local north east perspective. In Bonner, A. (ed) *Local Authorities and the Social Determinants of Health*, Bristol: Policy Press, pp 121–148.

Liddle, J. (ed) (2016a) *Contemporary Issues in Entrepreneurship Research: New Perspectives on Research Policy and Practice in Public Entrepreneurship*, Bingley: Emerald.

Liddle, J. (2016b) Public value management and new public governance: Key traits, issues and developments. In Ongaro, E. and van Thiel, S. (2016) *The Palgrave Handbook of Public Administration and Management in Europe*, London: Palgrave Macmillan, pp 967–990.

Liddle, J. (2020) New public governance, general civil society. In List, R.A., Anheier, H.K. and Toepler, S. (eds) *International Encyclopaedia of Civil Society*. New York: Springer.

Local Government Association (2019) *Measuring Social Value in Local Government Procurement: TOMS Guidance*. London: LGA.

Local Government Association (2020) Measuring social value in local government procurement: TOMS guidance-COVID 19 plus, in LGA (ed) *The Community Right to Bid* (Localism Act, 2011). Available at: https://www.gov.uk/government/publications/social-value-act-information-and-resources/social-value-act-information-and-resources (accessed 28 August 2020).

Meynhardt, T. (2019) Public value: Value creation in the eyes of society. In Lindgreen, A., Koenig-Lewis, N., Kitchener, M., Brewer, J.D., Moore, M.H. and Meynhardt, T. (eds) *Public Value: Deepening, Enriching and Broadening Theory and Practice*, Abingdon: Routledge, pp 5–22.

Moore, M. (1995) *Creating Public Value: Strategic Management in Government*, Cambridge, MA: Harvard University Press.

Moore, M. (2006) Recognising public value. ANZSOG Public Lecture, 9 November, Shine Dome, Canberra.

O'Flynn, J. (2007) From new public management to public value: Paradigmatic change and managerial implications. *The Australian Journal of Public Administration*, 66(3): 353–366.

OECD (2013) *Public Governance Reviews, Together for Better Public Services: Partnering with Citizens and Civil Society*, Paris: OECD. Available at: https://wpi-strategy.com/levellingupmap/ (accessed 18 November 2020).

Osborne, S.P. (2010) *The New Public Governance?*, Abingdon: Taylor and Francis.

Parnham, A. (2018) Wholistic well-being and happiness: Psychosocial-spiritual perspectives. In Bonner, A. (ed) *Social Determinants of Health: An Interdisciplinary Approach to Social Inequality and Well-being*, Bristol: Policy Press, pp 29–40.

The Public Services (Social Value) Act 2012. Available at: https://www.gov.uk/government/publications/social-value-act-information-and-resources/social-value-act-information-and-resources (accessed 28 August 2022).

Smith, R. (2020) The power and value of relationships in local authorities' and central government funding encouraging culture change. In Bonner, A. (ed) *Local Authorities and the Social Determinants of Health*, Bristol: Policy Press, pp 205–206.

Stoker, G. (2006) Public value management: A new narrative for networked governance. *American Review of Public Administration*, 36(1): 41–57.

Talbot, C. (2008) *Managing Public Value: A Competing Values Approach*, London: The Work Foundation.

9

The effect of COVID-19 on the financial sustainability of local government

Aileen Murphie

Introduction

Local authorities deliver universal and specific services to their local communities and support vulnerable children and adults. Central government sets statutory duties for councils, from adult social care to waste collection. Local authorities also provide discretionary services according to local priorities set out by elected councillors and are independent bodies with their own democratic mandate and a range of statutory powers, including a 'general power of competence' under the Localism Act 2011 and independent borrowing powers.

Local authorities in England have made a major contribution to the national response to the COVID-19 pandemic, working to protect local communities and businesses, while continuing to deliver existing services. The pandemic has in turn placed significant pressure on local authorities' finances, which were already under strain going into the pandemic.

Going into the pandemic

Local government's financial sustainability (defined as their ability to set a balanced budget and deliver statutory services) has been weakened by ten years of funding reductions (Comptroller and Auditor General, 2014: 32 and 36). Since 2010–2011, central government has steadily reduced grant funding, introduced incentive-based mechanisms such as New Homes Bonus and Business Rate Retention, and encouraged local authorities to use their borrowing powers to invest and create their own income streams (Comptroller and Auditor General, 2014: 15). The Spending Review 2010 stated: 'Local people, communities, and frontline staff understand their local priorities and problems better than central government. This makes them better placed to allocate scarce resources and shape services' (HM Treasury, 2010: 32).

The Department for Levelling Up, Housing and Communities (DLUHC; formerly the Ministry for Housing, Communities and Local Government) measures the impact of reducing government funding on local authority income via 'spending power'. This indicator captures the main streams of government funding to local authorities alongside council tax. It also includes some funding streams that are not within the local government Departmental Expenditure Limit (Comptroller and Auditor General, 2018: 14). The result has been that at a sectoral level, local authority spending power has fallen by 26 per cent, equating to a reduction in government grant of 50 per cent (Comptroller and Auditor General, 2021b: 13).

Figure 9.1 illustrates these trends, showing spending power falling until 2016–2017 and then levelling off, supported by rises in council tax, with government grants maintaining a downward trend until an uptick in 2019–2020 (Comptroller and Auditor General, 2021b: 13).

Council tax

There are implications for the local government finance system and for individual authorities arising from these changes. System-wide funding reductions have had a proportionately greater impact on the spending power of authorities that depend more on government funding, although that pattern reversed slightly in 2021 (IFS, 2021). More grant-dependent authorities, like metropolitan districts, have had greater reductions in their overall spending power (Comptroller and Auditor General, 2014: 16). For individual authorities, relying more on council tax for revenue means that the amount they can raise is reliant on the types of properties within their boundary: if they have a preponderance of Band A properties, the amount they can raise is much less than an authority with a greater proportion of higher banded properties. There is no link between an authority's ability to raise council tax and need. Hence the introduction of the adult social care precept to fund adult social care services raises revenue differentially across the country and does not match yield. Lastly, council tax rises are limited by DLUHC (announced as part of the annual local government financial settlement); if a council wants to raise council tax by greater than the referendum limit, then they have to seek the permission of local council tax payers via a referendum. No council has held a referendum: the cost would far outweigh potential revenue.

Business rate retention

From 2013–2014, local authorities retained around up to half of local growth in business rates. The Department also stopped revising its distribution of annual grant funding according to updated assessments of need. The move to 50 per cent business rate retention was intended to lead to 100 per cent business rate retention by 2020 to make local government financially

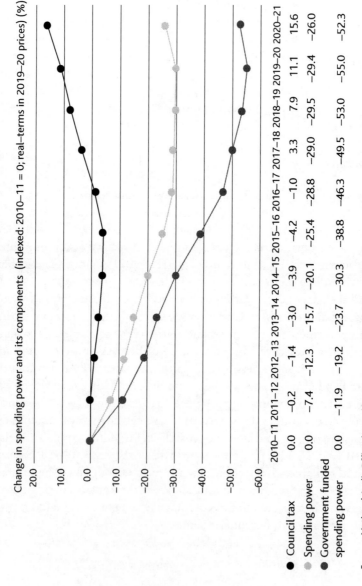

Figure 9.1: Changes in components of spending power in English local authorities, 2010–2011 to 2020–2021

Change in spending power and its components (indexed: 2010–11 = 0; real–terms in 2019–20 prices) (%)

	2010–11	2011–12	2012–13	2013–14	2014–15	2015–16	2016–17	2017–18	2018–19	2019–20	2020–21
Council tax	0.0	-0.2	-1.4	-3.0	-3.9	-4.2	-1.0	3.3	7.9	11.1	15.6
Spending power	0.0	-7.4	-12.3	-15.7	-20.1	-25.4	-28.8	-29.0	-29.5	-29.4	-26.0
Government funded spending power	0.0	-11.9	-19.2	-23.7	-30.3	-38.8	-46.3	-49.5	-53.0	-55.0	-52.3

Source: National Audit Office, https://www.nao.org.uk/other/financial-sustainability-of-local-authorities-visualisation-update/

Figure 9.2: Level of deprivation and gross rates payable per capita by billing authority

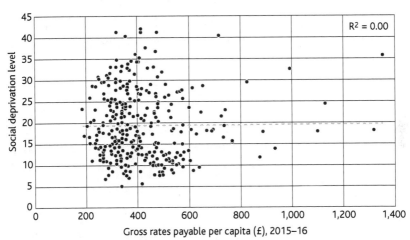

Source: National Audit Office, https://www.nao.org.uk/wp-content/uploads/2017/03/Planning-for-100-local-retention-of-local-business-rates.pdf

self-sufficient; to contribute to making places more successful and for local authorities to lead 'place shaping'. In fact, owing to lack of parliamentary time, 100 per cent business rate retention never happened.

Business rates are charged on most types of commercial property in a local area, according to a national rate set by DLUHC against property valuations set by the Valuation Office Agency. Business rates are a charge on most non-domestic properties. Business rates are essentially a property tax on commercial property, levied on most buildings with some exemptions.

Reliance on business rate retention raises challenges for local government, the main one being need versus yield. Business rates yield varies between areas through accidents of history and geography. Important factors for rates yield include how built up an area is, the proportion of commercial versus domestic property, how rural it is and wider economic activity. Social care spend relates to need and is connected to deprivation (Murphie, 2018). Need and business rate yield are not correlated, as Figure 9.2 shows (Comptroller and Auditor General, 2017b: 14).

Increased sales, fees and charges income

Total council spending is funded by income generated within service areas (such as planning and development) and reserved for use within the service, including income from sales, fees and charges. Growth in income from sales, fees and charges means that a greater share of the cost of service provision is falling on the service user. By 2017–2018, across all non-social-care service areas, income from sales, fees and charges increased from 16.1 per cent to

21.9 per cent as a share of total spend. Within service areas, the effect is marked: net current spending on development control fell by 52.9 per cent in real terms from 2010–2011 to 2016–2017. However, due to an increase in income from sales, fees and charges, total spend fell by only 6.7 per cent (Comptroller and Auditor General, 2018: 32).

Growth in commercial income

Since 2010–2011, local authorities have faced less pressure on resources to support capital expenditure relative to revenue. The use of other forms of capital resource, such as capital receipts, has also increased and, in 2016, DLUHC allowed the use of capital receipts to fund transformation schemes. Authorities can and do borrow to support capital spending. However, the revenue and capital sides of local authority spending interact and the primary challenge facing authorities in managing their capital spending and resourcing has been to minimise the revenue cost of their capital programmes as authorities meet debt servicing costs from revenue spending. The short-term need to reduce revenue pressure needs to be balanced with the longer-term need to maintain capital assets and invest in new assets (Comptroller and Auditor General, 2016: 9).

The acquisition of commercial property has become a significant area of activity for some authorities. While authorities have held properties for investment purposes for many years, the period 2016–2017 to 2018–2019 saw a step-change in scale: authorities spent £6.6 billion on commercial property from 2016–2017 to 2018–2019: 14.4 times more than in the preceding three-year period. This is shown in Figure 9.3 (Comptroller and Auditor General, 2020: 21 and 23).

Local authorities acquire commercial property for a variety of reasons, but yield is an important factor. A substantial amount of spending is on property outside authorities' boundaries, including 47.9 per cent of all acquisitions by value in 2018–2019, likely to be predominantly for yield (Comptroller and Auditor General, 2020: 23). Spend on the acquisition of office and retail property accounted for the bulk of local authorities' recent investment (£3.1 billion and £2.3 billion, respectively).

The government has discouraged borrowing to fund purchases of commercial property due to concern about disproportionate borrowing and risk. The Department issued a new capital framework; HM Treasury has stopped local authorities from accessing the Public Works Loan Board funding if they make commercial purchases and the Chartered Institute of Public Finance and Accountancy published a strengthened Prudential Code in 2021 (Comptroller and Auditor General, 2021b: 31).

Nevertheless, the growth in borrowing for investment means that debt servicing costs, as a proportion of net revenue expenditure, is increasing over time as Figure 9.4 shows (Comptroller and Auditor General, 2020: 45).

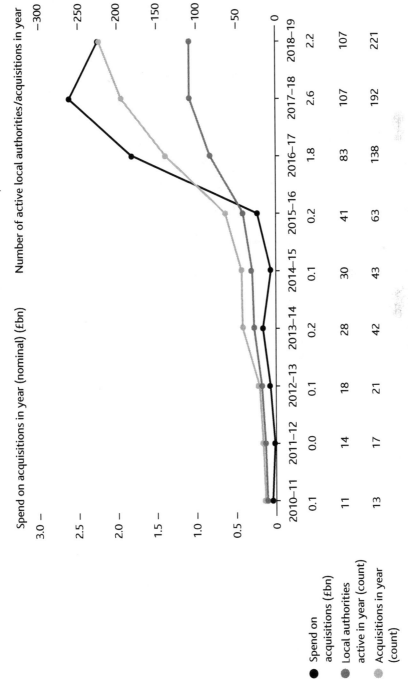

Figure 9.3: Commercial property purchases by English local authorities, 2010–2011 to 2018–2019

	2010–11	2011–12	2012–13	2013–14	2014–15	2015–16	2016–17	2017–18	2018–19
Spend on acquisitions (£bn)	0.1	0.0	0.1	0.2	0.1	0.2	1.8	2.6	2.2
Local authorities active in year (count)	11	14	18	28	30	41	83	107	107
Acquisitions in year (count)	13	17	21	42	43	63	138	192	221

Source: National Audit Office, https://www.nao.org.uk/wp-content/uploads/2020/02/Local-authority-investment-in-commercial-property.pdf

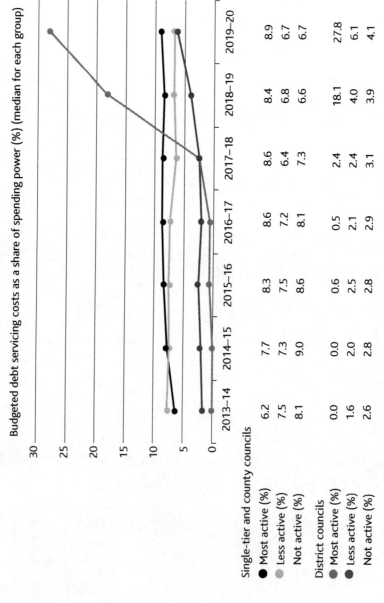

Figure 9.4: Debt servicing costs as a share of spending power in English local authorities, 2010–2011 to 2018–2019

Budgeted debt servicing costs as a share of spending power (%) (median for each group)

	2013–14	2014–15	2015–16	2016–17	2017–18	2018–19	2019–20
Single-tier and county councils							
Most active (%)	6.2	7.7	8.3	8.6	8.6	8.4	8.9
Less active (%)	7.5	7.3	7.5	7.2	6.4	6.8	6.7
Not active (%)	8.1	9.0	8.6	8.1	7.3	6.6	6.7
District councils							
Most active (%)	0.0	0.0	0.6	0.5	2.4	18.1	27.8
Less active (%)	1.6	2.0	2.5	2.1	2.4	4.0	6.1
Not active (%)	2.6	2.8	2.8	2.9	3.1	3.9	4.1

Source: Comptroller & Auditor General, 2020: 45

Effect on services from funding reductions

Increase in demand

Pressures on key areas of local services have increased since 2010 as Figure 9.5 illustrates (Comptroller and Auditor General, 2018: 20). From 2010–2011 to 2016–2017, the total population grew by 5 per cent. There was also growth in the adult population in need of care; growing homelessness and increasing demand for children's social care. All measures of homelessness have risen, meaning growing demand. Elements of welfare reforms have contributed, notably the freezing and capping of local housing allowance (Comptroller and Auditor General, 2017c: 21). There have been increases in the number of referrals to, and the complexity of cases in, both adult and children's social care and the pace of growth in demand for children's social care has accelerated (Comptroller and Auditor General, 2018: 19). Possible reasons include reductions in spending on early intervention services and the long-term effects of austerity on deprived communities. There is also rising demand for services for children with special educational needs or disabilities, or both. Some authorities are facing cost pressures linked to asylum-seekers with no recourse to public funds.

Coping with increasing demand

Despite pressures from increasing demand, to cope with funding reductions and balance their books each financial year as is necessary under the tight legal framework governing local authorities, from 2010–2011 onwards councils adopted various strategies, including cutting service spend and drawing down reserves (Figure 9.6). In the first three years, reductions in service spend were greater than reductions in main income streams. This strategy allowed authorities to increase their reserves and increase other spending. In the next three years, there was a marked switch, where the use of reserves and reductions in other spend become more important (Comptroller and Auditor General, 2018: 22).

The effect on individual service areas has been reductions across all service spend apart from children's social care. Authorities have tried to prioritise and protect services for the vulnerable but despite that, spend on adult social care fell to 2017–2018. After that point, a one-off adult social care grant and the adult social care precept meant that spend began to rise again. Figure 9.7 shows the impact to 2019–2020 of funding reductions across service areas (Comptroller and Auditor General, 2021b: 27).

Protecting social care spend

Social care spend has been relatively protected, with reductions in service spend including the Better Care Fund to 2017–2018. Other services have been cut

Figure 9.5: Change in demand in key local authority service areas in England

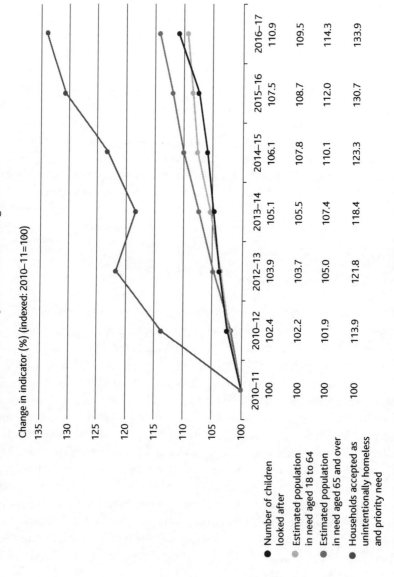

Change in indicator (%) (indexed: 2010–11=100)

	2010–11	2010–12	2012–13	2013–14	2014–15	2015–16	2016–17
Number of children looked after	100	102.4	103.9	105.1	106.1	107.5	110.9
Estimated population in need aged 18 to 64	100	102.2	103.7	105.5	107.8	108.7	109.5
Estimated population in need aged 65 and over	100	101.9	105.0	107.4	110.1	112.0	114.3
Households accepted as unintentionally homeless and priority need	100	113.9	121.8	118.4	123.3	130.7	133.9

Source: National Audit Office, https://www.nao.org.uk/wp-content/uploads/2018/03/Financial-sustainability-of-local-authorites-2018.pdf

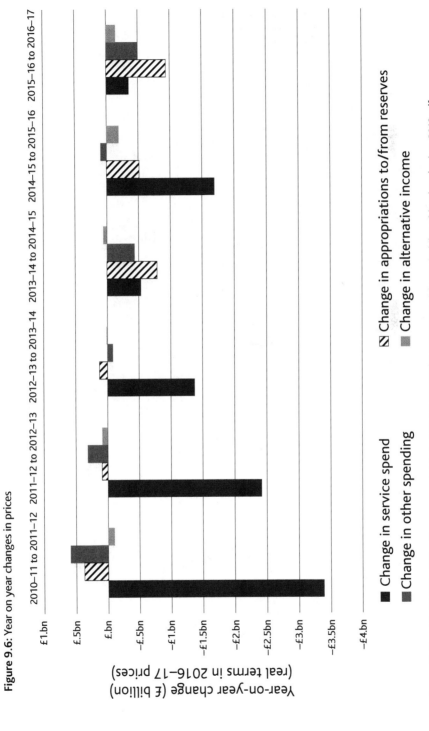

Figure 9.6: Year on year changes in prices

Source: National Audit Office,https://www.nao.org.uk/wp-content/uploads/2018/03/Financial-sustainability-of-local-authorites-2018.pdf

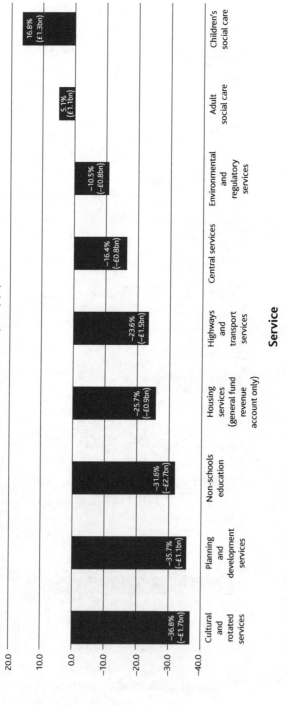

Figure 9.7: Change in service spend by English local authorities, gross of sales, fees and charges, 2010–2011 to 2018–2019

Change in service expenditure (indexed: 2010–11 = 0%, real terms in 2019–20 prices) (%)

Source: Comptroller & Auditor General, 2021a: 27

Figure 9.8: Social care as a share of service spend (percentage) (net current spend)

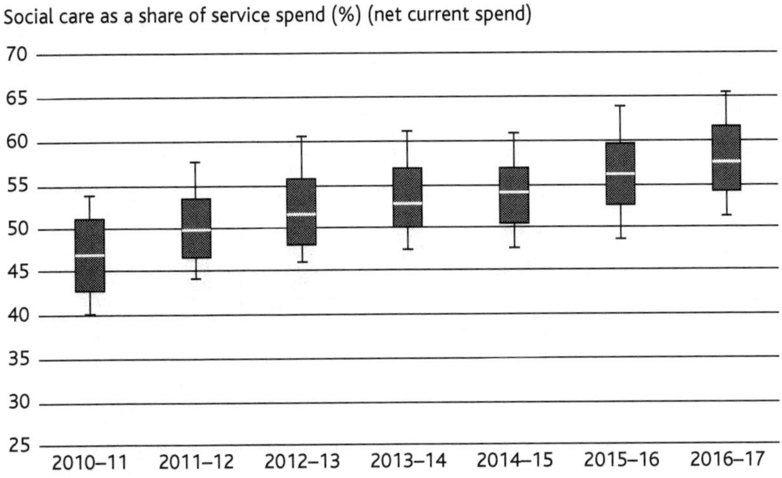

Social care as a share of service spend (%) (net current spend)

Source: Comptroller & Auditor General, 2018: 54

substantially; for example, a 35.7 per cent cut in planning and development (including fees and charges income) and a 25.7 per cent cut in housing services (Comptroller and Auditor General, 2021b: 23 and 27). One major implication from the increasing concentration on social care is that a greater proportion of council spend is now on social care which is more difficult to cut. Councils have not been able to reduce spending on social care to match their overall funding decrease so the room for manoeuvre for local authority finance directors is diminishing as Figure 9.8 shows (Comptroller and Auditor General, 2018: 54).

Conclusion on the sector going into the pandemic

Financial pressure on the sector has increased markedly over time with services other than social care continuing to face reducing funding despite increases in council tax. There is a pattern of growing service overspends and reducing reserves exhibited by some authorities which is not sustainable over the medium term. The sector needs a plan for long-term financial sustainability. But central government's approach via spending reviews has been characterised by one-off and short-term funding fixes, in an increasingly crisis-driven approach to local authority finances which has increased uncertainty and continues to risk value for money (Comptroller and Auditor General, 2018: 11). Local authorities budgeted for 2020–2021 on the basis of a one-year financial settlement once again. Major reforms such as the Fair Funding Review, the proposed move to 75 per cent retention of business rates and a reform plan for adult social care that could potentially have amounted to a long-term funding plan for local authorities have not been delivered and subject to repeated delay. Fragmented funding and the increasing use of competitive bidding creates uncertainty in both established and newer policy areas. Lastly, significant financial pressures create their own budget uncertainty (Comptroller and Auditor General, 2021b: 33).

The scale of the crisis: pressure from four directions

Increased cost from increasing demand for existing services and cost of provision

Local authorities have faced cost and income pressures as a result of the pandemic. Spending pressures have fallen most heavily on local authorities' adult social care, housing and public health services. Given the nature of the pandemic this is to be expected as authorities have moved to support the most vulnerable. Services are costing more because of increasing demand; for example in children's social care for looked after children. Spending on death management and domestic abuse services has also increased. Councils' own costs have increased too due to social distancing guidelines. Illness, self-isolation and shielding by staff across a range of services has meant spend on temporary staff has increased.

Cost pressures from responding to COVID-19

Local authorities have delivered specific programmes on behalf of central government. This includes infection control programmes in the adult social care sector, Test and Trace schemes and Everyone In to support rough sleepers. Local authorities are also a key part of Local Resilience Forums supporting the most clinically vulnerable via the Shielding programme. Figure 9.9 shows the cost pressures across service areas: adult social care has seen the greatest absolute cost pressure during the pandemic but public health is experiencing the greatest pressure as a proportion of service expenditure (Comptroller and Auditor General, 2021a: 19).

Vanishing savings

All local authority budgets had planned savings built into their budgets for 2020–2021, both to cope with existing financial and service pressures and to carry out service transformation. Due to the pandemic, local authorities have been prevented from securing the savings included in their 2020–2021 budgets. The size of underdelivered savings varies across authorities but poses a risk to their individual financial sustainability. The effect was not be limited to the 2020–2021 financial year. Local authority finances have continued to be under significant pressure in 2021–2022. In addition to any ongoing costs and income losses due to the pandemic, local authorities

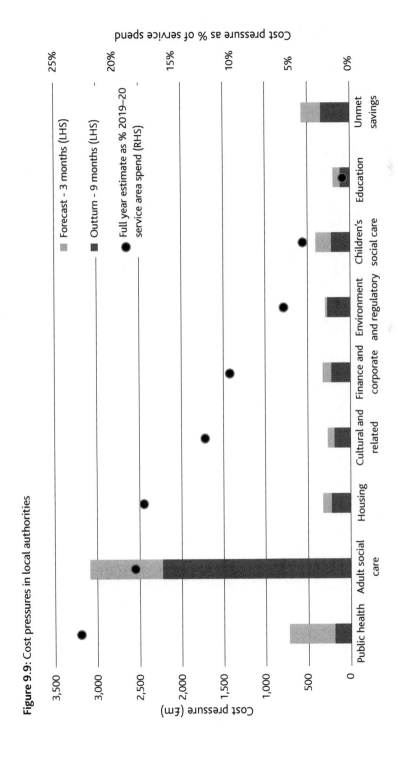

Figure 9.9: Cost pressures in local authorities

needed to replenish reserves, deliver delayed savings programmes and address tax deficits from 2020–2021.

Falling locally generated income and tax losses

As regards sales, fees and charges, COVID-19 restrictions in place at different times have led to the closure of local authority owned facilities such as leisure centres, museums and theatres, and have substantially reduced demand for others like car parks. As already set out in this chapter, commercial income has been increasingly important to local authority finances over recent years. Local authorities' income from commercial investments such as rent from properties developed in regeneration schemes, or dividends from investments in local infrastructure such as airports, has reduced or disappeared. Authorities have also made investments in commercial property solely to secure yield: that income has been vulnerable to COVID-19 restrictions as footfall in shopping areas fell and demand for flights reduced. Estimates vary but the financial effect is estimated at £10 billion for 2020–2021 (equivalent to 20 per cent of net revenue expenditure). Pressures have varied across different authority types, with county councils being impacted most as Figure 9.10 shows but district councils have experienced the highest level of pressures as a proportion of spend (Comptroller and Auditor General, 2021a: 22–23, 2021b: 20).

The scale of the crisis: the Department for Levelling Up, Housing and Communities and central government action

Unringfenced grants

By July 2021, central government had announced £370 billion of COVID-19 response across 374 measures, with 21 lead organisations. Over £260 billion has been spent (National Audit Office, 2021). The effect of the pandemic on local government was immediate and substantial: DLUHC brought forward and allocated via the adult social care funding formula £1.6 billion of grants in March 2020, breaching its parliamentary control total and meaning that its annual accounts were qualified by the Comptroller and Auditor General (MHCLG, 2021: 21 and 95). This was the first of four tranches of unringfenced grant funding which amounted to £4.55 billion by March 2021, now allocated by a new relative needs formula, accompanied by floor funding for lower tier authorities (Comptroller and Auditor General, 2021a: 31–32). In October 2021 the Department estimated government COVID-19 funding for the sector for 2020–2021 at £10.8 billion. This is made up of £9.5 billion of grants and £1.3 billion in compensation for sales, fees and charges income losses (Comptroller and Auditor General, 2021b: 21). DLUHC has also offered exceptional support to local authorities facing unmanageable pressures.

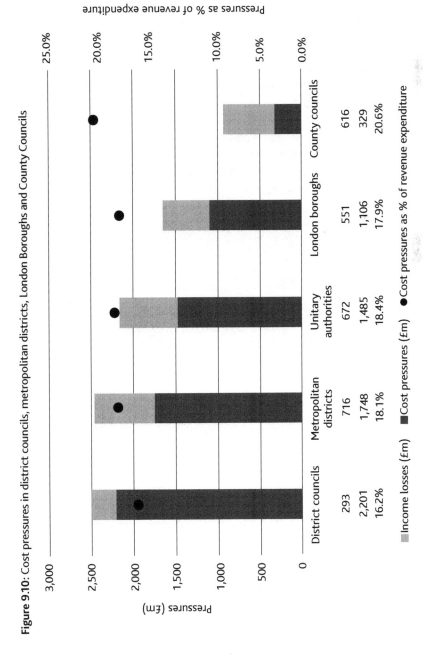

Figure 9.10: Cost pressures in district councils, metropolitan districts, London Boroughs and County Councils

Pressures as % of revenue expenditure

	District councils	Metropolitan districts	Unitary authorities	London boroughs	County councils
Income losses (£m)	293	716	672	551	616
Cost pressures (£m)	2,201	1,748	1,485	1,106	329
Cost pressures as % of revenue expenditure	16.2%	18.1%	18.4%	17.9%	20.6%

■ Income losses (£m) ■ Cost pressures (£m) ● Cost pressures as % of revenue expenditure

Source: Comptroller & Auditor General, 2021b: 19

Specific grants

Alongside unringfenced grants to local government, DLUHC and other departments have issued grants for specific purposes. These include local council tax hardship grant of £500 million, two Infection Control grants to support adult social care providers, grants to house rough sleepers under Everyone In and further funding for wider homelessness and a National Leisure Recovery Fund for leisure facilities (Comptroller and Auditor General, 2021a: 36–37).

Local authorities were also required to administer schemes on behalf of the Department for Business, Energy and Industrial Strategy to support local businesses and received funding from the Department of Health and Social Care (DHSC) for local test and trace schemes and other public health measures, including setting up test centres and vaccination centres. All come with administrative burdens: the sector has complained about onerous reporting requirements, central government announcing new measures without notice or consultation and the need to bid; for example, to the National Leisure Recovery Fund (Comptroller and Auditor General, 2021a: 35).

Reducing burdens on local authorities

The department lightened the burden on authorities including postponing local elections from May 2020, delaying the deadline for local authority accounts and delaying reform to the local government finance system. DHSC offered easements from duties under the Care Act 2015 and the Department for Education relaxed specific duties owed to children with special needs.

Compensating for lost income

DLUHC set up midyear a sales, fees and charges compensation scheme which disregards the first 5 per cent of shortfalls against budgeted income as a reflection of normal volatility and thereafter, compensates for 75 per cent of irrecoverable losses. The scheme does not provide compensation for any lost commercial income, reflecting the policy of discouraging investment solely for commercial yield but potentially impacts long-standing and policy-driven sources of commercial income. Shire districts have seen the greatest gap between income losses and compensation. The sales, fees and charges scheme has been extended into 2021–2022 (Comptroller and Auditor General, 2021a: 34).

As for tax losses, at October 2020, authorities forecast that business rates collected in 2020–2021 would be £1.6 billion lower than budgeted due to the pandemic. Council tax income would be £1.4 billion lower. Tax losses do not have a direct in-year impact and impact local authority budgets the following year. Before the pandemic, authorities were required to address the previous year's tax deficits fully in the following year. The government announced in July 2020 that 2020–2021 tax losses would be spread over three years. The government also committed to sharing part of irrecoverable local tax losses for 2020–2021, announced in the Spending Review at 75 per cent.

Authorities' tax bases are likely to shrink in 2021–2022 as the economic downturn affects local labour markets and economies. One sign is the number of council tax support claimants increasing: 6.0 per cent over the last year (Comptroller and Auditor General, 2021a: 54).

The situation with the pandemic is fluid and uncertain, and new funding streams continue to be announced, together with extensions of existing schemes. One big unknown is the effect on local authority tax income which will only become apparent over time.

The scale of the crisis: effect on economic development

The local growth landscape from 2010 to 2011

In 2010, the government set out a new approach for local economic growth, in the White Paper *Local Growth: Realising Every Place's Potential*. They closed the Regional Development Agencies and replaced them with new local growth organisations and funds, particularly Local Enterprise Partnerships (LEPs) and the first of several new funds: the Regional Growth Fund (Comptroller and Auditor General, 2013: 5).

LEPs were intended as private sector-led strategic partnerships to determine and influence local growth priorities. With the advent of the Local Growth Fund in 2012, central government funding to LEPs rose to £12 billion between 2015–2016 and 2020–2021 via locally negotiated Growth Deals based on local priorities to promote economic growth. This took place against a policy of increased localism, with a range of structures, including setting up nine combined authorities and elected mayors, forming alongside LEPs to support the devolution of funding and responsibilities from central government. By 2019, all LEPs had adopted a legal personality and all authorities had opted to belong to only one LEP clarifying the landscape considerably (Comptroller and Auditor General, 2016: 5, 2019: 5). However, LEPs have complained that they did not have the capacity to deliver what was asked of them, DLUHC did not evaluate the value for money of the Local Growth Fund's £12 billion, nor did it set specific quantifiable objectives for Growth Deals, meaning that it is difficult to assess how LEPs and the Growth Deals have contributed to economic growth.

Other problems affecting the local growth landscape including the complexity of structures and variation in powers between authorities. Of the mayoral combined authorities, only Greater Manchester displays the geographic alignment and co-terminosity which makes implementing policy very much easier (Comptroller and Auditor General, 2017c: 30; see Figure 9.11).

For combined authorities to deliver real progress they need to demonstrate that they are driving both economic growth and contributing to public sector reform (Comptroller and Auditor General, 2017c: 10).

The role of local authorities

Local authorities have a key role in 'place shaping' and in encouraging local economic growth to improve the lives of their citizens. However, since 2010–2011, as set out in Figure 9.7, spending on development had been cut by over 35 per cent by 2019–2020, including fees and charges income. In addition, the UK has had a long-standing problem with productivity, which lags behind Organisation for Economic Co-operation and Development comparators. Post the 2008 financial crisis, lagging productivity has combined with low wages (Department for Business, Innovation and Skills, 2012: 16). The underperformance historically of England's cities is another long-standing issue which has defied improvement, despite the creation of combined authorities (Comptroller and Auditor General, 2017c: 21).

The ongoing effects of the pandemic

The UK economy went through a double dip recession in 2020–2021, with the worst effects cushioned by the enormous scale of the government's response. However, unemployment is rising and the closure and curtailment of businesses and educational disruptions are affecting productivity. It is unclear how many businesses will survive and how long the damage to businesses and employment will last. The impact of the UK leaving the EU is becoming apparent too. Locally, the replacement of EU structural funds by the Levelling Up fund and the UK Shared Prosperity fund is still to be managed, against a backdrop of suspicion of partiality seeded by the botched launch of the Towns Fund (Comptroller and Auditor General, 2020: 6).

Conclusion

Short to medium term

Local authorities have played an important role in the public response to the pandemic, despite being under significant financial pressure after ten years of funding reductions. Local authorities are financially weaker than in 2010, with less capacity, more capital intensive, their income more volatile, the link with local need frayed and service pressures subject to continually

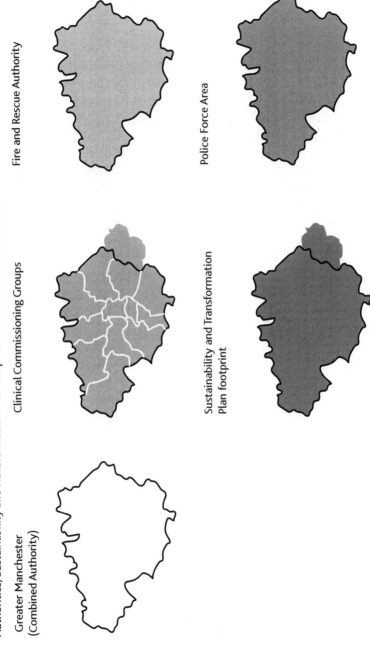

Figure 9.11: Great Manchester Combined Authority's geographical boundaries with Clinical Commissioning Groups, Fire and Rescue Authorities, Sustainability and Transformation Plan footprints and Police force boundaries

Greater Manchester (Combined Authority)

Clinical Commissioning Groups

Fire and Rescue Authority

Sustainability and Transformation Plan footprint

Police Force Area

Note: Greater Manchester Combined authority's boundaries are principally coterminous with other public administration boundaries

Source: Comptroller & Auditor General, 2017c: 10

increasing demand. Local authority governance is strained: risk profiles and risk appetites are higher and there is more complexity in local arrangements.

DLUHC supported authorities effectively and averted system-wide financial failure. Nonetheless, the financial position of the sector remains highly precarious. Many authorities relied on reserves to balance their 2020–2021 year-end budgets. The outlook for 2021–2022 is concerning. Across large parts of the sector, authorities set budgets for 2021–2022 in which they had limited confidence, and balanced only through cuts to service budgets and the use of reserves which will need to be replenished. There is a continuing trickle of individual financial failure of authorities and the consequences: increased cost to council tax payers; confusion while failure is addressed; restructuring which takes time and distracts senior leadership locally and nationally; and, lastly, undermines value for money.

Overall, the size of tax income losses to local government are not yet known and neither are other income losses which will depend on how the economy bounces back. Some income will never be recovered. On the service side, there are permanent increases in service pressures and costs which are not yet apparent. For example, homelessness was on the rise anyway and has only been damped down by the eviction ban and the effect of Everyone In. In adult social care, there is a risk to some providers' financial sustainability from the pandemic and the future shape of the service is undefined. On children's social care, the upward pressure in referrals is established.

It will be critical for national economic recovery that local economic recovery takes off and the needs of newly job impoverished areas are addressed along with historically left behind areas. Supporting economic recovery locally will entail local authorities being able to influence and adapt business support and job creation schemes; having real influence over improving infrastructure in their areas and being able to address skills shortages locally. This will mean devolution to local areas, a local/central partnership and an end to the differential approach of central government departments to devolution. The government should evaluate the current economic support schemes and merge the most effective measures into the plethora of new funds.

Long term

The overarching question is whether the local government finance system is viable. It is implausible that local government's future can be founded securely on a council tax system rooted in 1992 property values; a business rates system increasingly divorced from actual business activity hard hit by the pandemic; a diminishing and reactive grants programme, new grants dominated by competitive bidding and locally generated income dependent on the business cycle. These arrangements breed uncertainty, short-termism and financial instability and undermine good decision-making and longer-term value for money. Local government has survived thus far but it needs to flourish. The weaknesses in the system exposed by the pandemic need addressing urgently and there is an acute need for a long-term financial plan to secure the sector's future financial sustainability.

References

Comptroller and Auditor General (2014) *Financial Sustainability of Local Authorities 2014, HC 783, 2014–15*, London: National Audit Office.

Comptroller and Auditor General (2016) *Financial Sustainability of Local Authorities: Capital Expenditure and Resourcing, HC 234, 2016–17*, London: National Audit Office.

Comptroller and Auditor General (2017a) *Homelessness, HC 308, 2017–19*, London: National Audit Office.

Comptroller and Auditor General (2017b) *Planning for 100% Local Retention of Business Rates, HC 1058, 2016–17*, London: National Audit Office.

Comptroller and Auditor General (2017c) *Progress in Setting Up Combined Authorities, HC 240, 2017–2019*, London: National Audit Office.

Comptroller and Auditor General (2018) *Financial Sustainability of Local Authorities 2018, HC 834, 2017–19*, London: National Audit Office.

Comptroller and Auditor General (2019) *Local Enterprise Partnerships: An Update on Progress, HC 2139, 2017–2019*, London: National Audit Office.

Comptroller and Auditor General (2020) *Review of the Town Deals Selection Process, HC 576, 2019–21*, London: National Audit Office.

Comptroller and Auditor General (2021a) *Local Government Finance in the Pandemic, HC 1240, 2019–21*, London: National Audit Office

Comptroller and Auditor General (2021b) *The Local Government Finance System in England: Overview and Challenges, HC 858, Session 2019–21*, London: National Audit Office

Department for Business, Innovation and Skills (2012) *No Stone Unturned: In Pursuit of Growth*, London: Department for Business, Innovation and Skills.

HM Treasury (2010) *Spending Review 2010, Cmnd 7942*, London: HM Treasury.

IFS (2021) *An Initial Response to the Local Government Finance Settlement*, Institute of Fiscal Studies, December. https://ifs.org.uk/publications/15889. Accessed on 26 August 2022.

MHCLG (Ministry of Housing, Communities and Local Government) (2020) *Annual Report and Accounts 2019–20, HC929*, London: House of Commons.

Murphie, A. (2018) 'An exploration of the issues raised by the move towards to 100% Business Rate Retention', in *Governing England: Devolution and Funding*, London: British Academy, pp 53–62.

National Audit Office (2021) *COVID 19 Cost Tracker*, London: National Audit Office.

10

UN sustainability goals and social value: local authority perspectives

Rob Whiteman, Tim Reade and Dave Ayre

Introduction

In this chapter the concepts of social value reviewed by Liddle in Chapter 8 will be developed to include **environmental value** and, in particular, the wicked issue of climate change. Liddle critically reviews the literature on public and social value, and the historical development of these ideas in relation to New Public Management and the quantification of social value in relation to the relative importance that people place on changes experienced in their lives from a wellbeing perspective. Using a combination of accounting and economic measures, the Chartered Institute of Public Finance and Accountancy and Deloitte have used international accounting standards and UN Sustainable Goals.

Social value and environmental value is defined with reference to the different approaches through the lens of various organisations and, where focusing on environmental value in this chapter, it covers its impact at an international, national, regional and local level in particular with reference to climate change strategies and with references to housing. More detailed discussion of housing will be presented in Chapter 11, and youth employment in Chapter 12.

Global climate change concern

Concern and debate relating to climate change is not new. While provisions on climate change were adopted in the 'Declaration of the United Nations Conference' on 16 June 1972 in Stockholm, it was not until much later that decisive action could be said to have occurred. The size and scale of the problem was noted at the time within a statement released on 16 July 1992 by the Union of Concerned Scientists, a group of leading US scientists dedicated to raising issues around climate change. In its press release it noted that 'human beings and the natural world are on a collision course' and went on to outline specific areas of environmental concern, namely, the atmosphere, water resources, oceans, soil, forests and living species Union of Concerned Scientists, 1992).

The United Nations Framework Convention on Climate Change

In May 1992, underlining the need for a Framework Convention on Climate Change (FCCC), the UN stated that 'human activities have been substantially increasing the atmospheric concentrations of greenhouse gases, that these increases enhance the natural greenhouse effect, and that this will result on average in an additional warming of the Earth's surface and atmosphere and may adversely affect natural ecosystems and humankind' (UN, 1992). Following this, the UNFCCC was created. This was the first real act of relationalism on a global scale in relation to the **wicked issue** of climate change (United Nations Framework on Climate Change, 2021a).

Since the foundation of the UNFCCC, our understanding of the factors negatively affecting our climate have grown considerably as the complexity of climate modelling has increased and further scientific research has been undertaken. Alongside this has been further progress under the banner of the UNFCCC to galvanise and motivate those countries who are members to the convention. Principle among these activities has been the Kyoto Protocol and subsequent Paris Agreement.

Their construct and intent embedded the principles of relationalism in that they were designed to be agreements entered into through choice, requiring extensive debate and discussion ahead of contractual obligation. Their subsequent success, evidenced by their longevity and continuing relevance, is no doubt in part directly attributable to the relational process which resulted in countries signing the agreements. At their heart is trust, goodwill and a belief between signatories that the outcomes envisaged in the agreements provide mutual benefit for all.

The Kyoto Protocol

Created in December 1997 in Kyoto, Japan, the Kyoto Protocol was the next big step by the UN in driving forward its agenda on climate change. Seen as a means of 'operationalising' the instruments of the UNFCCC, arguably its biggest challenge was its ability to agree the specific measures and commitments signatories to the convention were prepared to agree to. This task best demonstrates the nature of the challenge we face as a global community in tackling climate change and perhaps highlights the extent of relational partnering required at a macro strategic level to deal with the truly wicked problem of climate change; it took four years and two months for the ratification process outlined in the Kyoto Protocol to be agreed by all signatories. The Kyoto Protocol also highlighted the difficulties that certain parties had in converting the relational partnering concept into tangible change. The most significant being the US, where attempts at ratification of Kyoto by the Clinton administration were thwarted by the US Senate, influenced by the fossil fuel lobby.

The Paris Agreement

The UN Paris Agreement entered into force on 4 November 2016. Its main aim has been 'to strengthen the global response to the threat of climate change by keeping a global temperature rise this century well below 2 degrees Celsius above pre-industrial levels and to pursue efforts to limit the temperature increase even further to 1.5 degrees Celsius' (UN, 2015).

The Convention of the Parties

A central pillar of the UNFCCC designed to maintain the momentum of activity by member nations in pursuance of activity to combat climate change has been an annual Convention of the Parties or COP. Acting as the 'Supreme Body' of the UNFCCC, signatories to the UNFCCC meet to ensure progress against the commitments outlined in the convention are being met. First established in Berlin in 1995, there have now been 26 COPs and in 2021 the UK hosted the annual Conference of the Parties in Glasgow, known as COP26 (UN, 1992).

The influence of the UN Sustainable Development Goals

On 1 January 2016, 17 Sustainable Development Goals (SDGs), agreed by world leaders at a UN Summit in September 2015, came into force. Their impact has been far-reaching, providing a high-level framework used by countries around the globe from which to develop policies and strategies to combat poverty, inequalities and climate change. They are not legally binding but add to the weight of influence exerted by UNFCCC agreements. In the UK they can be seen clearly in Scotland's National Performance Framework. Aligned to the 17 UN SDGs, its purpose is to reduce inequalities and give equal importance to economic, environmental and social progress. At a UK regional level too, it is now common to see examples of regional government aligning their policies and strategies with an inclusive growth framework that references the 17 UN SDGs such as that adopted by the West Midlands Combined Authority. At a local level, the development of local authority climate change strategies regularly reference SDG 13 on climate action as an underpinning motivation for detailed actions to reach their own organisation's climate change targets.

Historical perspectives on carbon emissions

In the last half century, our planet and the way we live our lives has changed beyond recognition. The rise of technology, the advent of globalisation and the increasing gap between the richest and poorest are all issues that have and will continue to create wicked problems that we must attempt to resolve. Arguably, it is the current generation that has had the biggest impact in these areas leaving us both morally and ethically responsible for their resolution. If left unchallenged, we are set to bequeath to our children and future generations a planet no longer able to support them and disparities in our economies that may never be closed.

Yet the seeds of some of our most significant challenges were sown even further back in history, and the roots of many of our present-day wicked issues are deeply embedded within that history. It is this fact that many opponents of climate change agreements conveniently ignore. Many conservative commentators justified Trump's announcement to withdraw from the Paris Agreement (British Broadcasting Corporation, 2020) by referring to the carbon emissions of China and India today.

It is the case that the world's countries emit vastly different amounts of heat-trapping gases into the atmosphere. Figure 10.1 and Tables 10.1–10.3 show data compiled by the International Energy Agency (The Guardian, 2016; International Energy Agency Atlas of Energy, 2018) which estimates carbon dioxide (CO_2) emissions from the combustion of coal, natural gas, oil and other fuels, including industrial waste and non-renewable municipal waste.

Figure 10.1 illustrates the stark differences in carbon emissions between the leading emitters and the rest of the world and Table 10.1 ranks the top 21 countries for emissions for 2018.

On the face of it, China is indeed the largest emitter of carbon, and this was the justification for the Trump position on the Paris Agreement. However, a straightforward comparison such as this ignores the significant differences in population and when these are factored in, the rankings change, as illustrated in Table 10.2.

The picture that emerges from these figures is one where, in general, developed countries and major emerging economy nations lead in total carbon dioxide emissions. However, developed nations typically have high carbon dioxide emissions per capita, while some developing countries lead in the growth rate of carbon dioxide emissions. These uneven contributions to the climate crisis are at the core of the challenges the world community faces in finding effective and equitable solutions to the wicked issue of global warming. Notably, this analysis relegates China from being the highest emitter to the 13th.

Figure 10.1: The difference in carbon emissions between the leading emitters and the rest of the world

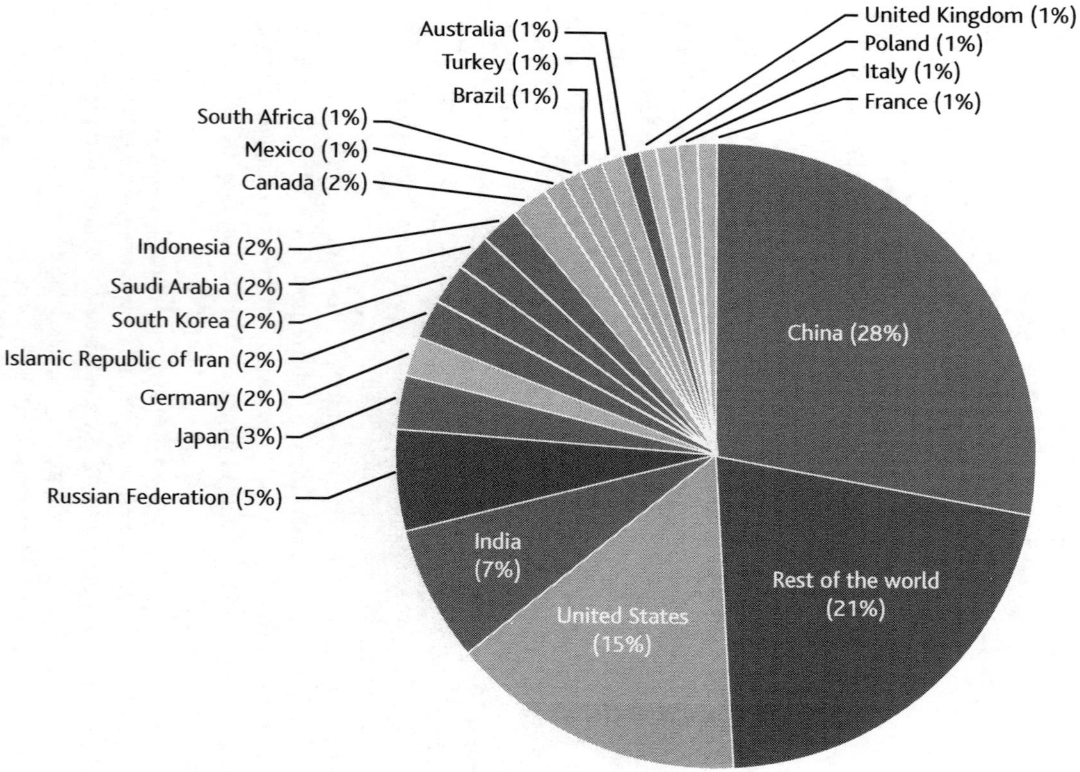

Table 10.1: The 21 highest emitters of carbon by nation-state, 2018

Rank	Country	CO_2 emissions (fuel combustion only, in metric gigatonnes)
1	China	10.06
2	United States	5.41
3	India	2.65
4	Russian Federation	1.71
5	Japan	1.16
6	Germany	0.75
7	Islamic Republic of Iran	0.72
8	South Korea	0.65
9	Saudi Arabia	0.62
10	Indonesia	0.61
11	Canada	0.56
12	Mexico	0.47
13	South Africa	0.46
14	Brazil	0.45
15	Turkey	0.42
16	Australia	0.42
17	United Kingdom	0.37
18	Poland	0.34
19	France	0.33
20	Italy	0.33
21	Kazakhstan	0.32

Then there are the historic contributions of carbon dioxide emissions. The UK may be the 17th highest nation–state emitter and the 14th emitter per capita in 2018, but when we take into account historic emissions, the UK ranks as the 5th highest after the US, Russia, China and Germany (The Guardian, 2016). This reflects the role of the UK as one of the first nations to move from a predominantly peasant economy to an industrial economy built in part by the deployment of steam technology powered by fossil fuels such as coal. This is illustrated in Table 10.3.

In summary, the UK's position in relation to emissions has seen considerable change since recording began in 1850. At this time, it was the top emitter of carbon dioxide, six times higher than the next ranked country, the US (Bolton, 2020). In 2019, it was subsequently ranked 16th globally, being responsible for 1.1 per cent of all global emissions, well behind

Table 10.2: The 21 per capita highest emitters of carbon by nation-state, 2018

Rank	Country	CO_2 emissions (fuel combustion only, in metric tonnes)
1	Saudi Arabia	18.48
2	Kazakhstan	17.60
3	Australia	16.92
4	United States	16.56
5	Canada	15.32
6	South Korea	12.89
7	Russian Federation	11.74
8	Japan	9.13
9	Germany	9.12
10	Poland	9.08
11	Islamic Republic of Iran	8.82
12	South Africa	8.12
13	China	7.05
14	United Kingdom	5.62
15	Italy	5.56
16	Turkey	5.21
17	France	5.19
18	Mexico	3.77
19	Indonesia	2.30
20	Brazil	2.19
21	India	1.96

the top five ranked countries of China, the US, India, Russia and Japan (IEA, 2019). The UK has undoubtedly done much to reduce its emissions. Since 1990 estimated UK greenhouse gas emissions have fallen 45 per cent (DBEIS, 2020).

A relational approach between countries can be said to have demonstrated progress through the UNFCCC, but world leaders must recognise both historical and per capita perspectives when it comes to the data when seeking to reach future agreements. From a position of improvements made demonstrated via empirical data on emission reduction, it is the UK's role to lead by example, by further reducing its emissions and achieving its carbon budget targets. However, as we will see later in this chapter, a lack of relationalism between central and local government in the UK is frustrating an ability to deal decisively with UK climate change commitments.

Table 10.3: Cumulative CO_2 emissions, 1900–2004

Country	CO_2 (million metric tons)
United States	314,772.1
Russia	89,688.3
China	89,243
Germany	73,625.8
United Kingdom	55,163.7
Japan	42,696.2
France	28,515.3
India	25,054.3
Canada	23,668.6
Ukraine	22,840.5
Poland	21,262.9
Italy	17,641.9
South Africa	13,241.7
Australia	11,929.4
Mexico	11,458.3
Kazakhstan	9,970.3
Spain	9,946.4
Czech Rep	9,399.6
Belgium	9,336.3
Brazil	9,136.3

Key risk areas from climate change

In the UK, the impacts and risks associated with and resulting from climate change have become more widely understood since the Climate Change Act 2008 created a legal requirement for a five-yearly risk assessment to be undertaken. Commissioned by the UK and devolved governments, the assessment sets out the risks, predicted impacts and opportunities facing the UK from climate change. In its latest assessment in 2017 it outlined six key areas of risk to the UK (Climate Change Committee, 2017):

1. Flooding and coastal change risks to communities, businesses and infrastructure.
2. Risks to health, wellbeing and productivity from higher temperatures.
3. Risks of water deficits in public water supply, and for agriculture, energy generation and industry, with impacts on freshwater ecology.

4. Risks to natural capital, including soils, coastal, marine and freshwater ecosystems, and biodiversity.
5. Risks from climate-related impacts on domestic and international food production and trade.
6. New and emerging pests and diseases, and non-native species, affecting people, plants and animals.

Supporting the risk assessment, the Adaption and Mitigation Committees, created as subcommittees within the construct of the Climate Change Committee, publish parallel reports further highlighting the work needed to tackle risks identified in the five-yearly assessments. Their latest findings have identified 'a substantial gap between current plans and future requirements and an even greater shortfall in action' (Climate Change Committee, 2019).

It is in this gap that relationalism has a key role to play. The example set through the UNFCCC at an international level is one which should be adopted at a UK national level between central government and local authorities. Up until now, the autonomy exercised by councils has meant they have been driven to declare climate emergencies through a combination of rising public concern, moral and ethical accountability. The often fractious relationship between central and local government is no doubt a key barrier in the adoption of a more relational approach. Given the current political, legislative and governance models adopted by the UK, through which intent manifests itself in obligatory action, one could argue that the current lack of progress in dealing with climate change at a national level can in part find its roots in our current reticence to adopt a more relational approach. Given this, redressing the balance in favour of an approach which accords with the principles of relationalism between central and local government adds a level of complexity which underlines the nature of the climate change challenge, further reinforcing its status as a wicked issue.

Extreme weather impact: flooding

In terms of human cost and impact, as our understanding of climate change effects become better understood, direct associations are now being drawn between climate change and the social determinants of health. Research has revealed that 50 per cent of people affected by extreme weather events such as storms or flooding are more likely to suffer from mental health problems, including depression and anxiety, while a quarter of people who have been flooded still live with these issues at least two and half years after the event (Environment Agency, 2020). Clearly, for those from lower income families and the elderly, the impacts of flooding are more greatly felt given the lack of financial resources and mobility restrictions.

For local authorities, the impact flood risk presents is growing as the effects of climate change rise in concert with sea levels and annual rainfall. Consequently, their ability to mitigate the risks presented by these changes is being degraded. The Public Accounts Committee have warned that councils, funded for local flood risk management, have found themselves spending more money than the agreed funding formula which central government allows for (Public Accounts Committee, 2021). The most recent decade (2009–2018) has been on average 1 per cent wetter than 1981–2010 and 5 per cent wetter than 1961–1990 for the UK overall, and the amount of rain from extremely wet days has increased by 17 per cent when looking at the same periods (Kendon et al, 2018). Along the English Channel coast, the sea level has already risen by about 12cm in the last 100 years. With the warming we are already committed to over the next few decades, we can expect a further 11–16cm of sea level rise by 2030. This equates to 23–27cm of total sea level rise since 1900 (Energy and Climate Intelligence Unit, 2016).

Extreme weather impact: heatwaves

In Europe, the 2003 heatwave caused an estimated 70,000 deaths, 2,000 of which occurred in the UK and in other regions such as the US and Russia research confirms that heatwaves increase the death rate, particularly among the elderly, children and those with pre-existing health conditions (Energy and Climate Intelligence Unit, 2014). In 2014, the Climate Change Committee said that health risks from heatwaves are not being taken into account sufficiently, with buildings such as old people's homes being designed for 'yesterday's climate' rather than the higher temperatures likely to materialise (Climate Change Committee, 2014).

Concern as to the extent of support available from central government on which local authorities can rely to deliver essential heatwave adaption measures is limited. In 2018 the Environmental Audit Committee noted that funding in this area had been withdrawn and was not being replaced and, despite government ministers emphasising the 'huge role' local authorities have in adapting to heatwaves, very little evidence has been seen of local authority activity in this area. With the average number of heat related deaths in the UK estimated to triple to 7,000 a year by the 2050s, with an ageing population who are more vulnerable to cardiac arrest and respiratory disease during heatwaves, the consensus of opinion is that more needs to be done at both a local and central government level to deal with this particular aspect of climate change and its effect on health (House of Commons Environmental Audit Committee, 2018).

The role of local authorities in dealing with climate change

Local authorities are key enablers in the nation's ability to deliver adaptive change to tackle both the effects and causes of climate change. Of great concern therefore is the lack of a statutory requirement at a local government level for climate change adaption measures to be delivered. Were these to be forced upon local government there is little doubt that due to the recent austerity period and the financial impact of COVID-19, councils would strongly resist their imposition without additional funding from central government. It is in areas such as this, that a more relational approach could be adopted.

The need to create adaption strategies that address the risks resulting from climate change is a relatively new challenge. The foundations of statutory obligations were laid via the Local Government Act 1929. Despite the lack of a statutory requirement to deliver adaptive change programmes, what has been seen across local government throughout the UK in recent years is a wave of **climate change emergencies** being declared. It is through these declarations that we are now beginning to see a more deliberate and purposeful approach by councils in their attempts to tackle climate change.

We are at a metaphorical crossroads and it is in this space that the concepts of environmental and social value become most relevant. If we are to tackle the wicked issue of climate change effectively, we need to see all things through the primary lens of sustainability in which environmental and social value are afforded better weighting.

A cultural and procedural shift is needed, and we have seen some movement through the introduction of the Public Services (Social Value) Act 2012. This requires procuring authorities to 'have regard' to social value, but is this enough? Since its introduction, we have begun to see a steady recognition by local authorities of a need to build into their procurement processes weightings related to social value. Indeed, the most forward leaning councils now separate social value from price and quality, giving it a weighting as high as 30 per cent, but these are few and far between. We have seen the private sector begin to react with the introduction of various tools such as the Social Value Calculator, concepts such as Social Return on Investment and the National Themes, Outcomes and Measures. While not perfect, and certainly lacking real 'teeth', given its need only to 'have regard' to social value, the Public Services (Social Value) Act 2012 appears to be having a positive effect which is gathering momentum. By comparison, in relation to environmental value, there is no equivalent of the Public Services (Social Value) Act 2012. Given the climate change crisis we are now in, this is perhaps one of the most prominent inadequacies frustrating our ability to deal more robustly with climate change. In its absence, perhaps an approach between parties seeking environmentally friendly outcomes and those able to provide them, could best be delivered via the principles of a relationalism approach.

Declaration of climate emergencies by local authorities

In March 2021 the Local Government Association reported that approximately 230 local authorities had declared a climate emergency (LGA, 2021), and across the spectrum of authorities making the declaration we have begun to see the many and varied ways they are seeking to achieve the net-zero targets they have set within their Climate Action Plans.

The approach taken by approximately half of all councils declaring a climate emergency has been to set a target for the achievement of net zero only in relation to their own operations, including their buildings, vehicle fleets and service operations. The remainder of councils declaring a climate emergency, and an associated Climate Change Action Plan, have set net-zero targets for both their own organisational footprint and the area over which they have jurisdiction. Clearly, the latter approach presents a greater challenge with councils having less leverage to achieve net-zero targets.

Local authority areas of focus to combat emissions

Across the spectrum of activity being undertaken by councils, initiatives have focused on areas including transport, housing, operational buildings, public awareness campaigns, regeneration projects and infrastructure.

In May 2020, the International Energy Agency reported that globally, 'transportation is still responsible for 24% of direct CO_2 emissions' (IEA, 2020). In the UK, we have seen road traffic increase 29 per cent between 1990 and 2018, and in 2017, greenhouse gas (GHG) emissions from road transport in the UK made up a fifth of the UK's total GHG emissions (ONS, 2019).

Clean Air Zones and transport related initiatives

One approach to curb vehicular GHG emissions, and so improve air pollutants that are harmful to health, is the adoption of Clean Air Zones (CAZs). The most notable has been London's CAZ implemented in 2008 and which covers most of Greater London. In addition, we are now seeing other major UK cities adopting similar initiatives, including Manchester, Leeds, Birmingham (Craglia et al, 2019), Oxford (Cromar, 2021b) and Bath (Bath and North East Somerset Council, 2021).

As well as seeing the introductions of CAZs in cities, some local authorities are seeking to reduce GHG emissions from vehicles in alternative ways. Several have begun to convert their vehicle fleets from diesel and petrol to electric or hydrogen and several are working with private sector partners such as bus operators to do similar. It is here that we are beginning to see the more relational aspects of partnering come to the fore as councils seek to find ways of tackling climate change and achievement of net-zero targets through commercially sustainable and mutually beneficial partnerships.

At a regional level Liverpool City Region Combined Authority and West Midlands Combined Authority (WMCA) are pursuing plans to deliver bus fleets that are net zero with the former set to agree funding for the provision of 20 hydrogen powered double decker buses and the installation of a hydrogen refuelling facility (Intelligent Transport, 2021). In the West Midlands, the WMCA is providing a £50 million investment in order to make Coventry the first city in the UK to operate an all-electric bus fleet (Coventry City Council, 2021). Leicester City Council are working in partnership with local bus operators to reduce emissions via the grant of £672,000 from the government-backed Joint Air Quality Unit that will see 42 buses adapted to reduce emissions (Leicester City Council, 2021). As well as buses, councils are looking more broadly at their own vehicle fleets (Cromar, 2021a), the provision of rental schemes for more environmentally friendly modes of transport such as e-scooters (Cromar, 2021c), public awareness campaigns that highlight the increased emissions produced when petrol and diesel engines are allowed to idle (Idling Action London, 2021), and funding for training to ensure enough mechanics will be available to meet the increased maintenance burden associated with the anticipated growth in electric vehicles (WMCA, 2021).

Reduction in housing related emissions

Alongside transport, initiatives in net-zero housing are becoming a major focus for councils, with many seeking to combine a need to deliver increased housing targets with a drive to build greener homes. Where new housing schemes are being delivered councils are increasingly partnering with private sector firms that deliver net-zero housing (Hailstone, 2020). Where existing housing stock is being targeted for refurbishment, net-zero retrofit solutions are being sought, most commonly where economies of scale can deliver commercially viable projects for those firms in the private sector who have recognised the opportunity to convert Housing Association and local authority housing stock (Energiesprong UK, 2020).

Clean energy technologies

In other areas related to housing and council operational buildings innovative clean energy technologies are being explored to heat premises in carbon neutral ways. In Aberdeen the council has already achieved a 34 per cent reduction in its own carbon footprint through various initiatives including the connection of 26 public buildings to district heating networks (Aberdeen City Council, 2021). In Welwyn, the local council has secured a £1.7 million grant to replace gas fired boilers with Air Source and Water Source Heat Pumps to heat leisure and entertainment venues (Powell, 2021). On a more novel level, Kingston Council is planning to heat 2,000 homes via a partnership with Thames Water that will see the use of a district heating system to utilise the energy and heat recovered from sewerage treatment facilities located nearby (Royal Borough of Kingston upon Thames, 2021).

Conclusion

The history of global collaboration in tackling climate change sets out clearly what can be achieved through a relational partnering approach between nations. It also shows the vulnerability of this approach to changes in the leadership of some of the most powerful nations who are also some of the largest emitters of carbon. World leaders should recognise the cumulative contribution to carbon emissions by the more developed countries when agreeing to strategies to work with developing countries to reduce the level of emissions for the future. If leaders fail to take this relational approach, they will be challenged by the growing climate activism of their citizens.

Setting targets is not enough on its own to deliver change. The UK government must heed the growing evidence from the Climate Change Committee, the Local Government Association and key environmental and professional organisations that it will not meet its 2050 net-zero target without a fundamental change in its relationship with local government. The response to the COVID-19 pandemic shows the success of local action to address street homelessness, contrasted with the centralised approach to test and trace. Government must recognise the unique role that councils can play in leading their communities through the changes that are necessary to secure a low carbon future, support them with funding and trust them to deliver. It can do this by establishing a joint task force with key players from central and local government who are committed to the relational partnering approach to achieving net zero and adapting to the inevitable changes in climate yet to come.

References

Aberdeen City Council (2021) 'Five-year climate change plan for council approved'. Available at: www.news.aberdeencity.gov.uk/five-year-climate-change-plan-for-council-approved/ (accessed 21 May 2021).

Bath and North East Somerset Council (2021) 'Bath's clean air zone'. Available at: www.beta.bathnes.gov.uk/bath-clean-air-zone (accessed 21 May 2021).

Bolton, P. (2020) 'UK and global emissions and temperature', UK Parliament House of Commons Library. Available at: www.commonslibrary.parliam ent.uk/uk-and-global-emissions-and-temperature-trends/ (accessed 21 May 2021).

British Broadcasting Corporation (2020) 'Climate change: US formally withdraws from Paris agreement'. Available at: www.bbc.co.uk/news/scie nce-environment-54797743 (accessed 24 May 2021).

Climate Change Committee (2014) 'Buildings and infrastructure ill-prepared for changing climate'. Available at: www.theccc.org.uk/2014/07/08/ buildings-and-infrastructure-ill-prepared-for-changing-climate/ (accessed 21 May 2021).

Climate Change Committee (2017) 'UK climate change risk assessment 2017 evidence report'. Available at: www.theccc.org.uk/uk-climate-cha nge-risk-assessment-2017/ (accessed 21 May 2021).

Climate Change Committee (2019) 'Reducing UK emissions 2019 progress report to parliament'. Available at: www.theccc.org.uk/publication/ reducing-uk-emissions-2019-progress-report-to-parliament/ (accessed 21 May 2021).

Coventry City Council (2021) 'All-electric bus city plan commitment by winter 2025'. Available at: www.coventry.gov.uk/news/article/3703/ all-electric_bus_city_plan_commitment_by_winter_2025 (accessed 21 May 2021).

Craglia, C., Gilmore, K., El Helou, I., Khouri, R., Ali, V.P.S. (2019) 'Reducing air pollution, congestion and CO2 emissions from transport across Cambridgeshire', Cambridgeshire County Council and Cambridge University Science and Policy Exchange. Available at: www.data.cambri dgeshireinsight.org.uk/sites/default/files/2019%20CUSPE%20Pol icy%20Challenge%20-%20Reducing%20Air%20Pollution%2C%20Con gestion%20and%20CO2%20Emissions%20from%20Transport%20acr oss%20Cambridgeshire.pdf (accessed 21 May 2021).

Cromar, C. (2021a) 'Manchester City Council's £10m electric refuse vehicle investment', Public Sector Executive. Available at: https://www.publicsect orexecutive.com/articles/manchester-city-councils-ps10m-electric-ref use-vehicle-investmentinvestment?utm_source=Public%20Sector%20Ex ecutive&utm_medium=email&utm_campaign=12235881_Newsletter%20 12%20Mar&dm_i=IJU,7A99L,VQF35Z,TJH6E,1 (accessed 21 May 2021).

Cromar, C. (2021b) 'Oxford's zero emission zone approved by Oxfordshire county council', Public Sector Executive. Available at: www.publicsect orexecutive.com/articles/oxfords-zero-emission-zone-approved-oxfordsh ire-county-council?utm_source=Public%20Sector%20Executive&utm _medium=email&utm_campaign=12252457_Newsletter%2019%20 Mar&dm_i=IJU,7AM21,VQF35Z,TL1ML,1 (accessed 21 May 2021).

Cromar, C. (2021c) 'West of England becomes first UK region to offer e-scooters for long-term rental', Public Sector Executive. Available at: www.publicsectorexecutive.com/articles/west-england-becomes-first-uk-region-offer-e-scooters-long-term-rental?utm_source=Public%20Sec tor%20Executive&utm_medium=email&utm_campaign=12157970_New sletter%20template%209%20Feb&dm_i=IJU,78L5E,VQF35Z,TC5CC,1 (accessed 21 May 2021).

DBEIS (Department for Business, Energy and Industrial Strategy) (2020) 'Final greenhouse gas emissions national statistics: 1990 to 2018'. Available at: www.gov.uk/government/statistics/final-uk-greenhouse-gas-emissi ons-national-statistics-1990-to-2018 (accessed 21 May 2021).

Energiesprong UK (2020) 'Energiesprong UK wins twice in whole house retrofit competition BEIS'. Available at: www.energiesprong.uk/newspage/ energiesprong-uk-wins-twice-in-whole-house-retrofit-competition-beis (accessed 21 May 2021).

Energy and Climate Intelligence Unit (2014) 'Climate change and health'. Available at: www.ca1-eci.edcdn.com/briefings-documents/Climate-cha nge-and-health.pdf?mtime=20190529130630&focal=none (accessed 21 May 2021).

Energy and Climate Intelligence Unit (2016) 'Flood risk and the UK'. Available at: www.ca1-eci.edcdn.com/briefings-documents/Briefing- flood-risk-and-the-UK-updated-for-website.pdf?mtime=20190529125 533&focal=none (accessed 21 May 2021).

Environment Agency (2020) 'The effects of flooding on mental health: Outcomes and recommendations from a review of the literature'. Available at: http://currents.plos.org/disasters/article/the-effects-of-flood ing-on-mental-health-outcomes-and-recommendations-from-a-review- of-the-literature/ (accessed 29 August 2022).

Environmental Journal (2020) 'District council to build its first zero carbon homes'. Hailstone. Available at: www.environmentjournal.online/artic les/district-council-to-build-its-first-zero-carbon-homes/ (accessed 21 May 2021).

The Guardian (2016) 'A history of CO2 emissions'. Available at: www.theg uardian.com/environment/datablog/2009/sep/02/co2-emissions-histori cal (accessed 24 May 2021).

House of Commons Environmental Audit Committee (2018) 'Heatwaves: Adapting to climate change'. Available at: www.publications. parliament.uk/pa/cm201719/cmselect/cmenvaud/826/826.pdf (accessed 21 May 2021).

House of Commons Public Accounts Committee (2021) 'Managing flood risk'. Available at: www.committees.parliament.uk/publications/4827/ documents/48528/default/ (accessed 21 May 2021).

Idling Action London (2021) 'Vehicle idling action'. Available at: www. idlingaction.london/ (accessed 21 May 2021).

IEA (International Energy Agency) (2019) 'World energy outlook 2019'. https://www.iea.org/reports/world-energy-outlook-2019

IEA (International Energy Agency) (2020) 'CO2 emissions from fuel combustion'. Available at: www.energyatlas.iea.org/#!/tellmap/1378539 487 (accessed 24 May 2021).

Intelligent Transport (2021) 'Double decker hydrogen buses to take big step forward in Liverpool'. Available at: www.intelligenttransport.com/transp ort-news/119188/liverpool-hydrogen-buses/ (accessed 21 May 2021).

Kendon, M., McCarthy, M., Jevrajeva, S., Matthews, A. and Legg, T. (2018) 'State of the UK climate 2018', Royal Meteorological Society. Available at: www.rmets.onlinelibrary.wiley.com/doi/abs /10.1002/joc.6213 (accessed 21 May 2021).

Leicester City Council (2021) 'Funding boost to further clean up bus emissions'. Available at: www.news.leicester.gov.uk/news-articles/2021/ february/funding-boost-to-further-clean-up-bus-emissions/ (accessed 21 May 2021).

LGA (Local Government Association) (2021) 'Climate change'. Available at: www.local.gov.uk/topics/environment-and-waste/climate-cha nge#:~:text=Around%20230%20councils%20have%20declared,cha nge%20on%20their%20local%20area (accessed 21 May 2021).

ONS (Office for National Statistics) (2019) 'Road transport and air emissions'. Available at: www.ons.gov.uk/economy/environmentalaccounts/articles/ roadtransportandairemissions/2019-09-16 (accessed 21 May 2021).

Powell, P. (2021) 'Council awarded £1.7m to support climate action commitments', Welwyn Hatfield Times. Available at: www.whtimes.co.uk/ news/welwyn-hatfield-council-decarbonisation-grant-7791120 (accessed 21 May 2021).

Royal Borough of Kingston upon Thames (2021) 'England's first sewage-powered heating scheme planned for Kingston'. Available at: www.kings ton.gov.uk/news/article/80/england-s-first-sewage-powered-heating-sch eme-planned-for-kingston (accessed 21 May 2021).

Union of Concerned Scientists (1992 'World Scientists warning to humanity'. Available at: www.ucsusa.org/sites/default/files/attach/2017/ 11/World%20Scientists%27%20Warning%20to%20Humanity%201992. pdf (accessed 21 May 2021).

Union of Concerned Scientists (2020) 'Each country's share of CO2 emissions'. Available at: www.ucsusa.org/resources/each-countrys-share-co2-emissions (accessed 24 May 2021).

United Nations (1992) 'United Nations Framework Convention on Climate Change'. Available at: www.unfccc.int/files/essential_background/back ground_publications_htmlpdf/application/pdf/conveng.pdf (accessed 21 May 2021).

United Nations (2015) 'Paris Agreement'. Available at: https://unfccc.int/ process-and-meetings/the-paris-agreement/the-paris-agreement (accessed 21 May 2021).

United Nations Framework on Climate Change (2021a) 'History of the convention'. Available at: www.unfccc.int/process/the-convention/hist ory-of-the-convention#eq-1 (accessed 21 May 2021).

United Nations Framework on Climate Change (2021b) 'The Paris Agreement'. Available at: www.unfccc.int/process-and-meetings/the-paris-agreement/the-paris-agreement (accessed 21 May 2021).

WMCA (West Midlands Combined Authority) (2021) 'New centre to train local people to work on electric vehicles opens in Wolverhampton'. Available at: www.wmca.org.uk/news/new-centre-to-train-local-peo ple-to-work-on-electric-vehicles-opens-in-wolverhampton/ (accessed 21 May 2021).

11

Housing policy and provision after COVID-19

Peter Murphy

Introduction

Adequate housing and shelter are undeniably a key factor in the social determinants of the health of the population, and the distribution of health inequality in the UK. The UK, and England in particular, is a densely populated nation and apart from agriculture, housing is the biggest user of land. Making cities and human settlements inclusive, safe, resilient and sustainable is the 11th **Sustainable Development Goal** of the United Nations. The latter sits alongside, inter alia, good health and wellbeing, quality education, decent work and the reduction of poverty and inequality, all of which are influenced by the quality and availability of domestic accommodation.

Housing is also an intrinsic part of the debate about how to tackle and reduce the factors generating climate change and the nature and control of energy. More recently, the physical layout and space standards of property and the family and social structures of those occupying domestic properties has been a key influence of the spread of the COVID-19 pandemic. As security of employment in the UK has weakened, investments in housing have increasingly been perceived as a 'safe haven' or buttress to increasing income insecurity and inadequate state assistance in provision for old age. The economic challenges of Brexit, the global pandemic and the emergence of more authoritarian regimes is exacerbating feelings of insecurity and falling confidence thus increasing already prevalent mental health issues (NHS Digital, 2021).

The complex multidimensional influences that housing has on the health and wellbeing of citizens is evident in the short-, medium- and long-term issues exemplified by the annual winter homeless crises, the response to COVID-19 and the need for long-term social and economic policies to avert the climate crises. This myriad of influences, reciprocities and interrelationships suggest and, in my view require, a comprehensive holistic analysis and a joined-up policy response to housing provision in the UK in the future. Our goal should be to provide appropriate types of accommodation across a range of tenures, for increasingly diverse social and family relationships within a national stock of accommodation.

To start on this long-term ambition, we need to take a comprehensive and holistic approach to evaluating what the country needs to provide in terms of its housing. We need to identify what policy and other systemic drivers need to be put in place to reach the goal of adequately accommodating all of our citizens, given the intention to optimise the contribution that housing makes to a healthy and prosperous society that is built on sustainable forms of development which reduce our impacts on the planet.

This ambition is far beyond the capacity of a single chapter and will require contributions from scientists, policymakers, think tanks, practitioners and academics across a range of disciplines from architecture to sociology. However, if we accept this goal as the purpose of housing in the future and we acknowledge that a comprehensive and holistic approach to policy and delivery is required, where do we start and what can this chapter contribute?

The aim of this chapter is to provide a high-level review of current housing policy across the main forms of domestic accommodation and identify the key drivers and mechanisms currently facilitating, enabling and/or contributing to the delivery of housing, shelter and accommodation in the UK.[1] Are these key drivers facilitating the achievement of the goals and ambitions for the future of housing or are they impeding, frustrating or inhibiting our progress? If the current approach continues where is that taking us to and will it provide the required contributions to both health and environmental sustainability identified by our revised ambitions?

A sectoral-based analysis

There are many ways we can approach this, and many that are both equally valid and important to our understanding of the policy debate. Traditionally, however, discourse in the UK has been conducted from either a social policy perspective (Clapham et al, 1990; Malpass, 2000; Malpass and Mullins, 2010; Madden and Marcuse, 2016) or an economic perspective (Barker, 2004; Marsh and Gibbs, 2011; DCLG, 2017) with increasing ascendency of the latter, particularly since the 2008/2009 recession. It would however be an unwarranted oversimplification to suggest that Labour governments and local authorities have tended to emphasise social policy considerations while Conservative administrations have favoured more economic approaches. Throughout the last century both approaches have had their advocates in all of the major political parties as they have in the more pluralist political party landscape associated with devolved governance of the UK in the 21st century (Anderson, 2020; Farrell et al, 2020). However, since the advent of the 1919 Addison Act, which provided significant subsidies for council house building, and the Homes Fit for Heroes[2] campaign of Lloyd George (1918), the state's duty to provide decent housing has been generally acknowledged across the political parties although what this has meant in practice has been continually contested within and between the parties.

Since 1919, this discourse has predominantly focused on the numbers and contributions of the public, private and third sectors to housing provision, and the regulatory regime and quality of housing to be provided. Successive governments have wrestled with the constraints on housing supply in a densely populated country with private ownership of land, which at the same time has been experiencing increased household formation and increased longevity of its citizens and hence growing long-term demand (Keohane and Broughton, 2013). As Glenda Roberts points out in the second volume of this series, the costs of housing and the ageing demography in the UK means the cost of care in old age can be 'profoundly influenced by housing provision' (Roberts, 2020: 229) and the Institute for Fiscal Studies recently calculated that Adult Social Care spending could rise from 30 per cent in 2018 to 50 per cent of all revenue from local taxes by 2035 (Amin-Smith et al, 2018).

Private sector

While Conservative administrations have generally favoured more economic approaches to housing policy and delivery this has become more explicit since the Conservative administrations of 1979–1997. The election of Margaret Thatcher was a watershed in terms of public housing as she facilitated one of the largest privatisations and transfer of public assets to private ownership through the sale of land and council houses (Meek, 2015; Edwards, 2017; Christophers, 2018). Her administrations also changed the approach to the provision of housing, re-emphasising the private sector as she sought to realise the 'property-owning democracy' first envisaged by Conservatives in the 1930s. The discourse on housing supply also became increasingly focused on the supply of available building land and the (alleged) inadequacies of the planning system in maintaining this supply, rather than the provision of a range of housing types and tenures to meet the needs of an increasingly diverse and expanding number of households. The result in terms of sectoral change is apparent in Figures 11.1a, b, and c.

A requirement on local planning authorities to have available (at least) a five-year land bank suitable for housing was introduced in the 1980s, albeit with a name change to 'sustainable housing land' from 2004. The issue dominates local planning inquiries as all local planning authorities are required to demonstrate that they have sufficient land that is suitable, available and achievable, and that any constraints to their sites can be overcome within a reasonable period. Much of this land is either owned or is under contractual 'options' by private landowners and in particular a decreasing number of

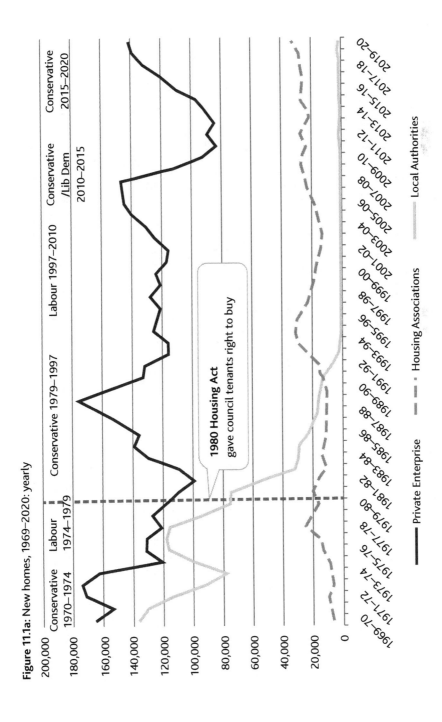

Figure 11.1a: New homes, 1969–2020: yearly

Figure 11.1b: New homes, 1969–2020: every three years

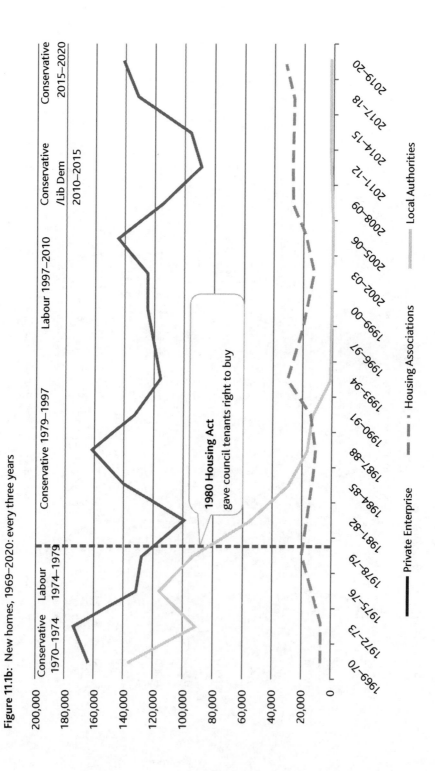

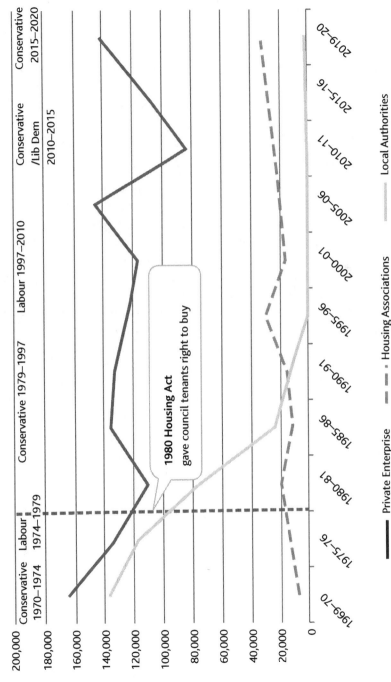

Figure 11.1c: New homes, 1969–2020: every five years

Source: MHCLG Housing Statistics. Ministry of Housing, Communities and Local Government is now the Department for Levelling Up, Housing and Communities. Figures 11.1a–c are live tables from the Office of National Statistics, available as part of Live tables on housing supply at https://www.gov.uk/government/statistical-data-sets/live-tables-on-affordable-housing-supply

'volume' housebuilders effectively operating within an oligopolistic market (Jenrick, 2020).

The Ministry of Housing, Communities and Local Government (MHCLG) conducts a Housing Delivery Test which is an annual measurement of housing delivery for which there is a methodological rule book (MHCLG, 2021a). These assessments have gradually moved to considering aggregate numbers as opposed to details of housing types. Similarly, there have been greater relaxations in changes of use and permitted development rights (Walker Morris, 2021). Housing demand has gradually come to be defined by market demand with a shrinking range of units and ownership models. Dwellings constructed by small and medium sized enterprises and by self-builders are a small and diminishing feature of housing provision in the UK (Jenrick, 2020) despite all the television programmes devoted to them.

One other long-term trend in housing provision that has been highlighted by the pandemic is the rising numbers of care homes and retirement villages and the change in their ownership status. There are now approximately 20,000 care homes in the UK catering for nearly half a million residents and predominantly owned by private companies or third sector housing associations (Competition and Markets Authority, 2017). The Office for National Statistics predicts a 36 per cent growth in persons aged 85+ between 2015 and 2025, from 1.5 million to 2 million. This is expected to lead to a substantial increase in demand for care and residential home services. The Competition and Markets Authority found that the current model of service provision cannot be sustained without additional public funding. The parts of the industry that supply primarily local authority clients are unlikely to be sustainable at the current rates that local authorities pay and 'significant reforms are needed to enable the sector to grow to meet the expected substantial increase in care needs' (HMG, 2017).

Affordability

The rate of housebuilding has lagged behind the UK's natural population growth and net immigration, with long-term household formation estimated as between 270,000 and 300,000 per year. Between 1979 and 1990 approximately 220,000 homes were constructed annually by private builders, local authorities and housing associations. That fell under the Major administration to approximately 190,000, rose slightly under Tony Blair but slumped because of the 2008/2009 recession. Prior to the COVID-19 pandemic it had recovered to approximately 170,000 completions in 2019 (although starts were only 151,020 in the same period), 79 per cent by private builders, 19 per cent by housing associations and less than 2 per cent by local authorities (MHCLG, 2021b). This has resulted in long-term upward pressure and above inflation increases in house prices.

One area where the government has therefore become more active is in the affordability of dwellings. In fact, since the 1980s affordability has become an enduring feature of housing policy in Europe and North America. Since the 2008/2009 financial crisis, the homes shortage has become more acute and ever more politically contentious.

Affordable housing includes social rented, affordable rented and intermediate housing, provided to specified eligible households whose needs are not met by the market. It can be a new-build property or a private sector property that has been purchased for use as an affordable home. The Department for Levelling Up, Housing and Communities (DLUHC, formerly MHCLG) publish annual statistics on affordable housing supply in England which show the gross annual supply of affordable homes, which includes new build and acquisitions from the private sector but does not take account of losses through demolitions or sales. The number of affordable homes delivered under the various government initiatives and schemes is shown in Figure 11.2. This has remained stubbornly low in overall terms despite the plethora of recent initiatives.

Since the recession low interest rates have meant land and houses became attractive investments not least because of the rise in prices. The UK-wide median house price rose to 7.7 times median annual earnings in 2017 – an all-time high and up from 3.5 times in 1998. The demand–supply mismatch is greatest in London and the South East – house prices were 12.2 times and 9.1 times earnings respectively in 2016 (Philip, 2017), and all evidence suggests this trend will continue.

Nevertheless, the government continues to promote ownership schemes over public rental provision. The most notorious recent scheme was the Starter Homes Scheme announced in April 2015. The government committed to delivering 200,000 Starter Homes to be sold at a 20 per cent discount and available exclusively for first-time buyers under the age of 40. It provided £2.3 billion to support the delivery of 60,000 of these planned homes. Not a single home was completed (Public Accounts Committee, 2020).

The other long-term change in housing provision has been in household tenure. Table 11.1 shows the latest figures available from the Department of Work and Pensions and although these figures are for 2017 there is little doubt this trend continues. It shows significant increases in private rented homes and decreases in buying with mortgages. It also shows a long-term shift away from public sector provision. The Office for National Statistics' Index of Private Housing Rental Prices indicates a long-term rise in average rental levels. Although tax allowances for 'Buy to Let' mortgages have reduced, borrowers are still entitled to credit on interest payments or other benefits if they choose to set up private limited companies.

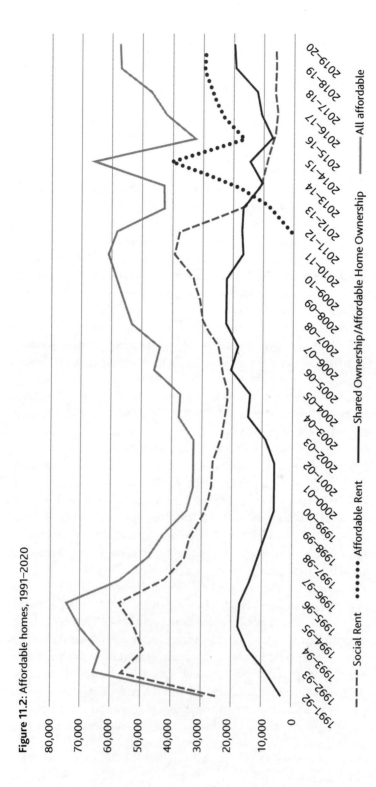

Figure 11.2: Affordable homes, 1991–2020

Source: Office for National Statistics 2022 Housing Statistics Live Table 1000: additional affordable homes provided by type of scheme, England part of Live tables on affordable housing supply at https://www.gov.uk/government/statistical-data-sets/live-tables-on-affordable-housing-supply

Table 11.1: Housing tenure, 2007 and 2017

Tenure	2007	2017
Owned outright	31	34
Buying with mortgage	37	28
Private rented	13	20
Social rented	18	17

Source: Department for Work and Pensions; compiled by author from annual Family Resources 'Tenure' statistics from ONS, 'Live tables on affordable housing supply', at https://www.gov.uk/gov ernment/statistical-data-sets/live-tables-on-affordable-housing-supply

Local authorities

Figures 11.1a, b, and c show the decline in the number of social houses built by local authorities, although the number of houses owned by local authorities in arm's-length trusts and commercial housing companies is larger. It is estimated as between 1 and 1.5 million, but the exact number is difficult to disentangle as some operate as housing associations. Broughton (2018) subtitled his book *Municipal Dreams* as *The Rise and Fall of Council Housing*. In it he traces the history of council housing and the contribution social housing has made to housing provision since the 1918 Addison Act.

Broughton, among others (Mullins and Murie, 2006; Lund, 2017), also provides a long-term view of housing policy under successive Conservative and Labour administrations. From the 1920s and 1930s he traces a policy shift that reflects broad divisions between the two main political parties in England, although he acknowledges that this is very broad and that there are many alternative views held at various times in both political traditions. He gleans a difference between Conservative politicians who believed council housing should properly be reserved for those most in need assuming that the market would provide for the rest, and those to the left who see social housing more broadly as making a contribution to general needs. The latter of course dominated the slum clearance eras before and after the Second World War and well into the 1960s.

Broughton sees the National Rent rebate scheme in 1973 (which became Housing Benefit in 1982) and the 1977 Housing (Homeless Persons) Act, which prioritised council housing for the most vulnerable and introduced or entrenched 'needs based allocations', as critical to the gradual hegemony of the Conservative approach which he characterises as 'residulisation'. Residualisation is the increasing confinement of social housing to the poorest. Right to buy and the cessation of new builds followed in the 1980s (see Figures 11.1a, b, and c).

However, he also detects a stronger variant emerging originally from the introduction of notions of 'welfare', which previously we had referred to as social security (Fitzpatrick and Watts, 2017; Broughton, 2018: 257):

> Since 2010 and more so since the return of single party Conservative Government in 2015 we've seen something further a welfarisation a conceptualisation of social housing as a very small highly residualised sector catering only for the very poorest and those with additional social 'vulnerabilities' on a short term 'ambulance' basis.

Welfarism has also attempted to end lifetime security of tenure for those in social housing (Parkin and Wilson, 2016). This occurred both under the Coalition government when it introduced short-term tenancies in 2011 (Shapps, 2010) and the bedroom tax in 2013, and the later Conservative government also attempted to introduce higher rents for tenants on higher incomes with the common assumption being that social housing should only be for the poorest sections of the population.

Housing associations

There are approximately 800 housing associations providing accommodation for approximately 6 million people in the UK. The National Housing Federation website, which is the national 'voice' of associations, provides an excellent summary of the history of housing associations from at least 1235, 'when an alms house in Cirencester was established to offer shelter for the seriously ill'. It goes on to note that '[t]he modern housing association movement was born in the late 19th century, when Victorian philanthropists set up charitable housing trusts to help homeless people and alleviate poverty, but for the first half of the 20th century, housing association homes made up a relatively small proportion of social housing overall' (National Housing Federation, 2022) although it often provided specialist provision for the poorest and most deprived (see also Malpass, 2000; Malpass and Mullins, 2010).

In the 1960s and 1970s, despite the boom in housebuilding, rising homelessness became more visible and the 1974 Housing Act provided public funding for associations to build social housing. In the late 1980s they could access private finance in addition to public funds. In 2000–2010 many local authorities transferred their social housing into housing association ownership through Large-Scale Voluntary Transfer agreements and improvements to this stock were provided through the Labour government's Decent Homes initiative announced in 2000. This sought to provide a minimum standard of housing conditions for all those housed in the non-private sector – that is, council housing and housing associations (DCLG Select Committee, 2010).

In 2010 the Coalition government, through its main funding agency (Homes England), reduced the support for affordable housing and housing associations had to generate their own income. Nevertheless, associations played a significant role in providing affordable homes to both rent and purchase through a variety of support schemes such as shared ownership models, care homes, low interest loans and sheltered housing schemes. However, from 1 April 2016 the Welfare Reform and Work Act and its regulations required registered providers of social housing in England to reduce social housing rents by 1 per cent a year for four years from a 'frozen' 2015/2016 baseline and to comply with maximum rent requirements for new tenancies. In each of four 'relevant years' registered providers of social housing must reduce the total rent payable by a tenant per year by 1 per cent. This reduced the resources available to associations to fund operations and investments.

In its response to the pandemic the government initially froze local housing allowances (LHAs) in real terms and later announced they would be frozen in cash terms in 2021. The Office for Budget Responsibility calculated that:

> [The government] has now decided that rates will be frozen in cash terms from 2021–22 onwards. This means the £1 billion cost of the measure in 2020–21 declines to £0.3 billion by 2025–26 (and that LHA rates will fall back below the 30th percentile of local rents over time). (Office for Budget Responsibility, 2020: 179)

The UK has a target to bring all its greenhouse gas emissions to net zero by 2050. Housing associations strongly support decarbonisation, as an essential part of tackling climate change, as 'it also saves residents money, helps combat fuel poverty, boosts the economy and creates jobs' but they face challenges such as lack of finance and skills shortages. Inside Housing (2020) reported the estimated cost of making social homes net-zero carbon by 2050 at £3.5 billion per year. The National Housing Federation campaigned for a Social Housing Decarbonisation Fund (SHDF) and in September 2020 the government formally launched the SHDF as a £50 million UK-wide 'demonstrator' scheme to provide government grants to upgrade the energy efficiency of over 2,000 of the country's worst-performing social homes with a further £60 million in 2021/2022. Seventeen projects were selected to receive a share of the SHDF. The second wave 'competition' (wave 2.1) to allocate this funding was published in July 2022 (DBE&IS, 2022).

Over the last decade, homelessness and rough sleeping has increased both nationally and in all the major cities in the UK. Long-term data is available through the Crises Homelessness Monitor (Crises, 2020), Homeless Link (2020) and the government's Official Statutory Homelessness Figures (MHCLG, 2020a), although the latter show that approximately half of the people who apply for help are judged to fall outside of the statutory definitions of those eligible for help. Government policy responsibility for tackling homelessness now sits with the DLUHC, while the delivery of services to support homeless people is the responsibility of local authorities.

People who experience homelessness, particularly those who are persistent rough sleepers, often also experience relatively poor health particularly in relation to respiratory and mental diseases. Increasing levels of poverty, the rising costs of accommodation and greater social and health inequalities have generated increased homelessness (Wilkinson and Pickett, 2009, 2018).

Pre–COVID-19 research suggests that people who are homeless experience barriers to accessing healthcare at three different but related levels (Campbell et al, 2015):

- Individual-level barriers which can include issues such as mental health (for example, anxiety and/or depression), emotional barriers (for example, fear or embarrassment) and/or alternative day-to-day priorities.
- Provider-level barriers which can include difficulties registering, negative attitudes of staff (for example, lack of empathy or understanding), time to address mental health concerns and geographical barriers (for example, proximity to services and transport).
- System-level barriers which can include the way healthcare services are or aren't integrated with other support services, and/or financial factors.

In an earlier volume Maguire (2018: 227) argued that 'an understanding of the relationship between the individual and their environment is necessary to understand the behaviours that lead to homelessness and rough sleeping'. He suggested that understanding these relationships, which are inherently complex, together with empirically based theory and practice are essential to make progress on reducing homelessness. An individualised approach with co-ordinated wraparound or integrated care and support generally known as 'Housing First' has been a relatively recent feature in Europe and North America (Bellis and Wilson, 2018) which has been spotlighted by the radical 'Everyone In' response to the pandemic in England (MHCLG, 2020b). It is an alternative homelessness intervention strategy, aimed at rough sleepers with complex needs, implemented during and since the first wave of the pandemic.

The Housing First approach does not require homeless people with complex needs to demonstrate 'housing readiness' before being offered permanent accommodation as in the traditional approach. Instead, homeless individuals are immediately rehoused in permanent accommodation and offered floating support services to tackle their other needs. The rationale behind Housing First is based on the idea that 'once the chaos of homelessness is eliminated from a person's life, clinical and social stabilisation occur faster and are more enduring' (Shelter, 2008; Blood et al, 2017). At its core is an open-ended offer of intensive high-quality holistic support and it cannot achieve the positive outcomes that it does without this intensive support being available. It also explains how it differs from other housing-led homeless projects (Homeless Link, 2015).

In 2018, the government Rough Sleeping Strategy (MHCLG, 2018) committed the government to 'halve rough sleeping in this Parliament and to end it for good by 2027'. It announced £28 million of funding to establish the Housing First programme. It also identified 83 local authorities it intended to work with on homelessness and commissioned three conurbation-wide Housing First pilot projects in Greater Manchester, Liverpool and the West Midlands (Blood et al, 2017). In December 2019 the Conservative manifesto committed to ending 'the blight of rough sleeping by the end of the next Parliament (2027)' through an extension of the Rough Sleeping Initiative, Housing First initiatives and using local services to meet the health and housing needs of people living on the streets. This would involve a significant increase in public expenditure.

In the first wave of the pandemic temporary accommodation was provided for rough sleepers as part of the government's Everyone In initiative (MHCLG, 2020b). People experiencing homelessness, particularly those who are rough sleeping, are clearly severely vulnerable during a pandemic. They are three times more likely to experience a chronic health condition including respiratory conditions such as chronic obstructive pulmonary disease. It is not possible to self-isolate or follow sanitation guidance if you are sleeping rough or living in shared homelessness accommodation. The successful Everyone In initiative provided hotel and emergency accommodation and adopted a public health approach, regardless of pre-existing tests as to who might qualify for statutory homelessness assistance. Funds of £3.2 million were allocated to local authorities in England to protect people who are homeless from COVID-19.

The government also raised the LHA rate to the 30th percentile of local rents to stem the rise of new homelessness cases. They suspended evictions from Home Office asylum accommodation and from the private and social rented sectors. In May 2020 Louise Casey was appointed to chair a taskforce on rough sleeping, which was to work with local authorities to ensure rough sleepers could move into long-term, safe accommodation once the immediate crisis was over – ensuring as few people as possible returned to life on the streets. In addition to announcing £52 million of additional funding, £160 million of rough sleeping services budget were brought forward and reprofiled over four years to stop a return to the streets. This funding was intended to ensure that 6,000 new housing units would be put into the system, with 3,300 of these becoming available 'within the next 12 months'.

Unfortunately, there was a partial return to the streets as the first wave of COVID-19 receded. In November the government provided a national briefing on the Rough Sleeping initiative entitled *Everyone In: Continuing to Reduce Rough Sleeping*, which included an update of the government's policies on the:

- continuation of funded services;
- delivery of new services;
- launch of the Next Steps Accommodation Programme.

This suggested that a social policy and health-based approach might continue to be part of the services provided to the homeless – within a broader based approach embracing the wider or 'social' determinants of health. In Scotland the Scottish Government (2021a) published its first long-term national housing strategy and its first anti-destitution strategy (Scottish Government 2021b), the latter specifically targeted at people with 'no recourse to public funds' (NRPF). NRPF designation restricts access to essential state support for groups such as those forced to seek sanctuary from violence and persecution, who are a significant group within both rough sleepers and the homeless generally. These strategies, which adopt a more holistic and joined-up approach, are underpinned by the assumption that decent housing is a fundamental human right (Scottish Government, 2021c).

In England the National Audit Office reported that in England, Everyone In had helped to house more than 33,000 people by the end of November 2020 and by June 2020 there had been only 16 deaths of homeless people linked to COVID-19. However, it also made clear that the scale of the rough sleeping population in England was far beyond the government's estimates. By November 2020, 23,273 people had been moved into more settled accommodation, with 9,868 people remaining in hotels and other emergency accommodation. When the Prime Minster made his original pledge to end rough sleeping by 2024 the 'official' count reported 4,266 people sleeping on the streets on any given night in England, not the 33,139 helped by Everyone In. 'Understanding the size of this population, and who needs specialist support, is essential to achieve its ambition to end rough sleeping' (NAO, 2021).

However, from June 2020 homelessness effectively became deprioritised. In August 2021, Shelter (Garvie et al, 2021) reported that 77 per cent of those helped by Everyone In where no longer in 'settled accommodation', Citizens Advice (2021) calculated that rent arrears were affecting over half a million privately renting households and although the temporary eviction ban on landlords was extended it was allowed to lapse later in the year. The ending of the temporary uplift to Universal Credit, the huge increase in demand for mental health and drug and alcohol services and the government's continuing underfunding of local authorities meant providing wraparound care was increasingly challenging. Everyone In was reintroduced immediately before the parliamentary recess in December 2021 but by then appeared to be a temporary response to the onset of the third wave of the pandemic caused by the Omicron variant rather than a fundamental shift in the government's approach.

Conclusion

If the long-term ambition is to provide, facilitate or enable appropriate types of accommodation across a range of tenures, for an increasing number of diverse social and family relationships within the national stock of accommodation, the government's policy and its preferred means of delivery needs to radically change. Increased dependence on private sector supply of accommodation, marketisation and the long-term privatisation of public assets has been pursued by all governments since it was introduced by Margaret Thatcher (Meek, 2015; Christophers, 2018). It has clearly and repeatedly failed. The pandemic has highlighted and exacerbated fundamental inadequacies in the policy and delivery of housing that has now persisted for decades, and these are growing not declining.

Everyone In and Housing First (properly implemented and funded) may be part of the solution to housing and homelessness (particularly rough sleeping) in England but poverty, inequality, insufficient and inadequate accommodation and housing policy and finance are longer-term drivers.

The contribution that housing and shelter makes to health and wellbeing has been obvious to social and economic reformers since before the Industrial Revolution. Sustainably built accommodation is a key part of the Sustainable Development Goals and has been technically feasible for many years.

Despite multiple policy initiatives and architectural demonstrations, the UK needs radical changes in the design and performance of current and future buildings to reduce energy consumption and its corresponding environmental impact. It needs a 'volte face' in housing policy and delivery and increased commitment to sustainable development of the kind seen in the US following the presidential election.

The UK government's purely economic approach continues to fail even on its own terms and the focus must return to a social policy perspective. The objectives must be set within the long-term ambitions of reducing global warming and the use of limited non-renewable resources. The purpose should be to provide adequate and affordable housing in a variety of forms and tenures while reducing housing inequality, homelessness and the proportion of income that households are required to devote to their accommodation.

This will require fundamental changes in land ownership, planning and building control, as well as the encouragement and discouragement of more socially responsible behaviours and activities and changes in the goods and services we produce and consume. This radical agenda will require changes in the key financial levers and a greater role for local authorities and the public sector. England needs a sea change in its approach to both policy and delivery of housing.

Notes

[1] For the purposes of this chapter, 'housing' will be used as a generic term to embrace all forms of shelter, accommodation lodging and places to live, both domestic and institutional.

[2] He referred to '[h]abitations fit for the heroes who have won the war' but Homes Fit for Heroes was how the press presented it at the time.

References

Amin-Smith, N., Phillips, D. and Simpson, P. (2018) *Adult Social Care Funding: A Local or National Responsibility? Briefing Note BN227*. London: Institute for Fiscal Studies.

Anderson, I. (2020) Devolution and the health of Scottish housing policy. In A. Bonner (ed) *Local Authorities and the Social Determinants of Health*. Bristol: Policy Press.

Barker, K. (2004) *Review of Housing Supply: Delivering Stability: Securing Our Future Housing Needs*. London: TSO.

Bellis, A. and Wilson, W. (2018) *Housing First: Tackling Homelessness for Those with Complex Needs*. House of Commons Briefing Paper Number 08368.

Blood, I., Copeman, I., Goldup, M., Pleace, N., Bretherton, J. and Dulson, S. (2017) *Housing First Feasibility Study of the Liverpool City Region*. London: Crises.

Broughton, J. (2018) *Municipal Dreams: The Rise and Fall of Council Housing*. London: Verso.

Campbell, D.J.T., O'Neil, B., Gibson, K. and Thurston, W. (2015) Primary healthcare needs and barriers to care among Calgary's homeless population. *BMC Family Practice*, 16(139).

Christophers, B. (2018) *The New Enclosure: The Appropriation of Public Land in Neo-liberal Britain*. London: Verso.

Citizens Advice (2021) Half a million renters in arrears as evictions set to resume. Available at: https://www.citizensadvice.org.uk/cymraeg/amda nom-ni/about-us1/media/press-releases/half-a-million-renters-in-arre ars-as-evictions-set-to-resume/. Accessed on 29 August 2022.

Clapham, D., Kemp, P. and Smith, S.J. (1990) *Housing and Social Policy*. London: Palgrave.

Competition and Markets Authority (2017) *Care Homes Market Study: Summary of Final Report*. London: CMA. Available at: https://www. gov.uk/government/organisations/competition-and-markets-authority. Accessed on 29 August 2022.

Crises (2020) *Homelessness Monitor*. Available at: https://www.crisis.org.uk/ending-homelessness/homelessness-knowledge-hub/homelessness-monitor/england/homelessness-monitor-england-2020-covid-19-crisis-response-briefing/. Accessed on 29 August 2022.

DBE and IS (Department of Business, Energy and Industrial Strategy) (2022) *Social Housing Decarbonisation Fund Wave 2.1 Competition Guidance Notes*. London: TSO

DCLG (2015) *Accelerating Housing Supply and Increasing Tenant Choice in the Private Rented Sector: A Build to Rent Guide for Local Authorities*. London: TSO. Available at: https://assets.publishing.service.gov.uk/government/uploads/system/uploads/attachment_data/file/416611/150323_Accelerating_Housing_Supply_and_Increasing_Tenant_Choice_in_the_Private_Rented_Sector.pdf. Accessed on 29 August 2022.

DCLG (2017) *Fixing Our Broken Housing Market*. London: TSO. Available at: https://homeless.org.uk/knowledge-hub/2020-annual-review-of-single-homelessness-support-in-england/ Accessed on 20 August 2022.

Edwards, C. (2017) Margaret Thatcher's privatization legacy. *Cato Journal*, 37: 89–101.

Farrell, C., Law, J. and Thomas, S. (2020) Public health and local government in Wales: Every policy a health policy – a collaborative agenda. In A. Bonner (ed) *Local Authorities and the Social Determinants of Health*. Bristol: Policy Press.

Fitzpatrick, S. and Watts, B (2017) Competing visions, security of tenure and the welfarisation of English social housing. *Housing Studies*, 20(3): 1021–1038.

Garvie, D., Rich, H., Berry, C. and Brown, R. (2021) *Everyone In: Where Are They Now? The Need for a Roadmap out of Street Homelessness in England*. London: Shelter.

HMG (2017) Competition and markets annual concurrency report. Available at: https://www.gov.uk/government/publications/competition-and-markets-authority-annual-concurrency-report-2017. Accessed on 28 August 2022.

Homeless Link (2015) *'Housing First' or 'Housing Led'? The Current Picture of Housing First in England*. London: Homeless Link.

Homeless Link (2020) Facts, Figures and Information. Available at: https://homeless.org.uk/knowledge-hub/2020-annual-review-of-single-homelessness-support-in-england/. Accessed on 29 August 2022.

Inside Housing (2020) Making social homes net-zero carbon by 2050 will cost £3.5bn a year, says Savills. *Inside Housing*, 2 December.

Jenrick, R. Rt Hon. (2020) Robert Jenrick's speech on planning for the future delivered at the Creating Communities Conference 2020, 21 September. Available at: https://www.createstreets.com/wp-content/uploads/2020/10/Creating-Communities-2020.pdf. Accessed 3 March 2021.

Keohane, N. and Broughton, N. (2013) *Hot House: The Politics of Housing.* London: National Housing Federation.

Lund, B. (2017) *Understanding Housing Policy*, 3rd edition. Bristol: Policy Press.

Madden, D. and Marcuse, P. (2016) *In Defence Housing.* London: Verso.

Maguire N., Towards an integrative theory of homelessness and rough sleeping. In Bonner A. (ed) *Social Determinants of Health: Social Inequality and Wellbeing.* Policy Press.

Malpass, P. (2000) *Housing Associations and Housing Policy: A Historical Perspective.* London: Macmillan.

Malpass, P. and Mullins, D. (2010) Local authority stock transfer in the UK: From local initiative to national policy. *Housing Studies*, 17(4): 673–686.

Marsh, A. and Gibb, K. (eds) (2011) *Housing Economics.* London: SAGE.

Meek, J. (2015) *Private Island: Why Britain Now Belongs to Someone Else.* London: Verso.

MHCLG (2018) The rough sleeping strategy. 13 August. Available at: https://www.gov.uk/government/publications/the-rough-sleeping-strategy. Accessed on 28 August 2022.

MHCLG (2020a) Statutory homelessness in England (live table). Available at: Live tables on homelessness - GOV.UK (www.gov.uk). Accessed on 27 January 2021.

MHCLG (2020b) Press release. Available at: https://www.gov.uk/governm ent/news/105-million-to-keep-rough-sleepers-safe-and-off-the-streets-during-coronavirus-pandemic. Accessed 5 March 2020.

MHCLG (2021a) *Housing Delivery Test: 2020 Measurement Rule Book.* London: MHCLG.

MHCLG (2021b) *Housing Supply: Indicators of New Supply, England January to June 2020 Housing Statistical Release.* London: MHCLG.

Mullins, D. and Murie, A. (2006) *Housing Policy in the UK.* Basingstoke: Palgrave Macmillan.

NAO (2021) *Investigation into the Housing of Rough Sleepers during the COVID-19 Pandemic.* London: NAO.

National Housing Federation (2022) The History of Housing Associations. Available at: https://www.housing.org.uk/. Accessed on 4 January 2022.

NHS Digital (2021)Mental Health Services Monthly Statistics Final November, Provisional, December. Available at: https://www.housing.org.uk/about-housing-associations/the-history-of-housing-associations/. Accessed on 29 August 2022.

Office for Budget Responsibility (2020) Economic and Fiscal Outlook. November 2020. CP 318. Page 179.

Parkin, E. and Wilson, W. (2016) Social Housing: The End of 'Lifetime' Tenancies in England? House of Commons Library. Briefing Paper 07173.

Philip, P. (2017) *Homes for Everybody.* London: Centre for Policy Studies.

Public Accounts Committee (2020) Starter Homes Thirty-First Report of Session 2019–21. HC 88.

Roberts, G. (2020) The cost of care if you don't own your home. In A. Bonner (ed) *Local Authorities and the Social Determinants of Health*. Bristol: Policy Press.

Scottish Government (2021a) *Housing to 2040*. Edinburgh: Scottish Government.

Scottish Government (2021b) *Ending Destitution Together*. Edinburgh: Scottish Government.

Scottish Government (2021c) *Ending Homelessness Together: Annual Report 2021*. Edinburgh: Scottish Government.

Shapps, G. (2010) Written Statement to Parliament: Localism and Social Housing. 9 December. House of Commons Hansard. Available at: https://hansard.parliament.uk/commons/2010-12-09/debates/10120948000017/LocalismBillAndSocialHousing. Accessed on 29 August 2022.

Shelter (2008) Housing First: Bringing Permanent Solutions to Homeless People with Complex Needs. Good practice: Briefing. London: Shelter.

Stilwell, M. (2017) Housing the returning soldiers 'Homes Fit for Heroes'. *Social Housing History*. Available at Homes_Fit_For_Heroes.pdf (socialhousinghistory.uk. Accessed 22 August 2022.

Walker Morris (2021) Planning Relaxations for Commercial Property. 10 February. Available at: https://www.walkermorris.co.uk/in-brief/planning-relaxations-for-commercial-property/. Accessed on 7 March 2021.

Wilkinson, R. and Pickett, K. (2009) *The Spirit Level 2009: Why Equality is Better for Everyone*. London: Penguin.

Wilkinson, R. and Pickett, K. (2018) *The Inner Level Review: How More Equal Societies Reduce Stress and Improve Wellbeing*. London: Allen Lane.

12

Employment and support

Elizabeth Taylor, Andrew Morton and Annie Dell

Introduction

In this chapter we will explore active labour market interventions in employment and health. We will look back at those interventions offered to people with health conditions as well as the role of local authorities and their place as partner with the employability sector. This chapter will conclude by focusing on those programmes that prioritise people. This begins with a mapping of those key employment support policies of the last 30 years or so, leading up to the current day.

Employment support interventions

Supported Employment: Traditionally, employment interventions targeting people with health conditions and disabilities were delivered by local authorities, often at a county council level, as part of their then statutory duties to provide services for people with learning disabilities. These were usually focused on Day Service facilities, but from this emerged the Supported Employment policy. Supported Employment had set the scene for all future health and disability provisions and became a model for supporting people with significant disabilities to secure and retain paid employment (Wilson and Finch, 2021). This was based on the premise that anyone could be employed if they wanted paid employment and if they were provided sufficient support. Supported Employment has sometimes been called the 'place, train and maintain' model of vocational rehabilitation. Supported Employment providers use a five-stage process itself based on a model of Customer Engagement, Vocational Profiling, Employer Engagement, Job Matching, In-work Support and Career Development.

In the contemporary period, many local authorities still fund Supported Employment services, others have ended these services due to lack of funding and, in some instances, has been picked up by national and local third sector organisations. There has been some Department of Work and Pensions (DWP) interest in Supported Employment with a DWP Proof of Concept Pilot which followed the publication of the 'Improving Lives: The Work,

Health and Disability Green Paper' consultation in 2017. This, however, has been overshadowed by nationally procured programmes and those of the devolved commissioners.

The District Managers Discretionary Fund: In the mid-1990s there were some locally procured Employment Service contracts (now known as DWP Jobcentre Plus), these contracts tested approaches by community-based organisations delivering services to people with health conditions and disabilities.

New Deal and the Flexible New Deal: In 1998, the Labour government introduced the New Deal funded by a one-off £5 billion windfall tax on privatised utility companies. Although originally targeting the young unemployed (18- to 24-year-olds), the New Deal programmes subsequently targeted other groups. This saw compulsory programmes for young people and the long-term unemployed and voluntary programmes for lone parents and disabled people. The mainstream New Deal had options including work experience with community and environmental organisations. The main New Deal contract became the Flexible New Deal in October 2009 in most locations, while New Deal remained in others, and all ended in 2011.

New Deal for Disabled People: The Labour government's New Deal programme ran from 1998 to 2011 but came with other attached 'New Deals' that ran alongside it. This included the New Deal for Disabled People (NDDP). After a NDDP pilot that ran from 1998 to 2000, this became a national provision in 2001 and ran until 2006. NDDP was Labour's main employment programme for people in receipt of a disability or incapacity-related benefit. Between September 1998 and June 2001 12 Personal Advisor Pilot schemes were run on an area basis where a personal advisor assisted people claiming incapacity benefits; six were run by the Employment Service (now known as Jobcentre Plus) and six were run by partnerships of private and voluntary organisations.

Workprep, Workstep, and the Job Introduction Scheme: From 2005 to 2010, the DWP funded Workprep, Workstep and the Job Introduction Scheme. This was replaced by a single 'Work Choice' programme in October 2010. The Workstep programme provided support to disabled people facing complex barriers to getting and keeping a job. Key figures from Workstep show 14,200 people in supported employment in April 2005 and 13,450 in June 2010. Workprep was a flexible, individually tailored programme that could help prepare individuals for a return to work. Workprep could help to: identify the type of work most suitable for an individual; gain work experience in a work environment; learn new skills or update old ones; and, lastly, build confidence. The programme did not last for a specific length of time and most participants were on it for between six and 13 weeks. At the end of a programme, the provider completed a final report and gave a copy to the participant and to their Disability Employment Adviser (DEA). Jobcentre

Plus DEAs are found in every Jobcentre in the country and work alongside Jobcentre Plus Work Coaches, specialising in finding the right support to help clients who have a disability or health condition into work. Jobcentre Plus DEAs identify and refer participants onto the DWP commissioned provisions. DEAs are key to making outsourced health and disability programmes a success. The participant and the DEA would agree an action plan, which may have included looking for work, training or further education.

Work Choice: In 2010 the DWP funded a new specialist health provision called 'Work Choice', which replaced Workprep, Workstep and the Job Introduction Scheme. Work Choice was for disabled people who could not receive help through other work programmes, Access to Work or workplace adjustments. Work Choice provided more specialist support and it ensured employers got the support they needed to employ disabled people. Work Choice was based on two modules: Pre-employment Support; and an In Work Support Module. There were 28 package areas for Work Choice delivered by nine prime contract holders and Remploy held one national contract. This, along with the Work Programme, constituted the launch of the DWP's 'prime' contractor payment-by-results model.

Work Programme: This programme was a payment-by-results scheme that replaced the New Deal in 2011. This had nine payment groups based on age, length of unemployment, benefits claimed, health conditions and prison leavers. The DWP's Work Programme commenced in a limited number of areas in November 2011 but was followed by a complete rollout in January 2012. The Work Programme ran alongside the Work Choice programme.

Work and Health Programme: The Work and Health Programme was introduced in 2018 to replace the Work Programme and became the DWP's leading national programme for outsourced provision. For a time, there was no long-term unemployed focus as for the first year it was all about health and disability. The Work and Health Programme retained the health and disability focus of the precedent Work Programme, with a long-term unemployed referral route, until the onset of the pandemic when a rapid policy response to surging numbers of Universal Credit claimants was required. In October 2020 Job Entry Targeted Support (JETS) was bolted on to the Work and Health Programme for anyone unemployed for three months or more yet is voluntary unless the person has been out of work and claiming unemployment benefits for 24 months. Participants do not however have to be receiving benefits to apply. Jobcentre Plus Work Coaches act as gatekeepers and a participant will be allocated their own advisor to discuss work options, match their skills to work that is available, introduce participants to employers, receive training and, most importantly, advice and support to manage health problems to reduce the impact of these on their work. The Work and Health Programme is delivered in England and Wales with Fair Start being the policy delivered in Scotland.

Fair Start Scotland: Fair Start Scotland is targeted at people with a disability or a health condition, possessing additional support needs, caring responsibilities, those who are single parents, care leavers, people from a minority ethnic community, refugees, people with a conviction and those who have been unemployed for a long time. Fair Start Scotland is different to other back-to-work-related services. Participation is completely voluntary, participants have tailored 12-month pre-work support with a further period of in-work support.

Intensive Personalised Employment Support: In September 2019 six-year-long Intensive Personalised Employment Support contracts were unveiled to provide those long-term unemployed persons requiring additional support with the assistance necessary to return to or enter meaningful work.

Restart: The government's Plan for Jobs was designed to assist people directly impacted by COVID-19 and was the flagship COVID-19 response outsourced programme. This is the largest contract procured by DWP to date, targeting 1.4 million people over three years. The first referrals to the Restart scheme came in July 2021 and had an initial focus on Universal Credit recipients on the intensive work search regime for between 12 and 18 months (Cosens, 2020). From January 2022, the focus was expanded to provide the opportunity for more claimants to benefit from Restart. Universal Credit claimants will be considered for Restart after nine months and with no upper limit.

Access to Work: Underpinning all of these schemes is Access to Work, administered by the DWP. Access to Work provides packages of support to enable people with health conditions and disabilities to enter and remain in employment. Access to Work is available to people with a paid job, which can be full- or part-time and can include employment, self-employment, an apprenticeship, a work trial or work experience, an internship or a work placement, but not voluntary work.

There has been considerable recent debate concerning the extent and nature of DWP control over employment support and welfare policy (see further comments in the 'Employment Support and Local Government' section). As a bridge to the next section addressing the role of the local level, some examples of specialist delivery outside of national DWP-led programmes are provided.

The first example concerns Health and Employment Partnerships within Social Finance. Social Finance designed and managed the world's first social investment-backed programme in health and work. This aimed to develop an evidence-based Individual Placement and Support (IPS) model in partnership with local partners. The programme started in three areas of London and the West Midlands in 2016 and now operates across 12 locations. Social Finance also manages IPS Grow, an NHS England-backed initiative to support the growth of IPS services across England.

The second example comes from the Greater Manchester Working Well project. Established in 2014, the Greater Manchester Working Well Pilot supported 5,000 people who were experiencing chronic/long-term unemployment. They had been jobless for at least two years and had left the National Work Programme without finding a job. The programme combined physical and mental health support and advice on drug and alcohol problems, skills, education and housing. This was a payment-by-results pilot with support organisations being fully paid when the programme participant had been in work for at least a year. On the pilot over 600 people found work, many of whom continued working for 12 months or more. Additional benefits, such as improved health and reduced antisocial behaviour, were among the positive outcomes seen in the programme. In November 2014, as part of a wider devolution agreement, Great Manchester expanded the Working Well project from 5,000 to 50,000 people.

From these experiences, successful policies and provisions targeting people with health conditions and disabilities must include the following:

- an ongoing relationship with Jobcentre Plus DEAs that puts what is best for the individual foremost and central;
- a belief that people can work, and that work is a good thing;
- a trusting relationship between the individual and their advisor;
- no coercion – the right steps at the right time;
- no coercion – the right job at the right time;
- support to manage health conditions, home life and in-work support for as long as it is needed;
- preparation for the work environment, including work placements if appropriate;
- engagement and ongoing relationships with employers, understanding employers' needs and routes to introduce candidates to employers;
- use of Access to Work;
- linkage between skills provisions and employability, pre-employment and in-work; and
- opportunities to upskill, and for in-work progression.

However, 'the role of government' prompts a more complex conversation about what government at what level, and namely what role local, regional and national government should play.

Employment support and local government

The local level is argued by many to be the most important in terms of understanding the nature of employment support, the problems that prompt it and what successful employment support looks like. The problems of unemployment and broader labour market disadvantage have much of their complexities bound in local level differences and local specificities. The relationships that need to be forged between the unemployed, employers, Jobcentres, schools and colleges and other stakeholders such as those of the third sector mostly need to be made at the local level. All this places local government in a critical place and role in the employment support landscape. However over the last 20 years or so the role of local government has been repeatedly undermined across a swathe of public policy areas where local governments would clearly have a key role, including housing, social care and education as well as employment support. Successful employment support requires strong local collaboration and strong local infrastructures, so our focus should be less upon local government and more upon its crucial role in facilitating local collaboration and building those local infrastructures that forge successful employment support policies.

A growing consensus has emerged in recent years around two broad sets of proposals: the first is the claim that there needs to be better integration between skills and employment support, and, with it, strong linkage and integration between the Department for Education (DfE) and the DWP, and the second is that these logically connected (but in reality – and curiously – divergent) skills and employment support realms need to be devolved much more to the local level. These two sets of proposals need to be brought together. In a 2017 report titled *Work Local*, Wilson et al called for the radical devolution of skills and employment support to forge a new integrated system (Wilson et al, 2017). The more recent report, *This Isn't Working*, by Pollard and Tjoa for the New Local think tank, argues for similar reforms that fully exploit key local relationships between various local services, employers and educators (schools and colleges) and the shared local knowledge of these practitioners and commissioners (Pollard and Tjoa, 2022). Finally, the influential House of Lords report *Skills for Every Young Person* published in November 2021 argued that 'more effective local and regional coordination of policies is the most effective way of addressing the issues facing those most in need' (House of Lords, 2021). Each of these important studies demand that the DWP and DfE be better integrated, however this line of critique of the 'role of government' is still rather *nation*-state centric and misses out the crucial 'third leg of the stool': the role of local government (House of Lords, 2021).

Local government needs more support from central government. With this – and firstly – the recognition that it is local government that is the locus of successful government intervention in employment support given that the unemployment problem is set locally around local labour markets, local services and local relationships. Centralised, top-down initiatives from a national government department will not achieve what localised schemes can, simply because the relationships required for these to be successful are forged at the local level. There are several potent examples that aid this point. The COVID-19 era 'Kickstart' scheme the UK government unveiled to address rising youth unemployment was beset by multiple and critical flaws in its administration and management due the overreliance on a central government department (the DWP) that was not equipped to deliver such a programme. In some local areas strong collaborative relationships between employers, councils (that often acted as 'gateways' that were critical to the Kickstart scheme) and Jobcentres were present to make the most of Kickstart, but were still far too reliant on DWP approval at various stages of the process. In some areas, conversely, where such collaborative relationships did not exist, the reliance on the DWP was all the greater and the scheme's failure was compounded in these examples. There are examples also of strong 'local' collaboration between different local councils, with the ten local councils of Greater Manchester (GMCA) coming together to forge a powerful demonstration of what a strong employment support regime across a UK city region can look like. Some in the GMCA, like Wigan, have had some success in 2021 in targeting care leavers to fill vacancies in local adult social care provision – a key responsibility of local government. This example demonstrates the role of local councils in linking different policy challenges like unemployment and adult social care through targeted employment support strategies. A less developed area of promise is found in the pandemic-era policy to create 'Youth Hubs' across the UK. These can provide a hugely useful complement to what Jobcentre Plus, councils and providers do and be a key part in the local infrastructures envisaged. The barriers to forging greater localised employment and skills support however are numerous and considerable. As a macrocosm of the Kickstart example, the current benefits system is centred on a top-down DWP running a Jobcentre Plus network from on high and focusing a sanctioning regime based around conditionality rather than personal development and tailored support. As Mark Cosens argued in 2020, the Jobcentre Plus network needs to be unshackled from such centralised control so they and their Work Coaches have the freedom to develop and exploit relationships at the local level. Additionally, as a Local Government Association study in 2021 described, the commissioning maps for DfE- and DWP-funded programmes are very different, which is cumbersome enough for local councils to navigate without their own maps and those of Local Economic Partnerships (LEPs) not aligning with these easily also.

At the centre of this are two fundamental truths: the unemployed will first reach out to local service points like local employers, the local Jobcentre who will assist in a job search and for obtaining benefits, and other available sources of support. Local employers may cast a wider net in geographical terms in trying to source labour, but most will also orientate themselves more towards the local labour market, thus will also require strong relationships with local stakeholders like Jobcentre Plus, private and third sector providers, schools and colleges and their local council.

This complex set of problems concerning skills and employment however must not merely focus on various organs of the state. The focus, again, must be about the relationships forged through local collaboration and strong local infrastructures. Local government is part of this, but only a part.

Employment support, funding and why the UK Shared Prosperity Fund matters

One of the most pressing policy concerns for contemporary employment support concerns how will EU funding for employment and skills will be replaced with Britain's exit from the EU. The UK Shared Prosperity Fund (UKSPF) has promised post-Brexit Britain another opportunity to rewrite the blueprint of support for disadvantaged communities (ERSA, 2022). As the replacement of the European Social Fund (ESF), the UKSPF must fulfil the government's manifesto pledge to deliver outcomes in 'getting people back into work and helping to improve their skills, by building networks between employers, local authorities and charities, or by working directly with disadvantaged or disabled people to help them move into work' (Conservative Party Manifesto, 2017). The ESF has previously enabled the UK to enjoy structural funding worth about £2 billion a year and as a result boasts a proud history of success stories. During the last round of funding, the ESF saw the enrolment of over 7 million participants in programmes within England. Of these over 700,000 found work, over 260,000 gained basic skills and over 650,000 gained full qualifications at level 2 or above. This exerts significant pressure on the government to ensure that the calibre of employment initiatives and social programmes available under UKSPF meet or exceed the precedent which has already been set, so that no one misses out (House of Lords, 2019).

The dangers of high demand versus limited supply: What differentiates UKSPF from other funding streams is the fact that its primary function is to create innovative pathways of support to those who are not currently served by mainstream services. These people are disproportionately faced with complex barriers such as physical and mental health conditions, disability, long-term unemployment, criminal records and housing issues. For instance, the difference in the employment rate between those who were disabled and those who were not reached 28.1 per cent in the third quarter of 2021. Data published by the Health Foundation also found that in January 2021, 43 per cent of those unemployed had underlying mental health conditions. Taking into consideration the effects of the COVID-19 pandemic on the economy, the degree of marginalisation which many of these demographic groups have encountered has evidently worsened and consequently had a spiralling effect on poverty levels (Wilson and Finch, 2021).

It is telling that there is a clear demand for service delivery owing to these significant gaps, however the scope and quality of supply is dependent on the administration of UKSPF. The ESF previously targeted action under initiatives such as the Solent Jobs Programme, which facilitated holistic health support, as well as intensive case management and cognitive behavioural therapy to individuals in need. It has had a noticeable impact in empowering individuals who would otherwise be overlooked in a very competitive job market. Even with these local-led interventions and the positive results produced, individuals are still being deprived of an equal opportunity to progress in life. With additional UKSPF delays, this problem will be exacerbated if services and projects are forced to shut down through lack of funding.

The government's mission to 'level up' the country must recognise the specific needs of communities and local growth agendas (Anon, 2022). As it currently stands, streamlined funding measures have put significant emphasis on place-based disparities and less focus on investment in the people who live within these areas. There is an inherent need for equilibrium between people and place in any policy regime, to ensure that future employment provision is achieved with utmost efficacy. The government has underscored that community-led activity and multisectoral stakeholder involvement is integral for shaping new outcomes. However, how it will go about improving life chances and re-engineering the country's social fabric through UKSPF is less obvious. It is prerequisite that those who are furthest behind need the most help. This can only happen when support is made widely available and accessible to the most vulnerable groups.

A call to prioritise people: In order to push forward an agenda that prioritises people, the government has a duty to ensure that UKSPF does not fall below the £2.4 billion annual pot the European Structural Investment Funds provided, and allocations must also be made in conjunction with local need. The gap in funding will inevitably limit the bandwidth of employment and skills support available to the most health-deprived communities, so it is imperative that the government is able to define what UKSPF will look like, how it will work and how third sector organisations can play its role in this agenda. UKSPF should also be less bureaucratic and more flexible by offering a mixture of short-term grant funding and longer-term financing options and allow for a broad range of expert providers to be able to access it, achieving enhanced longevity in the event of economic shocks such as the pandemic.

Introducing UKSPF swiftly and effectively is a gargantuan task, however the substantial gains it can generate can certainly overshadow this. It is estimated that the fund could see a 5 per cent rise in the employment rate of working-age disabled people, which would increase gross domestic product by £23 billion by 2030, as well as narrow the Black and minority ethnic employment gap, which could establish a £24 billion annual benefit to the UK economy. This strengthens the case for UKSPF as it cements the rationale that funding will not only help those who partake in these programmes, but on a broader scale will accelerate the post-COVID-19 recovery, productivity and economic growth.

References

Anon (2022) *Levelling Up the United Kingdom*. Available at: https://assets. publishing.service.gov.uk/government/uploads/system/uploads/atta chment_data/file/1052706/Levelling_Up_WP_HRES.pdf (accessed 8 February 2022).

Cosens, M. (2020) *Employment Response to Coronavirus: A Flexible Employment Programme for England and Wales*. Cosens Consult.

ERSA (2022) *Sharing Prosperity*. Available at: https://www.scribd.com/ document/437336680/An-ERSA-Report-Sharing-Prosperity-WEB (accessed 2 February 2022).

House of Lords (2019) *The UK Shared Prosperity Fund*. Available at: https:// researchbriefings.files.parliament.uk/documents/CBP-8527/CBP-8527. pdf (accessed 15 February 2022).

House of Lords (2021) *Skills for Every Young Person*. House of Lords Youth Unemployment Committee. Report of Session 2021–22.

Pollard, T. and Tjoa, P. (2022) This isn't working: Reimagining employment support for people facing complex disadvantage. *New Local*, 27 October.

Wilson, H. and Finch, D. (2021) *Unemployment and Mental Health*. London: The Health Foundation. Available at: https://www.health.org. uk/publications/long-reads/unemployment-and-mental-health (accessed 4 February 2022).

Wilson, T., Crews, A. and Mirza, K. (2017) *Work Local*. Leicester: Learning and Work Institute.

PART IV

The third sector

Claire Bonham

In the previous volume, *Local Authorities and Social Determinants of Health*, there was an acknowledgement that local authorities are increasingly developing partnerships that allow them to act as 'enablers' of change, alongside the recognition of the role of the third sector in providing the soft structures which are essential for reinvigorating healthier communities and individuals (see Introduction to Part IV and Chapter 16 of *Local Authorities and Social Determinants of Health*, and Chapter 16 in this volume).

Third sector is a term used to describe the range of organisations that are neither public sector nor private sector. It includes voluntary and community organisations (both registered charities and other organisations such as associations, self-help groups and community groups), social enterprises, mutuals and co-operatives.[1] As we will see in the chapters in this section, partnerships increasingly mean that the lines between public, private and the third sector become blurred.

The 'levelling up' agenda pursued by Prime Minister Boris Johnson resulted in a report by MP Danny Kruger, *Levelling Up Our Communities: Proposals for a New Social Covenant*, which was published in September 2020. Kruger notes that 'Civil Society, as individuals and organisations, when they act with the primary purpose of creating **social value**, are independent of state control. By social value we mean enriched lives and a fairer society for all. The government believes that social value flows from thriving communities' (Kruger, 2020).

The sector is often fragmented, with many small charities or groups focusing on a single issue or a particular community, and a number of larger charities that are well placed to respond to commissioning from local authorities or central government grants in a way that smaller charities are not. In 2017/2018 there were 166,592 voluntary organisations, with eight in ten of those having a turnover of less than £100,000.[2] For the third sector as a whole, government income as a proportion of total income was at 29 per cent.[3] Big funders such as the National Lottery and regional bodies such as the pan-London organisations (Greater London Authority, London Councils) are increasingly looking for charities to demonstrate added value through collaborative partnerships and will not fund individual organisations to deliver their big grants without these partnerships in place.

In addition to this lack of secure funding, the COVID-19 pandemic has also had a significant effect on the viability of smaller charities. A severe reduction in older volunteers manning charity shops and undertaking voluntary work due to 'shielding' means that they have not been available to help deliver community support and raise funds for their charities. Regrettably, not all charities have adequate financial reserves – the 2020 National Council for Voluntary Organisations (NCVO)Almanac reported that 23 per cent of charities had no reserves when going into the COVID-19 crisis. Some charities have responded to this situation by de-risking investment portfolios and selling assets to fund projects. Sixty per cent of community groups have closed or decreased their activities during COVID-19.[4]

A major feature of third sector organisations is their reliance on volunteers to deliver programmes. Volunteering has always been a strong tradition in the UK but has been dominated by certain sections of the population, namely older volunteers (people aged 65–74 are the age group most likely to volunteer on a regular basis) and people from a higher socioeconomic background. However, the benefits of volunteering for people from outside these particular groups can have manifold benefits for the individual and wider society in terms of building connections and social capital (Bonham, 2018).

In the first lockdown period there was an excitement by many who had not volunteered previously, with the *Civil Action* report produced by Pro Bono Economics (PBE) indicating that at that time, 18 million people in England helped neighbours with shopping, dog-walking and other activities. However the PBE report estimated that 6 million fewer people volunteered or supported their neighbours in the second wave of lockdowns, with only 26 per cent having done so since October 2020. The surge of volunteering was noted by the government, which, working in crisis mode to organise personal protective equipment, testing equipment and respirators, had a range of critical resource procurement issues, saw the third sector as an important untapped resource.

Local authorities have also understood that the third sector and voluntary organisations can be a skilled partner in helping them address **wicked issues** that require collaboration and innovation to deliver lasting change. The role of local authorities and the third sector in responding to the needs of their local communities has been highlighted in our response to the COVID-19 pandemic; and responses to COVID-19 form a main theme within this book.

In the initial wave of the pandemic, lockdown of the UK population caused a crisis in food supply. There was stockpiling of food (and toilet paper) by some people and lack of access to food for others, either because they were isolating and shielding, or due to lack of money to buy food. An immediate response to this situation was the setting up of food hubs by local councils. In many cases, but not all, council food hubs collaborated with established food banks. Distribution of food into the community was largely undertaken by volunteers. Chapters 13 and 14 review food banks and volunteering, respectively.

COVID-19, itself a **wicked issue**, exacerbated a number of pre-existing wicked issues, including a rise in **domestic abuse**. This is discussed in Chapter 15, from the perspective of a local authority working in partnership with third sector organisations.

The Kruger Report made a number of observations and proposals, including a 'covenant between the government and the faith-based organisations'. This is addressed in Chapter 16. The role of faith-based organisations is an important one, as they are often able to reach different groups of society who may be more comfortable accessing support through their existing faith communities than through central or local government sources.

Kruger also pointed out the lack of philanthropic activity in the UK compared to the US. As noted earlier, many organisations within the third sector lack access to sustainable sources of income.

What all the chapters in this section have in common, however, is the recognition that wicked issues require innovative solutions that involve a number of stakeholders across a range of sectors. The global nature of the COVID-19 pandemic means that we should also draw on the experiences of diverse communities, learning from innovation across the world and being brave enough to experiment with radical partnerships that may lead to unexpected outcomes – good and bad – but without which these wicked issues will continue to prevent everyone in our communities from having access to health, wellbeing, wealth, justice and opportunity.

Notes

[1] National Audit Office, 'What are third sector organisations and their benefit for commissioners?', https://www.nao.org.uk/successful-commissioning/introduction/what-are-civil-society-organisations-and-their-benefits-for-commissioners/ (accessed 12 July 2021).

[2] NCVO UK Civil Society Almanac, 2020, https://data.ncvo.org.uk/ (accessed 12 July 2021).

[3] NCVO UK Civil Society Almanac, 2020, https://data.ncvo.org.uk/ (accessed 12 July 2021).

[4] https://www.civilsociety.co.uk/news/over-60-of-community-groups-have-closed-or-decreased-services-during-covid-19.html

References

Bonham C. (2018) Building an inclusive community through social capital: The role of volunteering in reaching those on the edge of community. In Bonner A. (ed) *Social Determinants of Health: Social Inequality and Wellbeing*, Bristol: Policy Press.

Kruger, D. (2020) *Levelling Up Our Communities: Proposals for a New Social Covenant. A New Deal with Faith Communities.* A report commissioned by the Prime Minister. Available at: https://www.dannykruger.org.uk/files/2020-09/Levelling%20Up%20Our%20Communities-Danny%20Kruger.pdf (accessed 14 November 2020).

13

Relational collaboration and innovation in responding to need and austerity: food banks

Alex Murdock

Introduction

Maslow in a seminal work talked of a hierarchy of needs whereby the most basic needs were physiological. The need for food was placed in the most basic category (Maslow, 1943). The need for some security in the availability of food is rooted in the concept of life itself. The responsibility of government to meet such basic needs is a measure of whether it is fulfilling its essential obligation to citizens (Alaimo, 2005). International aid efforts to respond to famine typically emanate from a failure of government in the country to address this need. In the UK the rapid emergence of food banks was seen by some as a measure of government failure to respond in the face of clear evidence of unmet need (Garthwaite, 2016).

This chapter examines, through the medium of responses to food insecurity, the range of responses in terms of collaboration and innovation. Though the image in the UK is the phenomena of food banks we will take a broader approach and will explore aspects such as technological responses and the growth of social supermarkets and food recycling initiatives. We will draw upon examples in a range of countries and upon concepts of collaboration and partnership which reach beyond the traditional charity model driven by fundraising/grant approaches. Social enterprise and social innovation will be explored together with mechanisms which significantly derive from private sector initiatives. Reference will be made to emerging trends which may impact on food insecurity and the potential implications going forward.

Collaboration and innovation

Collaboration in the context of social welfare has a well established literature (Hudson, 1987). It typically envisages collaboration between organisational entities (such as between state agencies and the private and third sector).

The UK policy agenda on linking health and social care is a reprise of a long established discourse (Leathard, 1994). The language of 'partnership working' is commonplace though this has been influenced by the use of 'partnership' in contexts such a Public Private Partnership to enable infrastructure projects (Delmon, 2011). The language of partnership and collaboration has long been inherent in relationships between the state and the third sector. However this has typically been closely related to service delivery under either a contractual or a grant aided funding regime in which the third sector is often in a subordinate role (Milbourne, 2009).

The area of contracting is obviously there but the notion of the 'collaborative citizen' also emerges. This has an eminent link with the 'co' agenda (co-commissioning, co-delivery, co-evaluation, etc) (see Bovaird and Loeffler, 2013). This concept of collaboration, which explicitly involves the recipient of a service being involved in some or all aspects associated with the development, delivery and evaluation of the service, reaches across into various other discourses such as active citizenship.

As we will see there are some issues in linking this to aspects of the responses to food insecurity especially where the most obvious provision – that of food banks – is concerned. Possibly this may be associated with the nature of food insecurity itself – namely that it replaces a situation where the individual implicitly did have a degree of choice and control over what, when, where and how their food needs were met (Lang, 1999).

The concept of collaboration possibly sits less easily with responses to food insecurity where the recipient is concerned at least in the UK and US context. Individual budgets are reasonably well established in enabling personal choice in areas such as disability, mental health and ageing. However where food insecurity is concerned the discourse is of a 'failure' by the individual (or family) to adequately provide food through their own or state allocated resources. Hence there may be an implicit sense of responding to a need which cannot be simply met by replacing one source of 'free income' with another.

In the area of food insecurity collaboration is an active and essential construct in terms of gaining access to food sources and also in terms of the appropriate distribution of food and food related provision to people who are judged to be qualified to receive it. Here the concept of collaboration is core to effectiveness and efficiency in responding to food insecurity. The presence of food insecurity is for some evidence of state failure in meeting a basic need of citizens but the response to this requires the active participation of a range of non-state (and in many cases) state actors.

Innovation (not necessarily social innovation) is often a rationale for collaboration. In the context of so-called 'wicked' problems the ability to find a solution is sought through engagement with different stakeholders. The argument which is often made by voluntary organisations and social enterprises is that they can offer creative and efficacious solutions which, for various reasons, are not within the capability of the public sector. The example of the introduction of digital hearing aids on a large scale is one such example where the particular expertise of a national voluntary organisation was critical but without the collaboration with both the UK National Health Service and the private sector little would have been achieved. In effect collaboration was the solution to a 'wicked problem' (Murdock and Lamb, 2009).

LeRoux and Goerdel suggest that there are four types of collaboration respondents engage in with other non-profits and the state (LeRoux and Goerdel, 2009):

- piloting new programmes or services;
- collaborating to reduce costs;
- collaboration as a requirement of funding;
- other type of collaboration.

This is generally useful in considering collaboration in the context of food insecurity. However it is not comprehensive, as the category labelled 'other type of collaboration' implies. Though developing and piloting new programmes/services is a significant part of the response to food insecurity the essence of much of the response to food insecurity is ensuring the reliability of ongoing and proven programmes.

Aspects such as costs are significant but the implication of 'costs' are the costs involved in a programme delivery. In food banks, for example, the challenge is typically to obtain the necessary resources and these are often obtained via donation as opposed to purchase. The cost is typically of storage and distribution as opposed to acquisition.

Le Roux and Goerdel's model does not appear to encompass collaboration with the private sector and also, perhaps because it is organisationally based, does not explicitly encompass collaboration with citizens and beneficiaries of services.

The argument here is that responses to food insecurity open up collaboration to a wider definition. In December 2012 in parliamentary questions the Prime Minister was implicitly linking food banks and the associated volunteering to the 'Big Society', which was a much contested policy beloved of the then Prime Minister, David Cameron.

Arguably this hit upon a significant point that the nature of food banks as represented by the Trussell Trust and similar initiatives was of citizens responding in a collaborative fashion to a perceived need. The question as to whether this need was a consequence of government policy (or of a government failure) is a separate debate. It also brought into play the concept of innovation as a factor in such collaboration.

Innovation

In terms of innovation in a managerial or enterprise context consider the conventional Schumpeterian notion of innovation which encompasses the following:

- *Product*: The introduction of a new good.
- *Process*: The introduction of a new method of production.
- *Business model*: The opening of a new market.
- *Source of supply*: The conquest of a new source of supply.
- *Mergers and divestments*: The carrying out of the new organisation. (Schumpeter, 1934)

The area of food insecurity itself raises some interesting examples which would evidence a response to all these in respect of innovation. During war time when food was rationed this led to consequent innovation such as powdered egg. The food industry is itself a model of innovation with new products, processes, markets and sources of supply.

The need to examine and report on innovation in ways to meet food insecurity would appear to be self-evident. However, given that the focus is on the role of innovation in resolving food insecurity primarily from the perspective of not for profits and the third sector it is reasonable to argue that the focus should be on innovation for social benefit. This brings in a definition or concept of innovation with a social goal – typically described as 'social innovation'. Such innovation brings with it a societal and often a political dimension. It is seen as 'correcting inequalities and injustice' and bringing about a better societal outcome (Nicholls and Murdock, 2012). It differs from the purely enterprise construct of innovation which may be indifferent to social benefit as a prime objective. Therefore in the context of food insecurity innovation has to be construed as 'innovation aimed to bring about a better world'.

In examining social innovation, and drawing on Nicholls and Murdock, three levels of innovation can be described (see Table 13.1).

The levels of innovation set out do offer a mechanism to approach innovation in respect of positive societal responses to food insecurity. The incremental level can be seen in the provision of food to people in need, such as via soup kitchens and food banks. The obtaining of food by more efficient means through collaboration (whether it be with private sector, government or citizen donation) sits well with this level.

The institutional level represents a more systemic approach to food insecurity. Here responding to 'food deserts' (areas of inner cities which are economically unattractive for the private sector) through not simply giving food handouts but seeking to change the market structures to encourage provision (a so-called bottom of the pyramid approach).

Table 13.1: Levels of social innovation

Level	Objective	Focus	Example organisation (sector)
Incremental	To address identified market failures more effectively: for example, negative externalities and institutional voids	Products and services	Kickstart (low-cost irrigation foot pump) Aurolab (low-cost intraocular lenses) Afghan Institute of Learning (female education)
Institutional	To reconfigure existing market structures and patterns to create new social value	Markets	MPESA (mobile banking) Institute for One World Health ('orphan' drugs) Cafedirect (Fair Trade)
Disruptive	To change the cognitive frames of reference around markets and issues to alter social systems and structures	Politics (social movements)	Greenpeace (environmental change) BRAC (micro-finance) Tostan (human rights)

Source: Nicholls and Murdock (2012: 4)

The disruptive level is more societal in nature and involves changing fundamental mindsets. For example, the Trussell Trust, which engages in strong campaigning aimed at changing the perception of food insecurity and the political landscape. However (pace Schumpeter) the disruptive level also may involve aspects of behavioural change and fundamental changes to the nature of the food value chain.

Constructing a frame for examples of collaboration and innovation

Based on the preceding discussion a two-dimensional space can be created in which the two constructs of collaboration and innovation form the parameters (Table 13.2).

Discussion and examples of collaboration and innovation

The following section will explore innovation and collaboration not just from food banks but will also draw on the general arena of social innovation and collaboration in the context of relieving or resolving food insecurity.

Incremental innovation
In existing products and services

The traditional soup kitchen model is an example of a long-standing service. It has evolved to move away from purely 'soup' delivery based on institutional

Table 13.2: Framework for examples of collaboration and innovation

Innovation and collaboration	Incremental	Institutional	Disruptive
In existing services/ products	Food banks and soup kitchens	Partnerships with suppliers and supply chain	Food distribution, usability and sources
In new services/ products	Linked community facilities health, education and training	One-stop shops Food regulations regarding use-by/sell-by dates	Farming technology (LED internal vertical 'farms')
In reducing costs	Volunteers and corporate partnerships	Food recycling Bartering Imputing costs to partners	Fareshare Gleaning
As a requirement	Regulations of networks and rules of eligibility and practice	Assessing for eligibility to wider provision than food	Regulations about wastage and use of waste food

Source: Nicholls and Murdock (2011: 4)

setting to a more flexible approach, 'the soup run', and also offers other foods such as sandwiches.

The 'food bank' model is an incremental development from an earlier soup kitchen run by the charity St Vincent de Paul. However the food bank approach is itself an incremental development and typically what starts as an occasional distribution of a limited number of products evolves into a more complex operation with facilities to store cold goods.

The Trussell Trust model, which is in effect a concession or franchise to run a food bank using the Trussell Trust approach, enables a fast rate of growth. However it is predicated on a degree of conformity to set down rules not too dissimilar to the McDonald's approach.[1] The conformity to the 'franchise' rules creates an interesting potential discourse as to the extent to which it is a 'disruptive' innovation. In this respect it is akin to the Feeding America network which also sets out a series of rules governing both the relationships and procedures (Feeding America, 2011).

In new products and services

The Trussell Trust provides an obvious UK based example of the development of new products and services. They initially provided food which was to be prepared and cooked by the beneficiaries. However, it became apparent that some who were referred actually did not have access to full cooking facilities or had no electricity due to an inability to pay the bill. Therefore the Trussell Trust produced 'cold packs' of food products which did not require cooking. The Trust also recognised that some people did not have access to full cooking facilities but did have hot water which led to a 'kettle pack' with tea, coffee and 'pot noodles'.

In reducing cost

The area of food insecurity where it involves not-for-profit and third sector organisations typically makes use of donated goods and volunteer labour. The role of collaboration with the for-profit sector is typically seen in the context of donated food and related products through either direct donations by supermarkets and parts of the food chain.

Where the role of the private sector is less recognised (especially in the UK) is in the aspect of volunteering (Agostinho and Paço, 2012). In the US in particular food banks offer extensive options for corporate volunteering. This will typically involve a company bringing a significant number of staff to the food bank to sort food, pack food parcels and so forth. This aspect is now emerging in the UK with an example of a relationship between a social enterprise (Benefacto) and Kensington and Chelsea Food Bank. Significantly the link for the volunteering is on the social enterprise website – not the food bank's.[2]

As a requirement

The key place which food plays in life means that in any society with a functioning and evolved government any organisation involved in distributing food to people in need cannot operate without reference to some kind of regulatory framework even at the most basic level of observing food safety precautions as indicated by use-by dates and hygiene.

However where the food provision by third sector has become institutionally linked to aspects of the state welfare support then this brings about a further set of requirements (Gundersen et al, 2011). In the US is probably found the most developed form of requirement in which regulations for the Supplementary Nutrition Assistance Program (SNAP) serve to set the detailed requirements for eligibility as to what food banks (which are not state entities) can provide.

Federal eligibility for SNAP is limited to those with gross incomes up to 130 per cent of the federal poverty line. Participants must further show a net income of less than or equal to 100 per cent of the poverty line and are subject to an asset test. Able-bodied adults without dependents may only receive three months of benefits during any three-year period if they are not working a minimum of 20 hours per week or participating in a training program.[3]

Institutional innovation

In existing products and services

The collaboration between private sector and community organisations and US food banks furnishes ample examples of how food drives, volunteering and actual financial donations have become part of the normal environment. The relationships established are ongoing and typically multifaceted. They are mutually beneficial in that the private company derives a positive corporate image and that the staff volunteering is encouraged as a part of 'team building' for company employees.

In the US such collaborations sometimes extend to use of inmate labour through the use of volunteers from nearby correctional institutions. The author observed that this was welcomed by food bank staff as inmate labour sometimes represented a high skill level.

In new products and services

At the Global Foodbank Leadership Institute Conference in Houston held in March 2015 the author was impressed by the synergy shown by the corporate organisations and the food banks with which they were associated.

Griffith Laboratories, a major private research company which develops ingredient systems for food companies, had worked with the Bangalore Food Bank in India to develop and produce a food product called khichdi. The company noted (October 2014) that:

> Five hundred kilograms of khichdi, a nutritionally balanced meal containing a mixture of lentils, rice, vegetable, nuts and seasoning will be produced and donated to the Bangalore Food Bank. This will provide 5,000 meals to the hungry in Bangalore.
>
> We saw an opportunity to create something different – not only are we producing to stop hunger, but also improving the quality of life of those who are hungry. ... It was important for us to utilize our culinary and R&D expertise to create an enjoyable experience for those we are helping.
>
> Griffith's research & development and culinary teams worked together to develop a meal that was easy to cook, is nutritious and satisfies the local tastes.[4]

In reducing cost

The cost aspects of food banking relate to administrative, storage and distribution costs. In food donation drives involving supermarkets where customers purchase food to donate then there is clearly an element of actual profit going to the supermarket itself. In the UK Fareshare and the

Trussell Trust secured an agreement with a major supermarket chain that it would donate a sum of money based on the weight of goods bought and donated by customers as a simple means of apportioning the profit made by the supermarket. This now functions smoothly, with the third sector organisations concerned 'weighing' the donated goods and electronically notifying the supermarket, which then pays within six weeks. It has in effect become institutionalised.

As a requirement

The extent of institutional impact was demonstrated to the author in one US food bank when the food bank indicated that it had been given delegated powers to function in a quasi-state capacity to assess and judge the eligibility of applicants for SNAP (which involved more than eligibility for the food bank provision). In effect, the food bank had taken on de facto functions of the state welfare system.

Disruptive innovation
In existing products and services

The disruptive aspect in existing products and services is found where the existing mode or practice is challenged. This can take place where there is a de facto 'social movement' which changes the way people perceive the world.

A good example is Incredible Edible.[5] It began in 2007 in a small town in the UK where people started to identify places where food could be grown in community areas such as roadside verges. The food was not sold nor was it distributed. Rather a social movement grew up whereby people came together to grow food. There was initially no formal structure, no legal structure and no board of trustees as would normally be found in a third sector organisation. People brought things for common consumption and there was no obligation other than a degree of social pressure to 'do one's bit'.

In 2012 with some foundation funding a network was established and there are (currently) over 100 groups in the UK. It is clearly a disruptive model in that it does not conform to any market model nor does it comply with a regulated distributive model such as might be found in a food bank such as the Trussell Trust.

Incredible Edible now has networks in the US, Australia, Canada and France.[6] Perhaps significantly, these mirror the countries where food banking took hold and it is the power of a social movement as opposed to a regulated and governed innovation which has allowed such a rapid expansion. Conceivably in food terms the Incredible Edible model may come to surpass the food bank model in a global setting. In some respects it is allied to the gleaning concept – a long established practice of scouring field of crops after harvest for what has been left (Wong and Bank, 2012).

In new products and services

The original food bank model envisaged that people would receive food according to a determination of need made by the food bank and also that it would be free of charge (Riches, 1986). This model operated in North America and Australia and is the model of Trussell Trust in the UK.

However, in the Tafel in Germany – which in terms of numbers is possibly the largest food bank network in Europe – some interesting variations were found (Selke, 2010). Known as the Stuttgart model it involves providing a supermarket setting where 'customers' who had defined eligibility (such as being on low income) were issued with a membership card and then were able to shop and choose what products to buy at a very significantly discounted price. The model represents both a change in the service concept with the user having free choice and also in offering a wider range of products.

There is also considerable evidence of diversification in services provided by food banks. Possibly the most diversified model encountered was that in Hong Kong where a major social service provider, St James Settlement, operates both a food bank and a canteen in the context of a multiservice 'one stop shop' offering a diversity of services ranging from kindergarten through to funeral services. The food provision was seen as being part of an enormously rich tapestry of provision which served to remove any stigma associated with entering the building. In effect the food bank was in a vast collaborative network of services probably beyond the most imaginative and ambitious plans of any food bank anywhere else in the world.

In technological terms one of the most significant developments is 'vertical farming' in which the concept of land usage and distance from end user is radically changed through the use of hydroponics and low cost/low power usage LED lights to promote growing. This technology has emerged significantly in private sector contexts, for example a former nightclub in urban New Jersey is now a very productive vertical farm.[7] It also offers a solution to the growth of urbanisation which has restricted the availability of nearby farmland as shown by a Singapore example.[8] When vertical farming methods and technology link with inner-city urban farming projects then the potential is not hard to see.

In reducing cost

The potential to reduce cost through a disruptive approach is found in a range of collaborative examples. In the UK, Fareshare is a charity which seeks to obtain food for distribution to other agencies which then are the final source of distribution. Fareshare realised that it would be more efficient to move back up the value chain, away from the retail setting to the actual factory floor.[9] Therefore, via a partnership with the supermarket Asda, Fareshare worked to divert food further back up the supply chain through locating within the food depots. It is now diverting a large amount of food (which would otherwise have gone to waste before it reaches the retail setting).

As a requirement

An interesting evolution focused upon food insecurity is where the disruption is through actually introducing a regulation which disrupts the status quo. The Real Junk Food project which emerged in the UK in 2014 assumes the mantle of a social movement. Nesta regards it as one of the New Radicals in terms of innovation.[10] The concept is simple requiring that the food used in a café or restaurant should be discarded food which would otherwise have gone to waste. Subsequently this movement has been clearly linked to positive impact on public health issues (Williams et al, 2018).

Perhaps the largest project to recycle food, which was, in effect, taken from the table leftovers, is to be found in Egypt through the Food Bank Regional Network (FBRN). Here the organisation gathers food from hotels and from private homes to recycle to people in need. The hospitality expectation in the Arab world is that a plentiful supply of food is available for a banquet, which involves inevitable potential waste. The FBRN diverts such food from waste and through training and certification of its staff is able to comply with food handling regulations. The organisation reports that in Egypt it feeds over 1 million people.[11]

Conclusion

We have sought to illustrate how food insecurity is amenable to analysis and in a global as opposed to a national context.

Food banking is now well established as a global phenomenon and as such is worthy of detailed research from the perspective of the third sector. It spans boundaries between the sectors and offers a rich seam of potential for cooperation often to mutual advantage.

There are aspects of responses to food insecurity which are not impeded by national boundaries or indeed by cultural or governmental ones.

Perhaps of equal interest are the examples of social movements such as that offered by Incredible Edible and food recycling where the concepts and ideas can spread rapidly and be adopted with relative ease.

Notes

[1] In an interview where the author was present a very senior member of staff of the Trussell Trust agreed that the model of franchising could be compared (in that respect) to McDonald's.

[2] See http://benefacto.org/product/kcfoodbank/ (accessed 22 August 2015).

[3] See http://www.feedingamerica.org/take-action/advocate/federal-hunger-relief-progr ams/supplemental-nutrition-assistance-program.html (accessed 20 August 2015).

[4] Global Food Bank Leadership summit (March 2015) and http://wwserver1.griffithlabor atories.com/public/US/English/SitePages/PressRoomBangalore.aspx?utm_source=The+ Global+FoodBanking+Network+Monthly+eNews&utm_campaign=d80edee76a-Octo ber_2014_eNews_10162014&utm_medium=email&utm_term=0_0e1754f5fd-d80edee 76a-181686437 (accessed 20 August 2015).

[5] See http://incredibleediblenetwork.org.uk/ (accessed 20 August 2015).

[6] See http://incredibleediblenetwork.org.uk/global-groups (accessed 20 August 2015).

[7] See http://www.nj.com/essex/index.ssf/2015/03/30m_vertical_farm_to_bring_jobs_ fresh_greens_to_ne.html (accessed 21 August 2015).

[8] See http://permaculturenews.org/2014/07/25/vertical-farming-singapores-solution- feed-local-urban-population/ (accessed 20 August 2015).

[9] See http://your.asda.com/press-centre/asda-and-fareshare-help-tackle-food-poverty-thro ugh-new-agreement-with-manufacturers (accessed 20 August 2015).

[10] See https://www.nesta.org.uk/feature/new-radicals-2014/the-real-junk-food-project/ (accessed 20 May 2021).

[11] See https://foodbankingregionalnetwork.com/en/about-fbrn/our-story (accessed 20 May 2021).

References

Agostinho, D. and Paço, A. (2012) Analysis of the motivations, generativity and demographics of the food bank volunteer. *International Journal of Non-profit and Voluntary Sector Marketing*, 17(3): 249–261.

Alaimo, K. (2005) Food insecurity in the United States: An overview. *Topics in Clinical Nutrition*, 20(4): 281–298.

Bovaird, T. and Loeffler, E. (2013) We're all in this together: Harnessing user and community co-production of public outcomes. Institute of Local Government Studies report Chapter 4. Available at: http://www. Birmingham. ac. uk/Documents/college-social-sciences/government-society/inlogov/publications

Delmon J. (2011) *Public-Private Partnership Projects in Infrastructure*. Cambridge: Cambridge University Press.

eRoux, K. and Goerdel, H.T. (2009) Political advocacy by nonprofit organizations: A strategic management explanation. *Public Performance and Management Review*, 32(4): 514–536.

Feeding America (2011) *Map the Meal Gap 2011, Preliminary Findings: A Report on County Level Food Insecurity and Food Cost in the United States in 2009.*

Garthwaite, K. (2016) *Hunger Pains: Life Inside Foodbank Britain*. Bristol: Policy Press.

Gundersen, C., Brown, J., Engelhard, E. and Waxman, E. (2011) *Map the Meal Gap: Technical Brief.* Chicago: Feeding America.

Hudson B. (1987) *Collaboration in Social Welfare: A Framework for Analysis.* Bristol University Press.

Lang, T. (1999) For hunger-proof cities: Sustainable urban food systems, in Koc, M., MacRae, R., Mougeot, L. and Welsh, J. (ed) *Food Policy for the 21st Century: Can It Be Both Radical.* Reading: Thames Valley University, p 216.

Leathard, A. (1994) *Going Inter-Professional: Working Together for Health and Welfare.* Routledge.

Maslow, A.H. (1943) A theory of human motivation. *Psychological Review*, 50(4): 370.

Milbourne, L. (2009) Remodelling the third sector: Advancing collaboration or competition in community-based initiatives? *Journal of Social Policy*, 38(2): 277–297.

Nicholls, A. and Murdock, A. (eds) (2012) *Social Innovation: Blurring Boundaries to Reconfigure Markets.* Basingstoke: Palgrave Macmillan.

Riches, G. (1986) *Food Banks and the Welfare Crisis.* Toronto: James Lorimer & Company.

Schumpeter, J.A. (1934) *The Theory of Economic Development: An Inquiry into Profits, Capital, Credit, Interest, and the Business Cycle.* Piscataway, NJ: Transaction Publishers.

Selke, S. (ed) (2010) *Kritik der Tafeln in Deutschland.* Berlin: VS Verlag für Sozialwissenschaften.

Williams, G., Robinson, C., Connell, S., Vella, G., Pope, D. and Verma, A. (2018) Junk food café's impact on public health, deprived communities and food waste in North West England. *European Journal of Public Health*, 1(28): 213–299.

Wong, S. and Bank, G.B.F. (2012) Gleaning: Capturing surplus to meet local needs. *Communities and Banking*, Spring. Available at: https://www. bostonfed.org/publications/communities-and-banking/2012/spring/glean ing-capturing-surplus-to-meet-local-needs.aspx

14

Volunteering and small charities

Chris O'Leary and Rita Chadha

Introduction

Emerging evidence from the voluntary sector in the UK provides an insight into the devastating impact of COVID-19 on charities' finances, staff, volunteers and service provision (Institute of Fundraising, 2020; Charity Commission, 2021). At the same time, many charities are reporting significant increases in demand for their services, with domestic violence, animal welfare, mental health and wellbeing, and homelessness charities being particularly affected in what has been described as a 'perfect storm' for the sector (Bradbury, 2020). Most charities expect ongoing challenges over the coming years in fundraising and of not being able to return to normal levels of service provision (Institute of Fundraising, 2020). But it is smaller charities that are really feeling the brunt of these pressures. More than 90 per cent of charities registered in England and Wales have an income of under £1 million. Used to surviving on nominal amounts of funding pre-pandemic, the demand for connection and support services at the local level and demand for specialist health support at a national level (particularly, for example, for people with rare health conditions) has definitely fuelled further demand.

We see this particularly in charities that play a vital local role in addressing health and social care need and the social determinants of health, through local service provision, but also importantly as engines of human and social capital (O'Leary and Fox, 2020). Disadvantaged communities – already disproportionately affected by the pandemic – face a longer and more challenging recovery because of the likely loss of local charities. This chapter has three objectives. Firstly, to set out the evidence around how charities – particularly through volunteering – play a significant role in addressing social determinants. Secondly, to review the emerging evidence of the impact of the pandemic on charities, focused very much on the resulting effect volunteering and also on the social determinants of health. Thirdly, the chapter will make the case for significant changes in the way the central and local government uses its commissioning and procurement functions to ensure that the voluntary sector is not totally decimated by the pandemic.

Background

Charities can and do play a vital role in addressing the social determinants of health (Boswell et al, 2017; O'Leary and Fox, 2020). Although most charities in the UK are not health-focused (NCVO, 2020), many nevertheless make significant contributions in areas of our lives that affect and are affected by our health (Boswell et al, 2017). They do so in a number of ways. They are information providers, signposters, referrers and gateways to health services (Daly and Allen, 2017). They can contribute to and shape health policy, research and delivery (Wood et al, 2011). Charities often provide services that generate social outcomes related to social determinants. They are social innovators, driving improvements in outcomes and changes in how and for whom services are targeted. Their services often focus on the individuals and groups experiencing significant disadvantage, in contrast to more universalist public services. And charities often engage with, and advocate for, people experiencing disadvantage in ways that the public sector often cannot do (Paten et al, 2007). They are also important engines of human and social capital, particularly in terms of volunteering (O'Leary et al, 2018).

There are, however, a number of factors that limit, or create barriers to, the role of charities in addressing social determinants. Firstly, many charities do not recognise the role they play in addressing social determinants, or struggle to evidence their impact in this area (Boswell et al, 2017). Secondly, there are significant place-based variations in distribution of charities (Mohan and Bennett, 2019). More affluent areas often have access to larger and more diverse range of charities, while more disadvantaged areas have fewer organisations with fewer resources (O'Leary and Fox, 2020). This uneven distribution of, and access to, charities can mean that the neighbourhoods that are most disadvantaged by health inequalities are also least able to benefit from the impact of charities on addressing social determinants. And finally, charitable funding is focused on a small number of large charities (NCVO, 2020). This is particularly the case in terms of funding from government commissioning and procurement; although around a third of income for the sector comes from this single source, most of it goes to a small number of large charities (O'Leary and McDonald, 2019).

The role of charities in addressing social determinants of health was increasingly being recognised before the COVID-19 pandemic. But there is a real danger that, in the aftermath of COVID-19, local authorities reduce their engagement with, and procurement of, charities, and that this will have a devastating effect on more disadvantaged areas.

Charities, volunteering and social determinants

Charities are a fundamental part of civil society, touching every aspect of our lives (O'Leary and McDonald, 2019). Before COVID-19, evidence suggested that the charitable sector was a growing part of the UK's economy (Keen and Audickas, 2017), and was increasingly a key partner for the delivery of a wide range of public services (Han, 2017). There is also a significant and growing body of evidence that charities play a key role in addressing the social determinants of health and tackling health inequalities (James, 2017). As information providers and educators, as policy influencers, as service providers and as social innovators, charities can and do make a substantial and significant impact. Charities are also part of the social fabric of civil society, and play a key role in social cohesion, connectedness and social capital. It is through these routes – and particularly the role that volunteering plays in social capital and thereby in addressing social determinants – that is the focus of this chapter.

Volunteering is a broad concept, which covers a wide range of activities that 'help or benefit those beyond one's immediate family or environment' (Lee and Brudney, 2012). It is an important part of our civil engagement (Goth and Smaland, 2014); it can take many forms, and takes place through organisations (formal) or with friends and neighbours (informal) (James, 2017). A key component of most definitions of volunteering is that it is done without remuneration, and for the benefit of others. Most small charities, even if they have a paid for staff team, will rely heavily in terms of both their governance and frontline service delivery on volunteers.

Much of the evidence base around volunteering focuses on formal, organisation-based forms of volunteering, undertaken predominantly through charities. There are a number of health and other benefits for individuals who volunteer. Southby et al (2019) set out a number of these individual-level benefits. They include improvements in the mental and physical health of volunteers, tackling social isolation, and reduced likelihood of hospital admission. Yeung et al (2017) further suggest benefits in terms of individuals' wellbeing and life expectancy. Volunteering can also increase individuals' human capital (O'Leary et al, 2018), and can have a number of other individual-level, non-health benefits. But volunteering also has wider social benefits, particularly because of its role in social capital. These wider benefits are increasingly being recognised by policymakers (O'Donnell et al, 2014), although there is a significant danger that the impact of COVID-19 will be devastating in this area.

Social capital is, of course, a complex and contested concept, but broadly involves social networks, civic and community participation, trust and reciprocity (O'Leary and Fox, 2020). It has been defined as 'the features of social organization, such as civic participation, norms of reciprocity, and trust in others, that facilitate cooperation for mutual benefit' (Kawachi et al, 1997: 1491). There are both community and individual-level dimensions of social capital. The inception of small charities is often spurred on by the feeling of isolation and marginalisation from the 'mainstream'. For many social entrepreneurs setting up charities, the act of establishing an organisation with a social purpose is precisely because they have been moved by a social injustice. On average the Charity Commission for England and Wales registers around 500 new charities a month, this has continued unabated during the pandemic. Small groups of individuals moved by their own or their collective plight have come together to do good. In so doing, they nearly always initially act as volunteers, either as trustees or at the operational level. It may be a year to three years before they get their first substantive input of funding, and they are fuelled in the meantime on high levels of mutual goodwill generating immense social capital.

Although both the concept of social capital and much of the empirical work around it was developed outside of healthcare (Pearce and Smith, 2003), social capital is recognised as playing a role in the social determinants of health. This role is an unusual one, and is contested (Solar and Irwin, 2010). It is a concept that has engendered much debate (Moore and Kawachi, 2017). There is a strong argument that social capital is a key factor shaping population health, and that policy interventions that seek to increase or improve social capital should be effective in addressing social determinants. For example, using data from the European Social Survey on 14 countries on the causal impact of social capital on health, Rocco and Suhrcke (2012) found that community-level social capital did not affect health, but that individual-level social capital did have an effect. They concluded that policy interventions should be targeted at individual social capital, but suggested this would also benefit the wider community. But there are also questions raised about the definition and measurement of social capital, its causal relationship to social determinants, and whether policy interventions can be effective in improving social capital and thereby addressing social determinants of health (Pearce and Smith, 2003). Southby et al (2019) stress that there is a growing body of evidence that shows a significant positive relationship between social capital and volunteering. This means that volunteering appears to improve the individual-level and community-level social capital, and is associated with individual- and community-level health benefits (Goth and Smaland, 2014).

This raises three important questions. Firstly, before COVID-19, were there differences in volunteering rates that might contribute to variations in the social determinants of health between different groups? Secondly, what is the likely effect of the pandemic on volunteering rates and the charitable sector more widely, and is this likely to affect social determinants? And, thirdly, what should policymakers take into consideration in their post-COVID-19 planning around charities and volunteering?

Variations in volunteering rates

There is a significant body of evidence that some groups and communities are less likely to engage in volunteering. Mandy James, in her report for Volunteering Matters, Barriers and Benefits: Tackling Health Inequalities through Volunteering (2017), puts this bluntly. She states that 'those who could benefit most from volunteering are the least likely to be able to take part in it', and sets out a number of barriers to volunteering faced by disadvantaged groups. James also argues that unless these barriers are addressed, the full benefits of volunteering will not be enjoyed by everyone. In a rapid review of the evidence around barriers to volunteering and their implications for addressing health inequalities, Kris Southby and colleagues (2019) find variations in volunteering, and that these variations result in 'unequal distribution of health and well-being benefits from volunteering'. They identify that different disadvantaged groups experience different barriers to participation. Goth and Smaland (2014) reference a wide, international literature that finds that most volunteers come from wealthier and more educated sections of society, echoing James' assertion that those who would most benefit are least likely to volunteer.

Yet this is an assumption that relies on a very visible, formal representation of volunteering. Volunteering as a trustee of a charity or in establishing an organisation are often not counted, because they do not form part of the formal lexicon of volunteering. Small charities that are volunteer-led will not count their founding personnel as volunteers, volunteer numbers are counted through formal infrastructure networks, as those that are brought into the system.

The other major omission from the volunteering lexicon is faith-based volunteering. All the major faiths in the UK rely heavily on relationism in service of their community and increasingly the broader community. During the pandemic many have become leading advocates at a local level in the distribution of food, medicines and befriending. Yet such volunteering features rarely in the official records of voluntary effort. In research for the All Party Parliamentary Group on Faith and Society around the role of faith-based groups, Chris Baker and Adam Dinham from Goldsmiths College, University of London, demonstrated how important the role of faith groups and their work had become to local councils during the pandemic (APPG Faith and Society, 2021). Beyond the immediate crisis, many faith organisations find it exceptionally difficult to secure grant and public funding, for the fear of the perception that such funds could be used for proselytising, yet they have been first responders and at the heart of early intervention for so much volunteering in health and social care.

While much of this literature identifies individual-level barriers to volunteering (time, skills, caring responsibilities, lack of support), there are also community-level barriers. Because there are significant variations between neighbourhoods in the size and quality of local charity economies (Mohan and Bennett, 2019), more affluent neighbourhoods tend to have larger and more diverse charity sectors, while more disadvantaged areas have fewer organisations with less resources.

Finally, it is also the case that previous experience of volunteering is a strong predictor of future volunteering, and that volunteering is a persistent lifetime activity for many. This is a finding of an analysis of data on 10,000 individuals aged 16 and over from the British Household Panel Survey by Chris Dawson and colleagues (Dawson et al, 2019). This suggests that policy interventions aimed at increasing first time volunteering in more disadvantaged areas are likely to have long-term benefits on volunteering rates and thereby address social determinants of health.

The impact of COVID-19 on volunteering and on charities

The full extent of the devastating impact of COVID-19 and the national and local lockdowns is not yet fully known. But there are already indications that the charitable sector has been very badly hit by the pandemic, suffering a 'triple whammy' of reduced fundraising/income, reduced levels of volunteering, and increased demand for services. Andrew Bradbury, in a piece in The Conversation in April 2020, called this a 'perfect storm' for charities (Bradbury, 2020), and things have deteriorated significantly since then.

The impact on funding is particularly significant. In a survey early on in the pandemic of 300 charities in England and Wales, New Philanthropic Capital (NPC, 2020) found that: firstly, more than half of all charities get income from public sector contracts (with 38 per cent of small and medium sized charities doing so, an increase of 18 points over three years); and, secondly, that 60 per cent were subsidising these contracts from other sources of fundraising. Most charities have seen a fall in their fundraising because of COVID-19, and expect it to be at least a year before fundraising returns to pre-COVID-19 levels (PBE, 2020). This means that, unless organisations find a way to ensure the costs of public sector delivery are covered by those contracts, many charities will need to severely cut their non-contracted activities to make ends meet. It will be challenging for many smaller charities to do this, and it is smaller charities that are most likely to engage with volunteering.

More recently, research by the Charities Commission (the UK's statutory regulator of charities) found that over 90 per cent of charities have been negatively impacted by the pandemic, with 85 per cent reporting negative impacts on service delivery, 72 per cent on their financial position, and two-thirds on staffing and governance (Charity Commission, 2021).

But the likely reduction in volunteering rates is also significant. During the early stages of the pandemic, anecdotal evidence suggested a significant number of existing volunteers have stopped working, and there has been a huge reduction in the flow of new volunteers. This is not surprising; the UK lockdowns would have prevented volunteering, and most volunteers are older people, the group suffering most from COVID-19. This anecdotal evidence has subsequently been backed up with survey evidence, with a third of charities reporting volunteering challenges. These challenges include loss of volunteers or volunteers not being able to work (reported by under a third of charities), not having the capacity to make use of volunteers who were available (reported by 12 per cent of charities), and increased need for mental health and wellbeing support for volunteers (reported by 17 per cent of charities). It is not possible from these survey data to understand whether and how smaller charities were differently affected. However, as with funding, this is likely to have a more significant impact on smaller charities, as these are more dependent on volunteers (Mohan and Bennett, 2019).

And we have yet to see the full impact of the crisis on demand for charitable services. The long-term social effects of the crisis – on mental health and wellbeing, on animal welfare, on poverty and on children – will likely see demand rising for years to come. Indeed, most charities in the UK expect demand for the services to rise significantly during 2020 (PBE, 2020).

In an ironic twist, the Small Charities Coalition, the leading national umbrella body in the UK for small charities, closed in Spring 2022 (Small Charities Coalition, 2021). The reasons for its closure are manifold, but should also be a reminder of the unique pressures that have also befallen trustees, who as volunteers with the ultimate responsibility for governance and the sustainability of the charitable objects of the organisation have also struggled. For relationism to be truly effective within the context of volunteering it needs to work both between organisations and within agencies. The Association of Chairs survey in November 2020 found that:

As a result of the challenges organisations have faced, Chairs found themselves giving significantly more time to their role: 62% of respondents reported spending four or more days a month on their chairing role compared with 43% before the pandemic. A total of 18% reported spending more than 11 days a month on chairing, compared with 10% before the pandemic.

The most common reason given for the increase was the time spent supporting staff, particularly the CEO (32%). Other common reasons cited were additional time spent in meetings, including more frequent board meetings and communicating generally (25%) and Covid-related funding and crisis management (24%). (AoC, 2021, p 3)

The landscape around the discussion of volunteering relies heavily on the recruitment of volunteers for service delivery. It relies on a narrative that looks at the individual volunteer as 'extra labour' for the execution of frontline services.

Conclusion

There is a danger of a significant and prolonged downturn in service delivery volunteering as a result of the COVID-19 crisis, with significant implications for social capital and for action on the social determinants of health. Before the crisis, there were already differing levels of volunteering between areas, with poorer communities being less able to enjoy the benefits of volunteering on individuals' and population health. There is a risk that more disadvantaged areas will see their already smaller pool of volunteers reduced more substantially than their more affluent neighbours. People and communities are still aspiring to establish small charities, but their ability to deliver sustainable and purposeful services for the long term is greatly diminished.

Concerted action is needed by policymakers and commissioners, and by charities, to minimise the impact of COVID-19 on volunteering and on the impact that charities have on addressing the social determinants of health.

First, concerted action is needed to address the funding gap between the cost of delivering public sector contracts and the price paid for these contracts. This is particularly important for smaller charities, who even before COVID-19 faced greater challenges in fundraising compared to larger charities (O'Leary and McDonald, 2019) and have seen their fundraising fall even further because of COVID-19.

Secondly, programmes are need to encourage people to start volunteering and to start measuring volunteering in its diverse formats. To have maximum impact in terms of addressing the social determinants of health, these programmes should be targeted at more disadvantaged areas and groups. These programmes need to address the barriers that disadvantaged groups and areas face that prevent volunteering. Encouraging a new cohort of volunteers will have long lasting effects on levels of volunteering, on the health and wellbeing of those involved in volunteering, on the wider community's health, and on levels of social capital. Finally, programmes are needed to get previous volunteers to return to volunteering.

References

AoC (2021) Chairing through COVID: Above and beyond. AoC Chairs' survey supported by CCLA.

APPG Faith and Society (2021) *Keeping the Faith: Partnerships between Faith Groups and Local Authorities during and beyond the Pandemic.* London: All Party Parliamentary Group on Faith and Society.

Boswell, K., Joy, I. and Lamb, C. (2017) *Keeping Us Well: How Non-Health Charities Address the Social Determinants of Health*. London: NPC.

Bradbury, A. (2020) Coronavirus is a perfect storm for charities – here's why the sector is calling for help. *The Conversation*. Available at: https://theconversation.com/coronavirus-is-a-perfect-storm-for-charities-heres-why-the-sector-is-calling-for-help-134088

Charity Commission (2021) COVID-19 survey 2021, Charity Commission. Available at: https://www.gov.uk/government/publications/charity-commission-covid-19-survey-2021

Daly, S. and Allen, J. (2017) *Voluntary Sector Action on the Social Determinants of Health*. London: Institute of Health Equity.

Dawson, C., Baker, P.L. and Dowell, D. (2019) Getting into the 'giving habit': The dynamics of volunteering in the UK. *Voluntas*, 30(5): 1006–1021.

Goth, U.S. and Smaland, E. (2014) The role of civic engagement for men's health and well being in Norway: A contribution to public health. *International Journal of Environmental Research and Public Health*, 11(6): 6375–6387.

Han, J. (2017) Social marketisation and policy influence of third sector organisations: Evidence from the UK. *Voluntas*, 28(3): 1209–1225.

Institute of Fundraising (2020) Impact on the charity sector during coronavirus – research report June 2020, Chartered Institute of Fundraising. Available at: https://ciof.org.uk/IoF/media/IOF/Policy/1coronavirus-impact-survey-report-june-2020-(2)_1.pdf?ext=.pdf

James, M. (2017) *Barriers and Benefits: Tackling Inequalities in Health through Volunteering*. London: Volunteering Matters.

Kawachi, I., Kennedy, B.P., Lochner, K. and ProthrowStith, D. (1997) Social capital, income inequality, and mortality. *American Journal of Public Health*, 87(9): 1491–1498.

Keen, A. and Audickas, L. (2017) *Charities and the Voluntary Sector: Statistics*. London: House of Commons Library.

Lee, Y.J. and Brudney, J.L. (2012) Participation in formal and informal volunteering: Implications for volunteer recruitment. *Nonprofit Management and Leadership*, 23(2): 159–180.

Mohan, J. and Bennett, M.R. (2019) Community-level impacts of the third sector: Does the local distribution of voluntary organizations influence the likelihood of volunteering? *Environment and Planning A: Economy and Space*, 51(4): 950–979.

Moore, S. and Kawachi, I. (2017) Twenty years of social capital and health research: A glossary. *Journal of Epidemiology and Community Health*, 71(5): 513–517.

NCVO (2020) *UK Civil Society Almanac*. London: National Council of Voluntary Organisations.

NPC (2020) *State of the Sector 2020: The Condition of Charities before the COVID Crisis*. London: New Philanthropy Capital

O'Donnell, G., Deaton, A., Durand, M., Halpern, D. and Layard, R. (2014) *Wellbeing and Policy*. London: Legatum Institute.

O'Leary, C. and Fox, C. (2020) Commissioning and social determinants of health: Evidence and opportunities. In Bonner, A. (ed) *Local Authorities and the Social Determinants of Health*. Bristol: Policy Press.

O'Leary, C. and McDonald, D. (2019) Procurement and commissioning in the social sector. In McDonald, D. (ed) *Innovation and Change in the Non-profit Sector: Case Studies in Survival, Sustainability, and Success*. London: Pavillion,

O'Leary, C., Baines, S., Bailey, G., NcNeil, T., Csoba, J. and Sipis, F. (2018) Innovation and social investment programmes in Europe. *European Policy Analysis*, 4(2): 294–312.

Paten, R., Mordaunt, J. and Cornforth, C. (2007) Beyond nonprofit management education: Leadership development in a time of blurred boundaries and distributed learning. *Nonprofit and Voluntary Sector Quarterly*, 36: 148S–162S.

PBE (2020) *COVID Charity Tracker November 2020*. London: Pro Bono Economics.

Pearce, N. and Smith, G.D. (2003) Is social capital the key to inequalities in health? *American Journal of Public Health*, 93(1): 122–129.

Rocco, L. and Suhrcke, M. (2012) *Is Social Capital Good for Health? A European Perspective*. Copenhagen: World Health Organization Europe. Available at: https://www.euro.who.int/__data/assets/pdf_file/0005/170 078/Is-Social-Capital-good-for-your-health.pdf

Small Charities Commission (2021) Small Charities Commission set to close. Available at: https://www.smallcharities.org.uk/post/small-charit ies-coalition-to-close

Solar, O. and Irwin, A. (2010) *A Conceptual Framework for Action on the Social Determinants of Health*. Geneva: World Health Organisation

Southby, K., South, J. and Bagnall, A.M. (2019) A rapid review of barriers to volunteering for potentially disadvantaged groups and implications for health inequalities. *Voluntas*, 30(5): 907–920.

Wood, L., Shilton, T., Dimer, L., Smith, J. and Leahy, T. (2011) Beyond the rhetoric: How can non-government organisations contribute to reducing health disparities for Aboriginal and Torres Strait Islander people? *Australian Journal of Primary Health*, 17(4): 384–394.

Yeung, J.W.K., Zhang, Z.N. and Kim, T.Y. (2017) Volunteering and health benefits in general adults: Cumulative effects and forms. *BMC Public Health*, 17(1): 736.

15

Creating added value: the third sector, local and national government working together to address domestic abuse

Emily Hodge

> For us to effectively tackle domestic abuse it is essential that we take a much more holistic approach. This means that we work together in partnerships across all agencies and sectors both on an operational and strategic level. We must put people who are affected by domestic abuse at the heart of this and treat them with trust and respect.
>
> Jacobs, 2021

Introduction

This chapter will explore the wicked issue of domestic abuse and the complex challenges faced by those providing support to people affected, including victim survivors, children and perpetrators.

It has long been considered that domestic abuse is a difficult and complex issue to address. Decades of changing political agendas combined with austerity have not only meant that legislation, funding and strategic frameworks have not reflected frontline work and the needs of communities in relation to domestic abuse, but have created barriers to putting the lived experiences of survivors at the heart of addressing the root cause of domestic abuse, which is so often the root cause of all other types of abuse.

This chapter will identify the roles of, and relationships between, different stakeholders in the public and voluntary sectors, including faith-based organisations, in addressing domestic abuse, and will argue that relationalism, partnership and a coordinated community response from strategic through to local levels are the only true way to address domestic abuse.

It will seek to explore some of the key challenges faced by these sectors, including the sustainability of services and the measurement of their impact. It will consider how the thought process about what 'good' looks like needs to change in order to fully gauge the difference made to individual lives affected by domestic abuse.

Domestic Abuse Act 2021

The landmark Domestic Abuse Act achieved Royal Assent in April 2021, and moves towards significant change for those affected by domestic abuse, including a comprehensive definition that recognises children as victims in their own right, names coercive control as abuse, and offers improved protections to victims. The statutory appointment of the Domestic Abuse Commissioner for England and Wales ensures that government and public bodies are held to account and have a duty to cooperate. Part 4 of the Act imposes a statutory duty on Tier One authorities to provide safe accommodation and support to all victims and children affected by domestic abuse.

Although the Act is a positive move forward and will enhance many provisions, there are some omissions, despite amendments being tabled, that would have strengthened the Act further, including protections for migrant survivors such as a firewall between police and immigration, a statutory duty for community-based services, and training for the judiciary.

Two women a week are killed by a current or former partner in England and Wales (ONS, 2018) and during Commons debates on the Bill, MP Jess Phillips read out the names of 118 women killed over the past year by a male perpetrator of domestic abuse (Anon, 2021).

Prevalence of domestic abuse and COVID-19

According to the Crime Survey for England and Wales (ONS, 2019) in the year ending March 2020, an estimated 5.5 per cent of adults aged 16 to 74 years (2.3 million people) experienced domestic abuse in the last year, and an estimated 8.8 million adults, aged 16–74, had experienced domestic abuse since the age of 16 years. This equates to a prevalence rate of approximately 21 in 100 adults. Women are much more likely than men to be the victims of high risk or severe domestic abuse.

Domestic abuse has a devastating impact on children and young people. Analysis by the Children's Commissioner in 2019 shows that 831,000 children in England are living in households that report domestic abuse and 62 per cent of children living with domestic abuse are directly harmed by the perpetrator of the abuse, in addition to the harm caused by witnessing the abuse of others (Caada, 2014). However, the problem is much bigger than official statistics, as many victim survivors and children don't report abuse, therefore it is not recorded.

The COVID-19 pandemic has worsened the situation, but it has not caused domestic abuse. Perpetrators must be held to account for their actions. During

2020, Women's Aid conducted research, resulting in the report, *A Perfect Storm* (Women's Aid Federation of England, 2020), which found that 60 per cent of survivors living with their abusers said their abuse had got worse from March to June 2020. Abusers have been able to use lockdown restrictions and the virus itself to induce further fear and control, and this is evidenced through the same report, which found that 67 per cent of survivors reported that COVID-19 was being used as part of the abuse they experienced. Furthermore, the pandemic has shone a light on existing inequalities and their impact on those they discriminate against, prompting all sectors to consider more fully the intersectionality of people they work with, or who work for them, to ensure inclusion is embedded. This is very much a work in progress, but something that the domestic abuse sector is speaking up about.

Partnership working: approaches and conflicts

The kind of partnership which should be sought in response to addressing wicked issues, and in particular domestic abuse, is the strategic-goal agreement model articulated by Osborne (2008). When there is a clear need, evidenced by partner responses, to understand different perspectives and motivations, it is these that should be made use of to reshape services.

Top-down approaches which have previously failed to resolve 'wicked issues' usually consist of an approach being applied by 'experts' in a way that narrows perspectives (Head, 2008) and not including service user perspectives (Kearns and Coen, 2014). Commonly, in seeking to address wicked issues, change or transformation programmes can easily fail to clarify what the issue truly is or if there is one (Snape and Stewart, 1996) and without this no solution can be agreed. When there is a lack of clear definition of the roles and responsibilities among partners, collaboration between different agencies is not enabled (Sullivan and Skelcher, 2002). Diverse voices and perspectives are missed or not brought to bear on the problem and partners do not then 'buy in' (Sullivan and Skelcher, 2002). The results of this type of approach are usually pre-prepared 'solutions' that add resources to existing services which only deal with 'components' of the whole system (Simon Breeze, Chief Executive Officer, Community Action Sutton).

In considering how this process sheds light on the use of partnerships to solve 'wicked problems' more broadly, a key learning point is that partnership work must be based on values. There is commonly a moral dimension to 'wicked issues' and this sometimes involves victims being seen as partly accountable (Wexler, 2009). Furthermore, a poorly recognised component of organisations (at least in practice) is the role of emotion (Fineman, 2000). As 'wicked problems' tend to be emotive and those who seek to solve them are often motivated by strong emotions and personal values (and sometimes experience) this recognition becomes crucial. Therefore in partnerships working on 'wicked issues' *how* things are done is as important as *what* is done.

This approach requires a deeper understanding of what motivates partners and investment in time to build trust. Simply put, in partnership working, relationships matter and 'securing accountability in a technical sense should not be seen as a replacement for the broader social process of creating (and embedding) trust and common purpose' (Lowndes and Squires, 2012: 404). This means that the individuals involved also matter and so creating a shared way of working, disagreeing and measuring is also essential. This is where 'boundary spanners', those who can work across sectors and organisational boundaries, are important (Williams, 2010). These individuals work as the 'glue' in partnerships and are able to find ways to create a shared purpose and maintain it. Sometimes, these will be internal people, other times they may be brought in as independent consultants who can take an objective view.

By seeking new models of partnership, and looking at how partnerships can function more effectively, positive improvements in relationships and the final output of programmes are generally seen to be transformative and the process that partners go through is collaborative. This suggests that the right way to 'do' partnerships is known. What is interesting is that despite this, organisational, sectoral, financial and personal factors militate against good practice. Chief among these would seem to be the effects of fragmented public services and funding cuts (Glasby and Dickinson, 2008) and the political/managerial expediency of focusing on more controllable, measurable interventions (Head, 2008).

While the right structures and organisations are essential to make a partnership work, when using such an approach to solve 'wicked problems' more than that is needed. Efforts to understand the moral and emotional motivations of different partners are essential. Through this process a shared definition of the issue can be produced and from this a shared plan and a sense of ownership will flow. People who can span boundaries and 'step outside' of their organisations are needed to achieve this. The complex nature of 'wicked issues' coupled with fragmented, often underfunded services mean that effective partnerships happen 'naturally'. As Kearns and Coen (2014: 5) put it, successful partnership working is 'not simply an infrastructure of coordination but entails an architecture composed of a set of processes and structures and a cultural appreciation of values and power'.

Figure 15.1: Standing Together Against Domestic Abuse, 2020

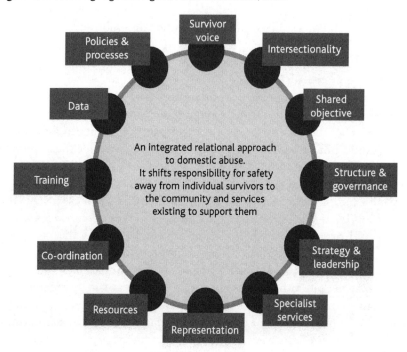

Best practice partnership models

The Coordinated Community Response

The most serious abuse can result in domestic homicides. Reviews of these murders and the surrounding circumstances (Domestic Homicide Reviews) usually highlight failures in information sharing, missed opportunities to intervene earlier, and gaps in services or provision to support people when they need it.

Standing Together Against Domestic Abuse (2020) is an organisation that aims to end domestic abuse by changing the way that local areas respond to it through an approach called the Coordinated Community Response (CCR), comprising 12 components (see Figure 15.1).

The fundamental notion of the CCR is that no single agency or person can see the full picture of what life is like for a family or individual, but working together, all agencies can bring insights and interventions to ensure safety and wellbeing. This model of a coordinated local partnership to tackle and ultimately prevent domestic abuse is now widely accepted as best practice, and encourages agencies to adopt a relational approach to partnership with each other, as described by Simon Breeze in the previous section.

A Whole Health Approach

In the year before getting effective help, nearly a quarter (23 per cent) of victims are at high risk of serious harm or murder. In the most extreme cases, victims reported that they attended accident and emergency departments 15 times. The Home Office estimates that every year domestic abuse costs the healthcare system over £2.3 billion, with the long-term emotional and physical health costs of domestic abuse estimated to be between £22,000 and £54,000 (Home Office, 2019) per person (not including the cost if homicide occurs). Only one in five victims calls the police – but many more access health services. Whether a GP surgery, a maternity unit or a mental health service, health providers are well placed to spot the signs of domestic abuse and provide immediate support and information.

In 2017, a coalition of domestic abuse specialist organisations, funded by the Department of Health and Social Care and the Department for Digital, Culture, Media and Sport, came together to deliver the Pathfinder Project (SafeLives, 2020), engaging nine CCRs and 18 NHS Trusts across England to implement wide-ranging and sustainable interventions in eight local areas. It built the case for a Whole Health Approach by working with health stakeholders, turning guidance into practice and providing interventions where a gap in provision was identified, embedding local health and domestic abuse governance structures and sharing learning.

A whole health model goes beyond the implementation of individual initiatives such as training; it requires systemic change and the strategic commitment of services. Figure 15.1 outlines the key components of this model. A robust strategic framework and governance structure is essential in creating the foundations for the implementation of this work and to ensure a coordinated and sustainable approach.

Commissioning domestic abuse services

Effective commissioning cannot be achieved in isolation and is best delivered in close collaboration with others, such as health partners, education, housing and the voluntary, community and social enterprise (VCSE) sector. Over the past decade, the focus of commissioning has moved from simply saving money, to focus on effective commissioning for people-centred health and wellbeing. The shift in perspective means commissioners and governing bodies aim to achieve good outcomes by using evidence, local knowledge, skills and resources to best effect.

This means working in partnership across the health and social care system to promote health and wellbeing, and to prevent, as far as possible, the need for health and social care. Effective commissioning plays a central role in driving up quality, enabling people to meaningfully direct their own care, facilitating integrated service delivery, and making the most effective use of the available resources. Examples of this are how Primary Care Networks connect into local place-based responses, but recognise the need for more Integrated Care Systems.

What Works Wellbeing describes wellbeing as 'how we're doing'. Commissioners need to be seeking not only to fill gaps and deficits, but to build on the strengths and assets of people and communities to improve the quality of life for people.

> Wellbeing is personal and subjective, but also universally relevant. ... Wellbeing encompasses the environmental factors that affect us, and the experiences we have throughout our lives. These can fall into traditional policy areas of economy, health, education and so on. But wellbeing also crucially recognises the aspects of our lives that we determine ourselves: through our own capabilities as individuals; how we feel about ourselves; the quality of the relationships that we have with other people; and our sense of purpose. (What Works Centre for Wellbeing, 2021)

A commissioning case study: London Borough of Sutton 'Transformation Programme'

In 2017, many local agencies came together to co-produce a place-based plan with residents. This is known as the 'Sutton Plan' (London Borough of Sutton, 2017). Four strategic priorities were identified through this process, one of which was reducing domestic abuse across the borough. From this process, the council invested a significant amount of money along with other partner contributions, and out of this came a multiagency strategic partnership board, with shared values and high level outcomes that underpinned the terms of reference.

For many years, as is so common across different local authority areas, domestic abuse services in Sutton were commissioned separately, meaning each provider worked to different measures and outcomes, and there was a lack of joined up working. In 2019, the Transformation Board hired a consultant to carry out a needs analysis, context and mapping exercise, and a commissioning review, with the intention to bring everything together under one commissioned specialist service. A tiered approach was deemed necessary, and so the service specification included universal awareness-raising among residents and training for frontline staff across the public sector, targeted work with families at risk of domestic abuse, specialist provision for victims, children and perpetrators, and interventions for those in crisis, including the continuation of Refuge provision.

Following market testing and engagement across the partnership, the VCSE sector, service users and residents, the procurement process took place. In

November 2019, a specialist service, 'Transform', was launched, as a VCSE lead provider model with five subcontracted partners. The elements of the provision included a single front door, the Independent Domestic Violence Advisor service and One Stop Shop coordination, Freedom programme and counselling for victims, group work and 1-1 support for children who have witnessed domestic abuse, group courses for young people at risk of becoming victims or perpetrators, a perpetrator programme to address and change behaviours, volunteer-led support for families with children under the age of five, and a Refuge. As well as this, the lead provider was responsible for the overall coordination of the service, capturing all data, meeting performance indicators, a single point of entry referral pathway and partner management.

Partners from other agencies were integral to the commissioning activity. Health, police, housing, education and VCSE sector colleagues in particular contributed to the process and each agency has done copious amounts of work as part of their membership of the Transformation Programme, through training their own frontline staff, raising awareness about recognising the signs of abuse, supporting staff through the implementation of staff policies about domestic abuse and incorporating elements of domestic abuse into primary and secondary curriculums.

As with many institutions set up within a local government framework, there were certain organisational and cultural barriers to overcome to achieve this effective partnership working. Whereas initially, a delivery plan was developed prior to the board convening, as a way to support partners and seemingly save time, it was soon identified that there was another piece of work around the emotive response to the issue, research, engagement and approach that needed to be established first, which in turn would lead to a more organic and effective delivery plan, and the recognition that domestic abuse is a gendered crime that disproportionately affects women also led to the decision to appoint a woman to chair the strategic partnership board.

The success of this programme and the commissioning of a specialist integrated service can largely be attributed to strong partnership working from the highest strategic levels or agencies through to frontline practitioners, underpinned by shared values and the desire to achieve the same outcomes for those affected by domestic abuse in the borough. The ongoing priority is always about evolving the service in response to need, maintaining and improving ownership of a CCR model across all stakeholders.

Co-production and the voice of lived experiences

It has been a primary priority of the strategic partnership board that domestic abuse services are co-produced wherever possible, and that the voices of lived experiences are paramount to all decisions that are taken. Only when the voices of people affected are truly heard can real change happen. The process of being involved also results in empowered communities who take an active role within their own lives to improve things for themselves and those around them.

The partnership recognises that better outcomes are achieved when services are shaped in person-centred ways through actively listening and responding to what is said, meaning fewer mistakes, less duplication and quicker solutions. Commissioning 'by and for' providers to deliver accessible services ensures that individuals' needs are met in an intersectional way.

Monitoring, evaluation and quality improvement

In order to truly monitor and evaluate the difference made through domestic abuse services in a person-centred and outcomes-based way, we must shift the question from 'What does good *look* like?' to us as a public sector commissioning body, to 'What does good *feel* like?' to the person we are commissioning services for.

For example, we may ask the person, 'How do you feel when you put your key in your front door at night, and how would you like this feeling to change through our help?' By measuring this kind of response, we can ensure we are actually meeting the outcomes that people themselves would like to see. The challenge to commissioners is how that is measured. There are a number of assets-based models that measure softer outcomes that can be used for this kind of service, such as the Developmental Assets Framework (Search Institute, USA, 2021), which is a robust, evidence-based model. This model was adopted by the London Borough of Sutton several years ago and is used as a way to measure added value to contracts above and beyond the contractual obligations, demonstrating additional benefits to residents within the borough.

The Transform partnership, made up of five voluntary organisations and one education setting, offers an inordinate amount of added value above the contract delivery. Transform users are often referred to other, non-commissioned services that the partners provide, such as 1-1 counselling, art therapy or English courses. All of these partners juggle several different funders and services within their organisations, as is so common within the voluntary sector, and so the people affected can usually access additional support, which is added value to the local authority contract. The success of Transform's work can be attributed, first and foremost, to the frontline workers providing genuine care and support as needed by each person through the building of supportive relationships, and underpinned by commissioning that is responsive and collaborative with stakeholders at strategic and operational levels. The tension that continues to be a challenge is that of person-centred and strength-based commissioning in a climate of efficiency savings and a global pandemic.

Faith and voluntary sector response

It is no surprise that the voluntary sector provides a vast amount of non-accommodation based provision for victim survivors of domestic abuse. In many circumstances, these organisations work with many people with complex needs, and domestic abuse may be one of many things that someone is experiencing at any one time, as well as often being the root cause of other problems, such as substance misuse, poor mental and/or physical health, debt and homelessness.

Interestingly, evidence suggests that levels of domestic abuse in church communities are reflect domestic abuse in wider society. In a survey carried out by the charity, Restored, 90 per cent of victim survivors are women with a male perpetrator. Therefore, faith communities, and more specifically, the church, are one of the few places that the whole family is present, whether together or apart.

When it comes to tackling the wicked issue of domestic abuse, faith organisations must promote good practice within their settings and communities, to ensure that they are not being complicit in the abuse, as it is known to have been in the past with other forms of abuse, such as child abuse and sexual abuse. If this is achieved, it provides a unique space and a wider model for other agencies and providers. For this reason, it is imperative that faith organisations connect in with local partnership responses to avoid responding, albeit with good intentions, in isolation (Restored, 2018).

The Salvation Army's national domestic abuse steering group is currently exploring a domestic abuse champions model across the UK, aiming to challenge perpetrators, while at all times upholding the safety and wellbeing of victim survivors as paramount. Captain Emma Scott, founder of The Salvation Army's 'The Link Cafe' (TLC) in Merton, says:

> In order to end domestic abuse, there needs to be a societal shift which can be done through relationship, awareness and challenge. If all our churches, whether through our theological teaching and/or our actions, overtly condemned violence against women and girls, and took steps to support those experiencing it, this would at the very least help. Domestic abuse won't ever go away until perpetrators stop abusing and while world views can seemingly support the abuse this also has to be tackled. (Scott, 2021)

Case study: the Link Cafe, Merton

The Salvation Army is an international denomination of the Christian church and is committed to supporting people to reach their full potential and to live a life of freedom. These values have been championed since The Salvation Army was founded in 1865, with their work including the set up of rescue homes for women fleeing domestic abuse in the 1800s. Today, The Salvation Army continues to help and support people from domestic abuse by providing confidential accommodation through to support programmes.

TLC began in 2016, by a new Salvation Army officer, Captain Emma Scott, who met a lady who had turned up on the church doorstep because she'd left an abusive partner and didn't know what to do. Emma was unsure how to help her in the moment, but promised the lady that she wouldn't leave her side until she was safe. Despite being inspired by the many domestic abuse services already available in the borough, Emma identified a possible gap in support, and through much work and collaboration, TLC was born.

TLC is a safe space where women who have left their abusive partners can be linked to services in the local community. TLC welcomes and works with women from all backgrounds, faiths and ethnicities.

The core objective as a service is to enable women to feel welcome and, at their own pace, to support women to find their worth through non-judgemental, impartial and unconditional support. TLC offers practical and emotional support, including a safe space to share feelings and experiences, and access to a group of volunteers who journey with people and signpost them to appropriate services and agencies.

TLC is funded fully through The Salvation Army, local donations and through the use of volunteers and local networks, meaning there are no ties to public sector bodies for dependency to sustain services, or pressure to meet specified targets or key performance indicators. This is a stark contrast to publicly commissioned services, which are underpinned by competitive markets, driven by price in many cases, and are dictated by thresholds and criteria. However, TLC is very embedded in the local partnership response by supporting the strategic board, referring into the Multi-Agency Risk Conferences, a statutory set of arrangements to assist with securing the right allocation of resources for high risk victims, and working closely with other frontline professionals to offer smooth pathways for the people they work with (HMG 2022).

At TLC, no one completes an assessment form. All of their work is relationship based, understanding what really matters to individuals and supporting them to reach their own goals.

'At a time of utter despair in my life, I was drowning with the weight of all my difficulties and struggles. I had lost all hope of just trying to survive when I found myself entering the haven, TLC. It was a moment that forever changed my life. The love, care, understanding and support shown to me is immeasurable without any judgement. For me TLC is my saviour, hope, courage, strength, my lifeline and light pulling me out from the darkness. In short, TLC is my everything.' (TLC attendee)

The makeup of volunteers and the supporting network is made up of a handyperson, experts on the law and other areas, and pastoral people. In some cases, people who were once helped through TLC now give of their own time to help others. This holistic approach based on a support network of genuinely caring and independent people is a lifeline to the many women it seeks to support on a weekly basis. In the five years that TLC has been running, not one person has returned to an abusive partner.

This grassroots model of support is one that clearly achieves the notion of meeting people where they are at through a pure relationships-based model. Public sector bodies can take a number of lessons from this, if they are prepared to think creatively and innovatively about what 'good' looks like, and whether 'good' is reflective of outcomes for the person living their experience.

Conclusion

Despite much research and evidence on the subject, domestic abuse continues to be a wicked issue that the public and voluntary sector work to tackle year upon year, decade upon decade. The complexities of the issues, relationships and needs of those involved in each individual situation cannot be underestimated and anyone involved in trying to find solutions or shape support services should have an in-depth understanding and knowledge of what these might be, they should listen to the stories of people with lived experience, and then understand how to take a trauma-informed approach to working with people affected by domestic abuse.

Relationships at all levels of a response to domestic abuse must be the first priority. People living through and recovering from domestic abuse regularly tell us about individuals who supported them, enabled them and cared for them. These relationships override the value of any course or service available to them, although these things do have their own merit and can often be enablers to developing those relationships. This is evidenced through examples such as The Salvation Army's relational approach at a national and local level, through initiatives such as TLC.

Partner relationships between agencies and stakeholders have to be based on shared values and objectives for true transformation to take place for individuals. Simon Breeze considers why and how partnerships that are based on trust, deep understanding of key issues and user voices are key, and the opposite of a forced, paternalistic, 'top-down' approach, to tackling wicked issues. The case study about the London Borough of Sutton offered insight into how this way of working resulted in an impactful service offer, through a CCR.

The Domestic Abuse Act offers a unique opportunity to continue to strengthen the response to victim survivors and their children, particularly through the statutory provision of safe accommodation. The Domestic Abuse Commissioner's Office is required, by the government, to carry out a mapping exercise of community-based domestic abuse services throughout 2021 in order to establish the make-up of what is available to people across England and Wales. It is anticipated and hoped that the findings of this work will result in recommendations for a statutory duty to also be placed on authorities to provide community-based services in future legislation, to scrap the postcode lottery that is the current situation. Authorities are required, under the Act, to monitor the impact of these services, and it would be fair to assume that the largest impact of these services on people affected by domestic abuse could be attributed to the people they meet and the relationships they form through those services.

References

Anon (2021) Jess Philips: Society has just accepted dead women. BBC News, 11 March. https://www.bbc.co.uk/news/uk-politics-56365827. Accessed on 26 August 2022.

Caada (2014) *In Plain Sight: Effective Help for Children Exposed to Domestic Abuse*. Bristol: Caada.

Fineman, S. (2009) *Emotion in Organizations*. London: SAGE.

Glasby, J. and Dickinson, H. (2008) Joined-up rationing? An analysis of priority setting in health. *Journal of Integrated Care*, 19(1).

Head, B.W. (2008) 'Wicked problems in public policy', *Public Policy*, 3(2): 101–118.

HMG (2022) Domestic abuse: How to get help. https://www.gov.uk/guidance/domestic-abuse-how-to-get-help. Accessed on 26 August 2022.

Home Office (2019) *The Economic and Social Costs of Domestic Abuse*. https://assets.publishing.service.gov.uk/government/uploads/system/uploads/attachment_data/file/918897/horr107.pdf. Accessed on 26 August 2022.

Kearns, N. and Coen, L. (2014) 'Charting the trajectory of domestic violence policy change in the Republic of Ireland since the mid-1990s: A path towards integration?', *International Journal of Integrated Care*, 14(28): 1–8.

London Borough of Sutton (2017) *The Sutton Plan*. http://www.thesuttonplan.org. Accessed on 26 August 2022.

Lowndes, V. and Squires, S. (2012) 'Cuts, collaboration and creativity', *Public Money and Management*, 32(6): 401–408.

Office of the Children's Commissioner for England (2019) *Childhood Vulnerability in Numbers.* https://www.childrenscommissioner.gov.uk/report/childhood-vulnerability-in-england-2019/. Accessed on 26 August 2022.

Osborne, S.P. (ed) (2008) *The Third Sector in Europe.* London: Routledge.

Restored (2018) *In Churches Too: Churches Responses to Domestic Abuse – A Case Study of Cumbria.* https://restored.contentfiles.net/media/resources/files/churches_web.pdf Accessed on 26 August 2022.

SafeLives (2020) *Pathfinder: Key Findings Report. Enhancing the Response to Domestic Abuse across Health Settings.* https://safelives.org.uk/sites/default/files/resources/Pathfinder%20Key%20Findings%20Report_Final.pdf. Accessed on 26 August 2022.

Scott, E. (2021) The Link Cafe in Merton. Personal communication.

Search Institute, USA (2021) *The Developmental Assets Framework.* https://www.search-institute.org/our-research/development-assets/developmental-assets-framework/. Accessed on 26 August 2022.

Snape, D. and Stewart, M. (1996) *Keeping up the Momentum: Partnership Working in Bristol and the West of England.* Bristol: Bristol Chamber of Commerce.

Standing Together Against Domestic Abuse (2020) *In Search of Excellence: A Refreshed Guide to Effective Domestic Abuse Partnership Work – The Coordinated Community Response (CCR).*

Sullivan, H. and Skelcher, C. (2002) *Working across Boundaries: Collaboration in Public Services.* London: Palgrave.

Wexler, M. (2009) 'Exploring the moral dimension of wicked problems'. *International Journal of Sociology and Social Policy,* 29(9/10): 531–542.

What Works Centre for Wellbeing (2021) Available at: https://whatworkswellbeing.org/about-wellbeing/what-is-wellbeing/

Williams, P. (2010) 'Special agents: The nature and role of boundary spanners', Paper delivered to the ESRC Research Seminar Series – Collaborative Futures: New Insights from Intra and Inter-Sectoral Collaborations, University of Birmingham, February 2010.

Women's Aid Federation of England (2020) *A Perfect Storm: The Impact of the COVID-19 Pandemic on Domestic Abuse Survivors and the Services Supporting Them.* https://www.womensaid.org.uk/wp-content/uploads/2020/08/A-Perfect-Storm-August-2020-1.pdf. Accessed on 26 August 2022.

16

Wicked issues: a faith-based perspective

Drew McCombe and Dean Pallant

Introduction

A response to the upsurge in community action in the initial wave of the COVID-19 pandemic, in 2020, was a request by the UK Prime Minister, Boris Johnson, for Danny Kruger MP to produce a report covering a number of issues including 'the contribution of faith groups in strengthening social capital and community resilience'.

The report *Levelling Up Our Communities: Proposals for a New Social Covenant* (frequently referred to as the Kruger Report) was published in September 2020 (Kruger, 2020). This report recognised that many of our public services, including the modern health, education and probation service systems, have their origins in Christian institutions. Prior to the establishment of the welfare state in 1946, independent charities provided social support for people in need. Bonner reviewed the work and research of 19th century social reformers including Joseph Rowntree (1836–1925), Lord Shaftesbury (1811–1851), Charles Booth (1840–1916), William Booth (1829–1912) and others (Bonner, 2006).

These significant philanthropic Victorian contributions to community resilience had their origins in Christian philosophy and belief. In 2021, the Joseph Rowntree Foundation (JRF), Livability (formed from a merger of the Shaftesbury Society and John Grooms) and Barnardo's play an important role as third sector organisations in addressing the unmet needs of people falling through the welfare net provided by the public sector in the UK. William Booth's Christian Mission (which became The Salvation Army (TSA) in 1878) (Booth, 2014 [1890]), now operates in more than 130 countries and is the only one of those Victorian social initiatives to maintain a strong Christian tradition through its 600+ community churches in the UK and Ireland, which work collaboratively with the 100+ Homeless Services Unit centres (see Case study 16.1). William Booth and others were concerned with the **social evils** causing distress in individuals and families in the 19th century. Joseph Rowntree (1908) identified the evils of war, slavery, excessive drinking, gambling and the drugs trade as the social evils which undermined individual and community wellbeing. A century later a JRF report on modern-day social evils (Harris, 2009) explored the views of people with learning disabilities, ex-offenders, carers, unemployed people, vulnerable young people, care leavers and people who had experience of homelessness in discussion groups across the UK. The main social evils reported by JRF in 2008 were: excessive use of drugs and alcohol, decline of family, decline of community, crime and violence, poverty, migration and unfairness.

Tony Blair (UK Prime Minister 1997–2007), a committed Christian, '[did] not do God' in the political arena (Petre, 2008). Kruger (2020) commented that:

> [P]ublic servants frequently believe that religious beliefs belong in the private sphere and that the public square is somehow a values-free zone ... however secular public servants bring their philosophy to work ... like religious people they have a moral vision. A recent survey indicated 53.5% of civil servants were Christian, 3.5% Muslim and 35.7% reported that they had no religion or belief (HMG, 2019). ... The lack of a relationship between faith based organisations, especially in poor and immigrant communities, and commissioners of public services, results from Faith illiteracy, and too often Faith phobia. (Kruger, 2020: 36)

Kruger (2020: 37) suggests that '[w]e need to form a coalition to tackle some of the *wicked social problems* that faith groups, working in partnership with the state, are best placed to tackle'.

It is worth noting that 'faith phobia', by some in the public sector, is not without justification. Ferris (2011: 609) reminds us of the legacy of Christian mission in assisting and driving Western colonialism, claiming that it is 'partly this evangelical, missional legacy that causes a sense of discomfort (ranging from vague to acute) in interactions between Christian organizations and secular ones, between Christian organizations and other faith-based organizations, and sometimes between Christian organizations themselves'.

There are also concerns that faith-based organisations may use the vulnerability of those they are serving through their charity and humanitarian work as an entry point to convert them (Fiddian-Qasmiyeh, 2011). Nevertheless, faith groups and organisations are seen as offering an approach that considers the whole human being, including their sense of spirituality. This is considered to be vital to solving poverty and other social evils (Marshall, 2007).

Tony Blair's **Third Way**, which aimed to unlock potential within society, promoted the idea that **social capital** should be recognised as providing added value to the state and financial markets, and recognised the role of faith groups' hard and soft assets available within the faith communities. These included buildings, activities, soft (social) support, the distribution of finances and the promotion of voluntary action. The Kruger Report noted that the Christian church in the UK (all denominations not just the established churches of England and Scotland) has an estimated 5 million members based in 20,000 local churches and supporting 15,000 charities. The combined revenue of these churches and charities is £11 billion per year, approximately 20 per cent of all charitable income in the country, and 4.5 million members of other non-Christian faith communities raised over £5 billion in 2016.

While faith groups and organisations can be very different from each other in structure, approach and connection to their faith tradition, there are certain general benefits that faith-based organisations are believed to offer. Organisations such as TSA that are still strongly connected to a network of churches are believed to be more sustainable than secular organisations, as individuals are invested in their own communities as well as being passionate about the charitable work being undertaken by the wider organisation (Chester, 2002). Secondly, faith-based organisations are believed to be 'closer to the grassroots' than their secular counterparts (Tomalin, 2013: 34) and therefore better equipped to listen authentically to the most marginalised within their communities articulate their own needs (see Case study 16.4).

The Salvation Army: a church and charity

TSA's faith-based response to contemporary social evils in the UK include innovative approaches to welfare reform and debt advice, unemployment, human trafficking and modern slavery, homelessness, supporting people with drug and alcohol problems in the community, children and youth priorities and providing for older person's care. These wicked issues have been addressed in the first two volumes of this Policy Press series on social determinants of health.

TSA is a multi-issue community-based faith-based organisation, with the capacity to respond to the complex multiple issues expressed by many of the people supported by the various TSA Mission Service Units, and has been working with **the whole person**. The social evils, a focus of TSA mission during the last 150 years and now across more than 130 countries, are now recognised as wicked issues (see Chapter 1, note 1, this volume).

In Local Authorities and Social Determinants of Health (Bonner, 2020), Chasteaneuf et al highlight the need for the soft structures, provided by organisations such as TSA, to work with the hard structures of public and private partnerships in promoting health and reinvigorating communities (Chasteauneuf et al, 2020). From the perspective of **relationalism** (see Chapter 2) 'soft structures' described by Chateauneuf et al, and Cook (Chapter 18, this volume), may be redefined as **relational support**. Supporting people with complex multiple issues can be challenging, requiring authentic listening, patience and often resulting in long-term relationship building in order to build trust. Many years of providing relational support by TSA has resulted in the development of psychologically informed environments in order to understand a person's real needs and agreeing on a journey of recovery with a focus on their personal strengths (see Case study 16.1).

This holistic support of people is based on an asset-based approach to supporting people in their communities. Many of the solutions to personal needs lie within the person themselves. With more than 600 community-based TSA community churches, a place-based approach underpins TSA's contribution to community needs assessment and insights in addressing the wicked issues noted. From Kruger's 'proposals for a new social covenant' TSA is well placed to work in partnership with the public and private sectors to collaborate in promoting a **relational dividend** (see Chapter 1 and Introduction to Part V). An example of this is the collaboration between TSA, a local authority and a private property business to deliver a solution to rough sleepers (see the Malachi Project, Case study 16.1; Figure 16.1).

Currently, the deep divisions within society, resulting from a decade of austerity policies, the process of the UK leaving the EU, the rise of popularist politics and ongoing socioeconomic issues related to COVID-19, are reflected in rises in the use of food banks (see Chapter 13), and the increase of the homeless population (see Chapter 11). These interrelated wicked issues are mirrored in increasing numbers of people presenting to health services with stress related, non-communicable illnesses (obesity, diabetes, circulatory issues, see Chapter 3), addictive behaviours (problematic alcohol and other drug consumption), mental health issues and suicide ideation. In reviewing the plight of 'underserved communities', resulting from contemporary political-economic policies and a decade of austerity, Professor Sir Harry Burns, former chief medical officer for Scotland, contributed a chapter on 'Deaths of despair', in *Local Authorities and Social Determinants of Health* (Burns, 2020), with reference to the Marmot Reviews (Marmot et al, 2010, 2020).

A detailed review of regional aspects of inequalities has been undertaken by TSA and the Institute of Employment Studies (Anon, 2021a). This report suggests that the levelling up White Paper provides an opportunity to reset the relationship between central and local government. The report notes that Whitehall calculations on implementation of the levelling up agenda in priority areas are based on three limited indicators: local labour pools; transport; and local infrastructure. These calculations are not enough to truly understand what is meant by being 'left behind'. An insight into what is meant by 'left behind' can be seen in the socially deprived in coastal communities (Anon, 2021a). Engaging and consulting with people who are 'left behind' would support a **relational commissioning** process as proposed in Chapter 18 and Chapter 12.

Social justice

The Kruger Report's main focus is on 'levelling up'. This might be viewed from a socioeconomic perspective, however there is a psycho-social-spiritual dimension to this as evidenced in the Marmot Reports (Marmot et al, 2010, 2020). This ongoing research led by Sir Michael Marmot clearly shows that health and social disadvantage in people at the lower end of the social gradient are exacerbated, particularly during the COVID-19 pandemic, by low self-esteem and poor self-image, significantly impacted by adverse childhoods, employment opportunities, poverty and other socioenvironmental factors. Burns (2020) rightly recognises the social and structural issues in society that lead to unequal health outcomes, exacerbated by COVID-19 lockdowns and the loss of social relationships.

In addition to the work of the Anti-Human Trafficking and Modern Slavery unit (see Case studies 7.3 and 16.3), TSA's approach to social justice includes support for asylum-seekers, as partners with the Home Office Community Sponsorship Scheme for Refugees. In responding to the many refugees fleeing the conflict in Syria, TSA works with the Home Office in the resettlement of refugees in pursuit of the Christian value of 'welcoming the stranger', as explored from a theological perspective by Luke Bretherton putting faith into action (Bretherton, 2006). In the case of asylum-seekers the following support is provided: English classes at no cost; safe spaces to make new friends or to enjoy a meal; carer and toddler groups open to everyone; Sunday worship; midweek activities such as sport sessions or intergenerational activities; and practical assistance through food banks and baby banks (TSA, 2020a, 2021a). The TSA Public Affairs Unit is currently involved in discussions on the controversial Nationalities and Borders Bill being debated in parliament.[1]

A number of TSA community churches work with local councils, other churches and faith-based organisations by participating in the Home Office Community Sponsorship Scheme. Local congregations raise funds to support families to provide accommodation and support families in settling into supportive communities, providing support in accessing schools for the children, training for adults and support in finding employment. TSA community groups, sometimes working with other faith groups, are providing refuge and resettlement support for individuals seeking sanctuary from unsafe living conditions in their home countries.

The energy, purpose and passion of TSA stems from a compelling imperative to 'Love God, Love Others'. The Christian motivation driving TSA, 150 years after its origins, has been significantly influenced by William Booth's challenge to 'go and do something':

> While women weep, as they do now, I'll fight
> While children go hungry, as they do, now I'll fight

While men go to prison, in and out, as they do now, I'll fight
While there is a drunkard left, as they do now, I'll fight
While there is a poor lost girl upon the street,
While there remains one dark soul without light of God, I'll fight
I'll fight, I'll fight to the very end. (General William Booth, 1918,
speech given at Booth's final public appearance)

Case studies 16.1–16.4 provide an insight into some of TSA's activities,
demonstrating the scope of this church and charity. TSA, comprising the
TSA Central and the TSA Social Trust, is one of the largest charities in the
UK (TSA 2021b).

Case study 16.1: Being homeless in a pandemic

Nicholas Redmore

The Salvation Army (TSA) is one of the largest providers of homelessness
services in the UK and Ireland. TSA Homelessness Services Unit (HSU)
portfolio consists of over 90 supported housing services, commissioned
addictions services, including a residential substance use service, floating
support services, housing first services, specialist services to support people
who are rough sleeping and day centres (Table 16.1).

The principal aims of HSU's Strategic Mission plan are transformation;
providing opportunity; enabling change; and promoting the strong belief
that both purpose and relationships are essential within an individual's life
to ensure their holistic wellbeing (TSA, 2021a).

The work of HSU has been underpinned with a **harm reduction** ethos
for many years and this is embedded in all expressions of the HSU's work.
This compassionate stance embraces a culture of unconditional positive
regard to support people to keep themselves as safe as possible. The current

Table 16.1: The current provision of The Salvation Army's Homelessness Services Unit
services in the UK

Country	Lifehouses	Outreach services	Day centres	Housing First
England	47	5	3	
Scotland	8	3	1	2
Wales	4	4		2
Northern Ireland	4			

HSU delivery model is based on the Psychologically Informed Environment approach, utilising a trauma–informed lens as our psychological framework (Maguire, 2018).

The HSU programme delivery is evidence based and underpinned by research. TSA Centre for Addiction Services and Research (Anon, 2020a) was established in February 2017 to take forward TSA's Drug and Alcohol Strategy through collaborative working between TSA and the Faculty of Social Sciences in the University of Stirling.

TSA's HSU is committed to delivering a high-quality service and has achieved ISO Quality Standard 9001 and 45001. HSU is registered with the Care Quality Commission in England, the Regulation and Quality Improvement Authority in Northern Ireland and the Care Inspectorate in Scotland.

Following the impact of the COVID-19 pandemic, the HSU 2019–23 Strategic Mission Plan was reviewed (TSA, 2021a).

The majority of people supported by HSU are single. Others may be people who have slept rough or who have been involved with the criminal justice system, and have physical or mental health issues and/or drug or alcohol issues. Services are also provided for young people and for families with children, specialised services for vulnerable women and people and for those who have served in the armed forces. In the UK, HSU provides support for people with no recourse to public funds and also to Syrian refugees sponsored to be in the UK through the UK government's Syrian Resettlement Programme.

In the Republic of Ireland TSA is well established, has a good reputation and significant role in addressing homelessness. There are six residential Lifehouses[2] in Dublin (see Table 16.2).

Table 16.2: The Salvation Army's Homelessness Services Unit services in Dublin

Service	Service type	Units
Coleraine	All male emergency accommodation	25
Granby Centre	55 residents with mental health issues 71 residents, in self-contained accommodation 30 residents with high support needs	101
York House	30 short-term residents (six months) 50 long-term residents (four years)	80
Houben House Family Hub	Large families and many without English as a first language	397 (by 2022)
Greencastle Parade Family Hub	Families experiencing homelessness	28
Clonard Road Family Hub	Families experiencing homelessness	25

Operating under different parliaments: central and local governments

TSA works with different central and local government partners and within different legislative frameworks. Despite some fairly comprehensive homelessness legislation across the territory, people still 'fall through the net' and become homeless.

In England the existing homelessness legislation was extended in 2017 by the Homelessness Reduction Act 2020 (HMG, 2020a). The Westminster government also made a commitment to eradicate rough sleeping by the end of this parliament – a promise accelerated through the 'Everyone In' initiative which saw the majority of people who were rough sleeping being offered temporary or hotel accommodation during the pandemic. This COVID-19-related response indicates that there could be an end to rough sleeping if sufficient funds were made available.

In Scotland, people have some of the strongest homelessness rights in the world with no distinction between priority and non-priority need. In 2020 the Scottish government updated its 2018 'Ending Homelessness Together: High Level Action Plan' and made a greater commitment to prevention; Housing First and the ending of night shelter provision (HMGScot, 2020).

The Housing (Wales) Act 2014 requires councils to focus on homelessness prevention and also expanded those eligible for help. The 2019 Strategy for Preventing and Ending Homelessness in Wales sets out a vision where homelessness is 'rare, brief and unrepeated' (HMG, 2014).

The main piece of legislation which deals with homelessness in Northern Ireland is the Housing (NI) Order (1988).[3] The Housing Executive is responsible for administering the legislation and for the homelessness strategy 'Ending Homelessness Together' published in April 2017.

Evidence of the impact of HSU on people's lives, empowering people to connect with others and to their community, is provided in Tables 16.3a and 16.3b.

Table 16.3a: User satisfaction survey of service users in November 2020 indicating very satisfied or satisfied

	Percentage of clients satisfied
Being made to feel welcome	94%
COVID-19 safety	90%
Mental health support	90%
Substance use support	86%
Physical health support	83%
Activities and learning	79%

Table 16.3b: User satisfaction survey February/March 2021 (710 responses)

	Percentage of clients satisfied
Being made to feel welcome	94%
Having choice and control	89%
Having the right staff	89%
Living at the service	83%
Help in moving on	82%

During the period of COVID-19 and lockdown restrictions in 2020–2021 TSA supported over 3,000 individuals reducing isolation for vulnerable people during the pandemic (see Tables 16.3a and 16.3b).

The HSU 2021 strategy aims to:

- build partnerships and influence;
- be sustainable;
- improve inclusivity and equality;
- nurture innovation;
- encourage resilience.

These aims are clearly demonstrated in the Malachi Project (Figure 16.1). This innovative interfaith approach to homelessness in the London Borough of Ilford, led by TSA, is a collaboration of local faith groups, supported by the local council. The adapted modular homes providing 42 units of accommodation for people with no recourse to public funds is staffed 24 hours a day, seven days a week by volunteers offering welfare support for homeless people. The Malachi Project is a contemporary initiative originating in a local community (Anon, 2020b).

A current development building on the success of the Malachi Project is a partnership between TSA, Citizens UK and the Hill Group, following a £12 million project by the Hill Group to gift 200 specially designed and fully equipped modular homes to organisations supporting people experiencing homelessness. TSA will provide homelessness support for those recovering from homelessness in a number of locations through this new exciting modular accommodation project.

Residents will be provided with opportunities that educate and empower them to establish their long-term independent living options, including private housing, local authority housing and other social housing. The priority is to create independence not dependence. This will be done while engaging with education, training and employment opportunities, building overall life skills.

Figure 16.1: The Malachi Project, a pop-up hostel

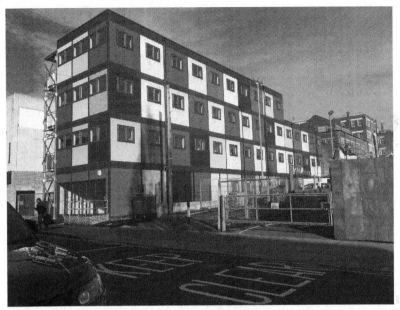

Source: Anon (2020a)

A new innovative approach to vulnerable rough sleepers is the development and roll-out of portable, structures called the Night-time Accommodation Project. These moveable structure are approximately the same size a shipping container comprises four COVID-19 secure "microflats" which offer dignity, privacy and safety for people who might otherwise be sleeping rough (see TSA

Providing a bed alone is not the solution to homelessness. TSA recognises that homelessness is often the secondary effect of a complex range of issues, as already noted. A non-discriminatory approach is adopted by TSA, which operates a resilient, bold and committed approach to each person, never gives up on anyone, and promotes hope through a person-centred approach. Staff work alongside individuals, to reach their goals, whether that be employment goals, getting back in touch with family, reducing or addressing a person's addictive behaviour. 'TSA does life with our people, in our communities, we don't do work for people, but do work *with* people' (TSA 2021a).

Case study 16.2: Older people, care homes and COVID-19

Jenny Pattinson

Data released by my former employer the Care Quality Commission (CQC) on 21 July 2021 showed the true scale of the impact of the pandemic on residents in care homes (CQC, 2021). More than 39,000 people died. Each loss a tragedy. They died unnecessarily, at a time of crisis. They will be sorely missed and the impact of their loss is felt every day as we continue to battle this terrible virus.

In March 2020, I was working for the CQC leading teams of inspectors regulating care homes in Essex. My team was responsible for driving improvement across over 450 locations caring for the most vulnerable in society, a challenging task under normal circumstances but we were just at the start of the first wave of a crisis in Adult Social Care.

In the early days of March 2020, we were receiving daily internal briefings on the spread of the virus and rapidly changing and contradictory guidance on how to advise the sector in ever changing circumstances. Our inspection programme was put on hold, unless the risk dictated a visit was necessary to keep people safe. We were advised to stay at home and to work closely with the local authorities, Clinical Commissioning Groups and care home providers to develop close working relationships. This would ensure rapid communication exchange and accurate information gathering for the Department of Health and Social Care (DHSC).

It became very clear from our briefings that DHSC's focus was entirely on preventing the National Health Service (NHS) from being overwhelmed. There were orders to ensure care homes did not delay in supporting admission from hospital and that vulnerable elderly residents were swiftly ejected from hospital beds. I felt at this time that the 'second-class' social care sector was seen as the place where the older population were out of sight, out of mind. It really felt like they didn't matter.

The CQC had worked tirelessly with the social care sector over a number of years to shift the culture from a task-focused, tick-box institutionalised care to true person-centred care, where who the person is and what they love drives the care provision, which is delivered with compassion and kindness. As we took calls from stressed care home managers pleading with us to help them to protect their residents from untested admissions from hospitals, I felt we had taken a giant leap backwards. This did not feel person-centred, it felt like system-led neglect.

The early days of the pandemic identified deep-rooted inequality between the health and social care sectors. In my position within the regulator at this time, I experienced first-hand the cries for help from care home managers who could not access personal protective equipment (PPE) yet were being told they could not operate without it. Sobs from care home staff who were exhausted, frightened and felt neglected by the government, and then from relatives desperate to see their loved ones and banned from doing so. Nervously waiting for the call to say there was an outbreak in the home. Fearful that their loved one would die without them being able to see them one last time. It was distressing and frustrating to hear as we, as CQC staff, felt helpless, unable to provide the practical hands-on support we were used to delivering.

From 26 May 2020 I found myself operationally responsible for 12 residential care homes owned and managed by The Salvation Army, my new employer. I joined a formidable leadership team supporting the 12 homes to continue to deliver care that meets the mission, vision and dream of The Salvation Army's Older People's Services as quoted to me during my induction during that first week by Elaine Cobb, who was director of Older People's Services at that time. Elaine told me: "My dream is that our homes, residents, families and staff have a sense of mutual love and support but much more than that, they will be reminded of or perhaps introduced for the first time to the wonder of God's love for them – whatever their age." I felt anxious in those first few weeks, coming directly from CQC where I had witnessed, from a desk, the desperation, the fear, confusion and chaos being experienced by care home providers. I tracked the media coverage of the care home sector. It depicted a tragedy. The so-called 'protective ring' did not materialise. It was only in July 2020 when parliament, through the Public Accounts Committee, finally acknowledged the failures (HMG, 2020).

I was leading a care provider through the pandemic. The first thing I noticed was the staggering amount of government and local guidance being issued almost daily in language that was not easily understood by care staff and changing daily or in response to differing circumstances. We focused on keeping on top of this guidance and interpreting it in a way our care home staff could understand and implement, communicating it with clarity and with the toolkits. This was to ensure our staff on the frontline could focus on delivering care to our vulnerable residents. At one point I recall having 12 different versions of guidance for our staff to ensure safe visiting considering the circumstances in each home and where it was located. We have conducted a root cause analysis of every outbreak in our homes and each one was linked directly to an admission or readmission from hospital. This evidenced that the drive to 'save the NHS' has an unbearable cost on care home residents. I expect most care home providers will be able to evidence the same.

At times during the last 15 months I have had the privilege to spend time in the care homes safely, following the guidance and subject to the gruelling testing regime and PPE requirements. In direct contrast to the media portrayal, inside the homes I found safe, loving communities, where joy, love and happiness were the overwhelming emotion. There was singing, dancing, communal mealtimes and socialising on a level now alien to me having lived with the rest of the population through various lockdowns. My amazing staff, dedicated, loving and passionate about the happiness of our residents, are tired. They have witnessed distressing outbreaks and been there holding the hands of our residents when they were sad, lonely and, tragically, when they passed away. They are grieving and some have not seen their families or had a holiday for a very long time. However, they love and care for our residents and each other so deeply that they have embedded the culture of person-centred care further than we or the CQC could have ever imagined. They have developed such familial relationships with each other that they now, better than ever, truly understand what each resident wants and needs to thrive.

At the time of writing (July 2021) the pandemic is far from over. Cases are rising again and we continue to be overwhelmed with frequently changing guidance issued at the last possible moment and the challenge of ensuring we keep safely staffed. This has been made yet more difficult as there is still a fear of working in the care sector. This is a consequence of our media industry focusing on the worst of care through the pandemic and the government's continued failure to ensure sufficient funding and parity with the NHS. I am proud to work in the care sector, I am immensely proud of my staff and we will continue to do everything we possibly can to deliver high quality care, in a Christian environment where each person is valued, achieves their potential and lives a truly fulfilled and joyful life. We are providing that 'protective ring' of love and my staff are the ones responsible for our residents living safely and happily through this pandemic (TSA, 2022).

Case study 16.3: Human trafficking in a pandemic: an international perspective

Anne Gregora and Anne Marie Douglas

Introduction

Modern slavery, 'the severe exploitation of other people for person or commercial gain', is widespread and in plain sight in the UK and other countries in 2021. Forty million people are estimated to be trapped in modern slavery across the world, one in four of them are children, 71 per cent are women and girls, and over 10,000 people have been identified as enslaved in the UK (Anon, 2021b).

The multiple dimensions of human trafficking and modern slavery include sociopolitical, community agencies, social networks, life opportunities and individual vulnerabilities. The projects supported by The Salvation Army's (TSA) Anti-Trafficking and Modern Slavery (ATMS) Unit focus on preventing modern slavery and trafficking of people; protecting individuals on their journey from victim to survivor; and ensuring the progress of the survivor to sustained freedom and promoting community resilience against trafficking.

The Salvation Army International Anti-Trafficking and Modern Slavery projects

The Salvation Army ATMS/UK International (UKI) programme is aligned to UKI international development programmes, including gender justice, clean water, food security and income generation, and supports the International Salvation Army Human Trafficking and Response Strategy.

The ATMS/UKI projects in Africa (Malawi, Tanzania, Nigeria, Ghana), Europe (Poland, Ukraine, Russia), and South and East Asia and South Pacific (Philippines, Bangladesh, East India, Nepal) are provided with technical and/ or funding support, implementing project teams and sharing best practice between projects. Improved communication, learning from these global responses to trafficking is underpinned by TSA co-chairing a subgroup on ATMS, within the Joint Learning Initiative (JLI). The JLI hub is a horizontal learning community linking academics, policymakers and practitioners to combat human trafficking (JLI, 2021). TSA works with a wide range of international partners to improve collaboration, sharing of resources and best practice including Stop the Traffic, the Anglican Alliance and Liberty Shared.

An example of the international collaborative work in which TSA is involved is given in Case study 7.3.

Impact of COVID-19 on communities supported by The Salvation Army in the UK and across the world

A recent report from JLI on the impact of COVID-19 on international trafficking has identified a number of constraints due to lockdown and social distancing, travel restrictions and limitations on social and economic activities. Although police visibility has increased, possibly discouraging crime, much criminal activity has continued behind closed doors. Despite travel restrictions criminals have adjusted their approach by exploiting modern technology, on the other hand trafficked victims have less chance of escape and receiving help (Gurung et al, 2021).

As an increasing number of countries are easing their lockdown, trafficking is increasing as traffickers take advantage of the reductions in job opportunities, deaths and economic stresses within families. The most vulnerable people are:

- Women who are more likely to lose their jobs or are unable to go to work.
- Migrant workers who are unable to return home due to the closure of country borders.
- Domestic workers confined indoors and forced to work longer hours.
- Children affected by school closures, unable to access food and accommodation.
- Disabled people subject to loneliness and those already in exploitation facing further abuse and violence.

The report concluded that:

- COVID-19 has exacerbated human trafficking activities, especially online exploitation and child labour. School closures and education moving online made children an easy target.
- Vulnerable families where parents had become unemployed or lost their livelihoods were also targeted.
- The additional support required by many families and communities meant there was a need for agencies to distribute basic necessities in order to prevent families from accepting risky opportunities.
- Face-to-face meetings between anti-trafficking networks and service users was a key challenge due to social distancing measures and travel restrictions.
- Online platforms were used to follow up and conduct counselling with survivors and additional resources were needed for this and for providing additional safety in safe houses and accommodation for migrant workers, for example, hand sanitisers, masks, gloves and so on. Additional funding such as government grants were difficult to obtain in some local contexts. Organisations who do not normally explore partnership opportunities with private companies should do so as additional resources, for example, phones and laptops, are now being sought.
- Responses to human trafficking and modern slavery should be strengthened and integrated within emergency responses to humanitarian crises such as pandemics.
- Encouragement should be given to the dissemination of awareness messages in the community that look at reducing health stigma especially among marginalised groups such as migrant and sex workers.
- Anti-trafficking organisations should seek ways of engaging with local faith actors beyond the Christian faith-based organisations and also should explore how non-faith actors at the local level also engage with faith activities in their communities.

The Salvation Army and Home Office victim support contract in the UK

The TSA ATMS Unit was, in 2020, awarded the Modern Slavery Victim Care contract from the Home Office. This contract, which has been renewed three times and is now in its tenth year, enables TSA to deliver a relational partnership approach to the wicked issue of human trafficking and modern slavery. As Prime Contractor of the Modern Slavery Victim Care, TSA/ATMS/UKI manages 13 subcontracting provider organisations to deliver support within the UK National Referral Mechanism (NRM) (TSA, 2021a). The Home Office Single Competent Authority has a target of five days from receipt of a referral to decide whether there are reasonable grounds to recognise that someone is a victim of modern slavery. If they are considered to be a potential victim, support will be offered if needed and a period of reflection and recovery will follow. In this period, a potential victim is able to access specialist support for up to 45 days, however this period can be extended if required. If the person is confirmed as a victim, TSA, working with its 13 subcontractors, will support the victim to move on from government funded support when the Home Office Single Competent Authority deems it appropriate to do so. This formal statutory work is linked to soft support in the rehabilitation of the victims. Transporting to safe houses and further support is provided by volunteers and highly trained staff. ATMS/UKI work in the UK is complemented by an extensive network of TSA units, working with TSA International projects and other non-governmental organisations across the globe (see Case study 7.3 and Figure 16.2).

Reforms to the UK Modern Slavery Act 2015 (HMG, 2015) have led to changes in the NRM, increasing the length of time support is provided from 12 to 45 days. An increased focus on identification is part of the new reforms (HMG, 2017b). Data from the NRM suggest an increase of 35 per cent, to 5,145 people, in 2017, potentially trafficked, in comparison with 2016.

It is concerning that 40 per cent of referrals into the NRM, in 2017, were children. Addressing this problem, the government has introduced Child Trafficking Advocates, aimed at building trust and improved decision-making. This approach across England has been recently evaluated. The report demonstrated significant relationship building, but there appears to be a lack of specialist support for vulnerable children.

Responses to trafficking include both criminal justice and health related approaches. The recruitment or movement of people by the use of threat, force, fraud or abuse of vulnerability is recognised as human trafficking. This is a crime which often occurs across countries and international borders, breaching a number of geographic and legal boundaries. Trafficking experiences can result in physical injuries, physical pain and illnesses, sexual health and mental health problems including mood disorders, such as depression and anxiety,

Figure 16.2: Nationalities of potential victims who entered support managed by The Salvation Army in 2019–2020

This year potential victims who entered support were of 96 different nationalities. 70% of all victims who entered support were of the ten nationalities in the map below:

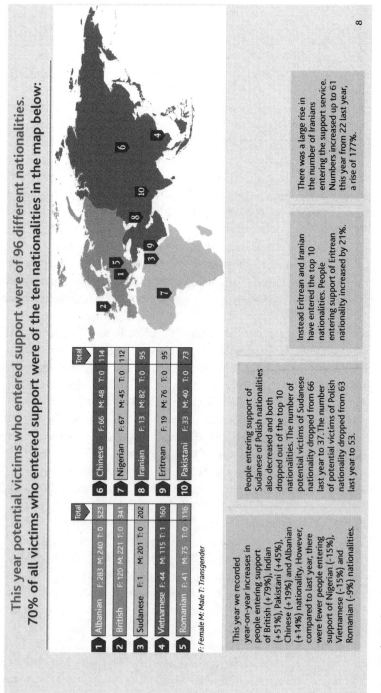

F: Female M: Male T: Transgender

						Total
1	Albanian	F: 283	M: 240	T: 0		523
2	British	F: 120	M: 221	T: 0		341
3	Sudanese	F: 1	M: 201	T: 0		202
4	Vietnamese	F: 44	M: 115	T: 1		160
5	Romanian	F: 41	M: 75	T: 0		116

						Total
6	Chinese	F: 66	M: 48	T: 0		114
7	Nigerian	F: 67	M: 45	T: 0		112
8	Iranian	F: 13	M: 82	T: 0		95
9	Eritrean	F: 19	M: 76	T: 0		95
10	Pakistani	F: 33	M: 40	T: 0		73

This year we recorded year-on-year increases in people entering support of British (+79%), Indian (+51%), Pakistani (+45%), Chinese (+19%) and Albanian (+14%) nationality. However, compared to last year, there were fewer people entering support of Nigerian (-15%), Vietnamese (-15%) and Romanian (-9%) nationalities.

People entering support of Sudanese and Polish nationalities also decreased and both dropped out of the top 10 nationalities. The number of potential victims of Sudanese nationality dropped from 66 last year to 37. The number of potential victims of Polish nationality dropped from 63 last year to 53.

Instead Eritrean and Iranian have entered the top 10 nationalities. People entering support of Eritrean nationality increased by 21%.

There was a large rise in the number of Iranians entering the support service. Numbers increased up to 61 this year from 22 last year, a rise of 177%.

Source: TSA (2020b)

and the more severe diagnoses of psychosis and post-traumatic stress disorder. Sexual violence and sexually transmitted infections have been reported by men and women trafficked for sexual exploitation and domestic servitude.

In order to address the complex needs of people who have been trafficked or enslaved a social determinants perspective should promote the development of networks within and between communities.

Case study 16.4: Supporting people in the community: the development of an evidence-based approach

Wendy Wasels and Tony Daniels

Volunteering with The Salvation Army (TSA) takes many forms and utilises many skill-sets from providing administration support, working in cafes and food banks, supporting victims of modern slavery to emergency response. Facilitating and empowering volunteers is one of a number of activities undertaken by TSA Community Services Unit (CSU) (TSA, 2020c). Much of TSA's work continued throughout the COVID-19 pandemic although it developed and adapted to include new ways of working to accommodate government COVID-19 restrictions. Measures to address COVID-19, in particular lockdown, have been responsible for the rethinking and reframing of some of our volunteer working practices – some of which will be retained going forward.

In the lead up to Volunteers Week 2021 (NCVO, 2021) a request was sent to TSA Community Engagement Specialists, across the UK, to identify stories of special interest relating to volunteer achievement over the past year. Stories that show a significant commitment to serving people in their local community and seen as part of their ministry and faith-based motivation. Together with TSA Officers (church ministers) and other members of the TSA community churches, regular volunteers happily switched from their usual duties, for example, to rally round to arrange food parcels and to support families who had been isolated during lockdown, to using the telephone and video conferencing tools to keep in touch.

New volunteers began to work with TSA as a result of being furloughed. One such volunteer joined the George Steven Community Hub volunteers to become a food delivery driver. The Hub delivers a variety of projects and programmes which serve the local community and includes specialist support for adults with learning disabilities (TSA, 2021b). The food delivery service was started to support service users who were unable to leave the house during lockdown. For this volunteer centre, like many others, volunteering fulfilled a dual purpose; helping to cope with the challenges of the lockdown and of being furloughed and provided TSA service users with much needed contact and support.

For TSA, as for many large and small third sector organisations, volunteers have been central to the delivery of essential services (Vibert, 2021). The challenge for volunteer managers has been to adapt to both the recruitment demands where volunteers have decided not to return and to ensure that processes are efficient but robust enough to ensure that volunteers can be onboarded quickly. An example of this has been the TSA volunteer recruitment campaign to support TSA charity shops. In anticipation of attracting younger volunteers as they complete college and school for the summer a volunteer recruitment campaign using social media and online recruitment tools was developed.

This culture change involved adapting to the changing requirements around volunteering and critically reviewing the processes of recruitment, retention and ongoing management of volunteers. TSA's volunteers are recruited both from within and outside the TSA church membership but all have to complete a thorough recruitment and induction process. With safeguarding central to TSA processes, this is a key but often time-consuming element and can delay starting in a role for up to four weeks. Greater agility was essential if TSA is to both compete to attract volunteers for its mission services in the future and provide a positive experience to the current volunteer base. The managers of TSA Anti-Human Trafficking and Modern Slavery Unit (ATMS), for example, have indicated a need to recruit approximately 250 volunteers (additional to the pre-COVID-19 numbers) to drive and chaperone trafficked victims with respect to the Home Office Victim Support service (see Case study 16.3). Recruiting, supporting and managing an additional 250 volunteers requires additional management support solutions from CSU.

In July 2020 a project commenced to further the development of the digitising of the TSA's volunteer data and to provide a digital solution to recruitment, retention and management of our data and most importantly enhance engagement with our volunteer force. The reasons were three-fold: firstly, the time was right; the pandemic had forced many people online and introducing a digital system during the pandemic would be easier than before the pandemic period, when engagement especially in older audiences was more difficult to achieve. Secondly, prior to the pandemic, TSA had no national oversight of its volunteer force, no way of telling how many people were volunteering for the TSA (for various reporting purposes), or whether volunteers were fully compliant with policy and process. Thirdly, recruiting and inducting a volunteer could take a number of weeks under manual processes (sometimes 6–8 weeks, or more) and with a new digital system the time could be reduced by a half.

The decision was made to explore the use of TSA's existing human resource system, iTrent, and a feasibility study into dedicated volunteer management software systems was undertaken. However, it appeared that the existing iTrent system, used by HR to support TSA Officers, managers and staff, had the potential to be developed to provide a volunteer recruitment and management solution. The decision was influenced in part by the financial pressure that the pandemic has put on TSA budgets, but also because there is a great deal of existing expertise and willingness to collaborate on this project across TSA (MHR, 2021).

Engagement with various services across TSA has been positive and has sparked a degree of curiosity and desire to be part of the pilot testing as we adapt and develop the iTrent functionality to facilitate the recruitment and management of volunteers. An important part of the project has been engaging with mission services to determine what they'd like from a new system: what processes we need to capture and how managers want to manage and engage their volunteers. A detailed pilot study was carried out with Debt Advice co-ordinators, ATMS Transportation, First Responder and Mentoring Teams, International Development as well as a number of corps including Regent Hall with their feedback used to further develop functionality. Regent Hall used the online system to successfully recruit volunteers for their new Welcome Hub. The International Development team recruited five entirely remotely based volunteers to help further their research work, website development and the Others project.

As the data management project progresses, the focus has moved to engagement and the need for a volunteer engagement bolt-on was identified. For any data management system to be successful it needs to be enticing enough to encourage people to use it. After the collection of data from TSA mission services and community church managers, the newly developed system will support recruitment and management of volunteers, generation of reports, facility to create rotas, reminders for refresher training and checks, and importantly give them the ability to engage with their volunteers, recognise them and request feedback. Volunteers will, via an app or for those less tech-savvy in situ with the support of their line manager or a volunteer buddy, have control of their data, be able to set their preferences, access all the relevant policies and training for their role and keep in touch with the latest news, their line manager and other team members.

The new system will help TSA plan and develop an agile volunteer strategy. Any system is only as good as the data it contains, but the insights that we will gather will provide significant management improvements on the pre-COVID-19 working arrangements. The technology will help facilitate and orchestrate a person's (volunteering) journey with TSA via personalised and seamless interactions. It will help TSA/CSU to understand those who volunteer and promote other TSA business and mission focused activities including fundraising. Importantly, it will help us facilitate the communication of TSA mission and engage with people in the community, many of whom have not previously been linked to the Christian church.

Conclusion

Chapter 16 and Case studies 16.1–16.4 are intended to provide an insight into key wicked issues, which were identified by Victorian social reformers as social evils. The Joseph Rowntree Foundation report in 2009 (Harris, 2009) indicated that these social evils still exist. Social evils might be reframed as wicked issues, and have been recently raised in the UK political agenda in the Kruger Report.

With reference to the interrelations of these wicked issues, from a social determinants of health perspective, faith-based approaches contribute to the (relational) soft support within the multicultural community, hopefully working in collaboration with the hard structures provided by local and national government (Chasteauneuf et al, 2020). Relational support requires a holistic approach, in many cases with specialist interventions, engaging with people, in a non-judgemental, safe environment, without a time-bound limit on support from this faith-based organisation.

Notes
[1] See https://www.gov.scot/publications/nationality-and-borders-bill-joint-letter-to-the-home-secretary/
[2] 'Lifehouses' were originally called hostels for the homeless.
[3] https://www.legislation.gov.uk

References
Anon (2020a) Salvation Army Centre for Addiction Services and Research. University of Stirling. Available at: https://www.stir.ac.uk/about/facult ies/social-sciences/our-research/research-areas/salvation-army-centre-for-addiction-services-and-research/ (accessed 14 November 2020).

Anon (2020b) The Malachi Project. Available at: https://www.redbridge. gov.uk/regeneration-and-growth/regeneration-and-growth-areas/ilford/the-spark-ilford/project-malachi/https://popuphostel-ilfordsalvationarmy. nationbuilder.com/about (accessed 14 November 2020).

Anon (2021a) Levelling up post-COVID Britain. The New Statesman. Available at: https://www.newstatesman.com/sites/default/files/ns_ salvation_army_supplememnt_june_2021.pdf (accessed 25 August 2021).

Anon (2021b) What is modern slavery? Antislavery International. Available at: https://www.antislavery.org/slavery-today/modern-slavery/ (accessed 25 August 2022).

Bonner, A. (2006) *Social Exclusion and the Way Out: An Individual and Community Response to Human Social Dysfunction.* Chichester: John Wiley & Sons.

Bonner, A. (2020) *Local Authorities and Social Determinants of Health.* Bristol: Policy Press.

Booth, W. (2014 [1890]) *In Darkest England and the Way Out.* Cambridge: Cambridge University Press.

Booth, W. (1918) General William Booth's speech given at his final public appearance. London: The Salvation Army Heritage Centre.

Bretherton, L. (2006) *Hospitality and Holiness.* Aldershot: Ashgate.

Burns, H. (2020) Deaths of despair: Causes and possible cures. In Bonner, A. (ed) *Local Authorities and Social Determinants of Health.* Bristol: Policy Press.

Chasteauneuf, T., Thorton, T. and Pallant, D. (2020) The role of the third sector working with the hard structures and soft structures of public-private partnerships to promote individual health and reinvigorated communities. In Bonner, A. (ed) *Local Authorities and Social Determinants of Health.* Bristol: Policy Press.

Chester, T. (2002) What makes Christian development Christian? Paper presented at Global Connections Relief and Development Forum, May. Available at: https://www.globalconnections.org.uk/sites/newgc.localh ost/files/papers/What%20makes%20Christian%20Development%20Ch ristian%20-%20Tim%20Chester%20-%20May%2002.pdf (accessed 25 August 2022).

CQC (2021) Data on notifications of COVID-19 deaths received from individual care homes expected to be published at July public board meeting. Care Quality Commission, 11 June. Available at: https://www. cqc.org.uk/news/stories/data-notifications-covid-19-deaths-received-ind ividual-care-homes-expected-publish-july (accessed 25 August 2022).

Ferris, E. (2011) Faith and humanitarianism: It's complicated. *Journal of Refugee Studies,* 24(3): 606–625.

Fiddian-Qasmiyeh, E. (2011) Introduction: Faith-based humanitarianism in contexts of forced displacement. *Journal of Refugee Studies,* 24(3): 429–439.

Gurung, T., Tomalin, E. and Sworn, H. (2021) How Has the International Anti-Trafficking Response Adapted to COVID-19? Joint Learning Initiative on Faith and Local Communities. Joint Learning Initiative on Faith and Local Communities. Available at: https://jliflc.com/resources/ how-has-the-international-anti-trafficking-response-adapted-to-covid-19- 2/ (accessed 25 August 2022).

Harris, J. (2009) 'Social Evils' and 'Social Problems' in Britain, 1904–2008. Joseph Rowntree Foundation. Available at: https://www.jrf.org.uk/rep ort/'social-evils'-and-'social-problems'-britain-1904–2008 (accessed 14 November 2020).

HMG (2014) Housing Wales Act 2014. Available at: https://www.goo gle.com/search?q=the+housing+(wales)+act+2014&rlz=1C5CHFA_ enGB855GB855&oq=The+Housing+(Wales)+Act+2014&aqs=chr ome.0.0i512j0i22i30l9.2526j0j4&sourceid=chrome&ie=UTF-8 (accessed 24 August 2021).

HMG (2015) Modern Slavery Act 2015. Available at: https://www.legislat ion.gov.uk/ukpga/2015/30/contents (accessed 25 August 2022).

HMG (2017a) Homelessness Reduction Act 2017. Available at: https:// www.legislation.gov.uk/ukpga/2017/13/pdfs/ukpga_20170013_en.pdf (accessed 26 August 2022).

HMG (2017b) Modern Slavery. Home Office. Available at: https://www.gov. uk/government/collections/modern-slavery (accessed 25 August 2022).

HMG (2019) Faith and Belief Toolkit: A Practical Guide Providing Information about Faith and Belief in the Civil Service. Cabinet Office, 31 July. Available at: https://www.gov.uk/government/publications/faith-and-belief-toolkit (accessed 14 November 2020).

HMG (2020) Public Accounts Committee: The UK Government Response to COVID-19 Pandemic. Available at: https://committees.parliament.uk/ committee/127/public-accounts-committee/content/136854/public-accounts-committee-the-uk-government-response-to-the-covid19-pande mic/ (accessed 25 August 2022).

HMGScot (2020) Housing First. Available at: https://www.gov.scot/coll ections/housing-first-publications/

JLI (2021) Joint Learning Initiative on Faith and Local Communities: Anti-Human Trafficking and Modern Slavery Hub. Available at: https://aht-ms.jliflc.com

Kruger, D. (2020) *Levelling Up Our Communities: Proposals for a New Social Covenant. A New Deal with Faith Communities.* Report commissioned by the Prime Minister. Available at: https://www.dannykruger.org.uk/files/ 2020-09/Levelling%20Up%20Our%20Communities-Danny%20Kruger. pdf (accessed 14 November 2020).

Maguire, N. (2018) Towards an integrative theory of homelessness and rough sleeping. In Bonner, A. (ed) *Social Determinants of Health: An Interdisciplinary Approach to Social Inequality and Wellbeing.* Bristol: Policy Press.

Marmot, M., Allen, J., Goldblatt, P., Boyce, T., McNeish, D. and Grady, M. (2010) *Fair Society, Healthy Lives: The Marmot Review.* London: Institute of Health Equity.

Marmot, M., Allen, J., Boyce, T., Goldblatt, P. and Morrison, J. (2020) *Health Equity in England: The Marmot Review 10 Years On.* London: Institute of Health Equity.

Marshall, K. (2007) *Religious Faith and Development: Rethinking Development Debates.* Oslo: World Bank. Available at: http://www.tanzaniagateway.org/ docs/religious_faith_and_development_rethinking_development_debates. pdf (accessed 25 August 2022).

MHR (2021) *iTrent HR and Payroll Software.* Available at: https://mhrglobal. com/uk/en/itrent?gclid=EAIaIQobChMIpu297ty88gIVibLICh05VAby EAAYAiAAEgI_q_D_BwE (accessed 19 August 2021).

NCVO (2021) NCVO *Volunteers Week*. Available at: https://volunteersw eek.org/ (accessed 19 August 2021).

Petre, J. (2008) Tony Blair reveals why he refused to 'do God'. *The Telegraph*, 4 August. Available at: https://www.telegraph.co.uk/news/uknews/1583 846/Tony-Blair-reveals-why-he-refused-to-do-God.html (accessed 14 November 2020).

Tomalin, E. (2013) *Religions and Development*. London: Routledge.

TSA (2020a) *Asylum Seekers*. The Salvation Army. Available at: https:// www.salvationarmy.org.uk/supporting-refugees/asylum-seeker-support (accessed 14 November 2020).

TSA (2020b) *Supporting Victims of Modern Slavery: Year Nine Report on The Salvation Army's Victim Care and Coordination Contract July 2019–June 2020*. The Salvation Army. Available at: https://www.salvationarmy.org.uk/mod ern-slavery/modern-slavery-latest-reports (accessed 26 August 2022).

TSA (2020c) *In the Community: Discover Our Work at the Heart of Communities*. The Salvation Army. Available at: https://www.salvationarmy.org.uk/ community (accessed 19 August 2021).

TSA (2021a) *Homeless Services Unit Mission Plan*. The Salvation Army.

TSA (2021b) The Salvation Army Trust Report and Financial Statements for the United Kingdom in the year ended 31 March 2021. Available at: https://www.salvationarmy.org.uk/sites/default/files/resources/2022-02/SA_Trust_Report_year_end_31Mar21.pdf (accessed 25 August 2022).

TSA (2022a) *NAPpads*. The Salvation Army. Available at: https://www. salvationarmy.org.uk/homelessness/nap-pads (accessed 25 August 2022).

TSA (2022b) *Older People: Life in All Its Fullness*. The Salvation Army. Available at: https://www.salvationarmy.org.uk/older-people (accessed 25 August 2022).

Vibert, S. (2021) Gentle and strong: Looking back on the role of the voluntary sector during the pandemic. NCVO, 24 March. Available at: https://blogs. ncvo.org.uk/2021/03/24/gentle-and-strong-looking-back-on-the-role-of-the-voluntary-sector-during-the-pandemic/ (accessed 24 August 2021).

PART V

The case for relationalism

Richard Smith

In order to prove, evidentially, the additional value/dividend that can arise from a **relational partnering** approach, the Centre for Partnering has initiated an Exemplar Projects Initiative. The purpose of this initiative is to create a partnering environment which incorporates the use of **relationalism** by the public, private and third sectors. On a practical note, this demands the establishment of a number of new projects and facilitating new ideas, innovation and thinking within a different cultural framework.

This will involve identifying a number of organisations prepared to approach a partnering opportunity in a different way. It demands key individuals with appropriate partnering experience to consider changes to a traditional partnering approach which has historically placed a high priority on compliance with procurement rules, including emphasis on value for money, meeting specifications and adherence to a contract framework. A future **relational culture** demands a partnership of equals with a clear focus on delivering enhanced social and commercial value combined to secure improved outcomes across a range of measures.

It is imperative that the Centre for Partnering takes account of previous and existing partnering arrangements in order to learn lessons as to previous successes and failures. These are in part reflected in the case studies described in this section. In establishing the new projects forming part of the Exemplar Projects Initiative, these lessons will be noted and become part of the Relationalism Knowledge Base (see Appendix). The case studies currently forming part of the Exemplar Projects will focus on the private sector and, in particular, a council's use of public assets. Other case studies will address renewable energy and homelessness. These case studies should be read in the context of lessons learned in the evolution of relational partnering and provide a perspective for the proposed changes that are discussed in Part VI.

These case studies raise a number of issues in connection with the underlying themes arising throughout this book with respect to the promotion of the concept of relationalism. Recurrent themes in each case study include fairness, a focus on outcomes, collaboration, communication, transparency and acknowledgement of the need to generate a profit while, at the same time, being socially and environmentally responsible.

There is a growing recognition that the age-old mantra that the sole purpose of a business is to deliver commercial value for its shareholders is no longer fit for these times. A new strain of responsible capitalism is emerging and growing in significance, driven, in part, by an increasing emphasis on the part of major funding institutions, as guardians of billions of pounds, euros and dollars of our pensions and insurance premiums, that business needs to do more for society as a whole.

The rise of corporate social responsibility, environmental, social and governance policies, B Corporations and activist shareholders suggests that the tide has firmly turned and that the triple bottom line of economic, environmental and social sustainability is now edging out of a purely financial focus. One of the great challenges, however, is in turning this direction of travel into practical actionable steps that can, indeed, put the focus on social and environmental matters in a way that ensures that effective outcomes are achieved for them alongside a viable commercial return.

This is where the adoption of relationalism can provide a framework for delivering meaningful change. The creation of a **relational dividend** from every pound spent will enable decision-makers to first identify and then measure both the commercial and social benefits that can arise from how they spend their money.

The Centre for Partnering's Exemplar Initiative is intended to make the case for such a change.

Case study: A relationalism exemplar

Richard Smith

To build the case for relationalism and its associated relational dividends, the following illustration shows the establishment of a knowledge base, see Figure 17.1.

The proposed projects through which relationalism can be researched include the use of public assets, renewable energy initiatives and addressing homelessness. It is intended to consider these projects in the context of their contribution to the social determinants of health as described in this volume and, specifically, their aim to tackle **wicked issues** affecting people, communities and inequality.

The Centre for Partnering will play a facilitating role in establishing, monitoring and reporting upon the projects forming part of the Exemplar Projects Initiative. The evidence collected will form part of the relationalism knowledge base.

The Working Groups forming part of the Centre for Partnering's governance arrangements will consider the various learning points arising from the Exemplar projects from a public, private, third sector and regional perspective. The groups will make proposals to continually improve the effectiveness of the Exemplar Projects Initiative where these can enhance the value of the knowledge base and research/monitoring activities.

One outcome from compilation of the knowledge base will be the need to accredit those organisations and individuals seeking relational dividends from partnering. This is especially important in terms of promoting a new partnering culture through which ideas and innovation can be introduced. For example, a proactive market will need to identify those public sector organisations (councils) who are willing and able to accept proposals and equipped to judge which forms of commercial enterprise are suitable for entering a **relational contract**. An accreditation model will provide evidence to all parties seeking to adopt a culture based on relationalism and its core principles.

It is the intention of the Centre for Partnering to develop a communication strategy through which its knowledge base will be disseminated. The Exemplar programme is intended to provide a practical perspective on the benefits of relationalism as it could impact upon the economic wellbeing of the country post-Brexit/COVID-19 and during the cost of living crisis. The

Figure 17.1: Centre for Partnering exemplar showing relational dividend

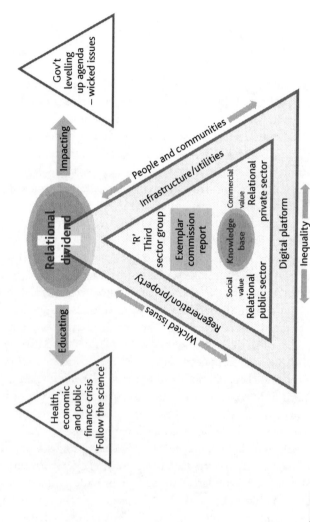

strategy will also address the impact of relationalism on the government's levelling up agenda.

It is anticipated that progress in the delivery of the Exemplar Projects Initiative and compilation of the knowledge base will provide evidence for any subsequent social determinants of health publications.

The future role of the third sector as an equal partner will also be addressed by the Exemplar Projects Initiative. The government's levelling up agenda is seeking to address a broad range of inequalities across sectors of society and regions of the country (see Part IV). To do this it will need to carefully target investment and seek to maximise the social benefits that arise from that expenditure. This is best achieved by mobilising the third sector in a way that has, hitherto, not proved possible and linking them to the wide range of projects that would traditionally be undertaken solely between the public and private sectors.

In setting up the Exemplar Projects Initiative and establishing the relevant principles to deliver relationalism, lessons will be drawn from past experiences. These include understanding the differences between an outsourcing of services versus an inward investment proposition based on improving the use of resources – people, assets, information and finance.

It also requires a focus upon a social outcome that would not otherwise arise through the application of market forces. For example, a regeneration initiative within a city's deprived areas can be improved where a council's assets are utilised from the point of view of optimising those assets held to achieve broader objectives.

An aim of the Exemplar Projects Initiative would therefore be to deliver a partnering outcome that would not otherwise exist, or be immediately viable, and could lead to reducing the cost of running, maintaining and holding assets and creating a future revenue stream. It could also kickstart further economic growth within the city centre and lead to new employment opportunities for local residents, in addition to a wider range of socioeconomic benefits.

The case studies within Part V of this book are dedicated to the memory of Denis Curran, of Hanson UK. Denis was a long-standing proponent of a more relational culture within public–private partnering, as is evidenced, in particular, with the Dorset Highways contract.

Over many years, Denis contributed his thoughts and ideas to the development of a new type of contracting behaviour focusing on the purpose and outcome of the contract activity. This thinking was invaluable in formulating principles and ideas that lie behind relationalism.

Denis sadly passed away on 10 July 2021, during the writing of this book, but he will be long remembered.

Case study: Housing and homelessness

Adam Cunnington

Introduction

Housing, or living in a decent home, is a fundamental part of the lives of each and every one of us. Ongoing failure to rise to the challenge of creating the right types of homes in the right places that are affordable to those that live in them, improve the quality of their lives and contribute to tackling climate change, has resulted in increasing levels of homelessness, inequality and cost of living. This chapter explores how, even if policy changes created an environment where housing delivery *could* meet demand, this might actually be achieved.

Context

In Chapter 11 Peter Murphy sets out the trajectory of housing delivery since the war and highlights the shortcomings in policy that have led to a continued shortfall in meeting housing need. For many years, it has been left very largely to the private sector to deliver the majority of the new homes this country so badly needs. The result of this has been the delivery of largely single tenure, market sale homes, in a cookie-cutter style across the country at a rate that suits the housing developers, with little in the way of product innovation. With limited exceptions, the majority of new homes built have ignored the pressing issues facing the sector, namely, building more homes, of better quality across a range of tenure types that face up to issues such as climate change, homelessness and fuel poverty.

Is it little wonder then that the country faces a continued housing crisis? Nominal house prices have risen dramatically since the early 1990s and continue rising today, even in the midst of the COVID-19 crisis. This historic trend can be seen in Figure 17.2.

For those who can afford it, the market offers a narrow choice of largely pastiche houses delivered to environmental performance standards, captured in the Building Regulations. These have changed in small increments at irregular intervals and to howls of complaints and threats of unsustainable extra build costs from developers who still build homes in largely the same way that our Victorian forebears did! These houses are frequently riddled

Figure 17.2: UK nominal house prices, 1991–2015

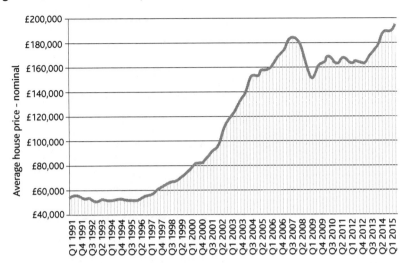

Source: Nationwide Building Society, https://www.economicshelp.org/blog/5709/housing/market/

with defects and struggle to even meet the standards set for them (HMG, 2017, 2020 a).

Solutions

A radical shift in housing delivery is required if the needs of those who aren't looking, or aren't able, to buy a new home with a mortgage are to be met. The answer to meeting this need sits with the very people who made the difference following the war; local councils and the public sector. It also requires an entirely new delivery capability to be created, since the market has clearly demonstrated that it is unlikely to deliver more than its long-term trend of 150,000 or so houses a year. The solution to this lies in off-site manufacture, modern methods of construction (MMC), pre-fabrication, call it what you like, but a new and better way of getting badly needed new homes built (HMG, 2017–2019).

The great advantage of MMC is frequently claimed to be the speed of delivery. In practice, this is probably, at best, a helpful by-product of the process. The real benefits of MMC are that it opens up new delivery channels, is attractive to a much broader workforce who would otherwise not be attracted to working in traditional construction, it produces an end product of a materially higher quality more consistently and, most importantly, by using non-traditional building techniques, it is significantly easier and cheaper to achieve high levels of environmental performance, reaching zero-carbon years ahead of broader government targets for the housing sector. And achieving this is important not just from a climate change perspective, but because new low or zero carbon homes can deliver huge savings in running costs for occupiers thus making meaningful steps towards tackling fuel poverty. However, the industry is in its infancy and is not cost competitive against traditional build, nor yet capable of delivering at the volumes required to meet the needs of the country (UK Essays, 2018; RIBA, 2019).

The sweeping changes to an entire industry that are tantalisingly drawn out here require a paradigm shift in thinking from funding, to planning, to delivery, to tenure and long-term ownership and management. It is not a small undertaking.

The forgotten 50 per cent

If the government's target is to see 300,000 new homes a year built and the market is delivering 150,000, where will the other 150,000 homes come from? And, crucially, how will they be paid for? If there was money to be made in building them, you can bet that they would be being built already. As a consequence, almost all the rules around current housing delivery need to be forgotten and a new approach put together from the ground up.

This is where Relationalism can come to the fore. Traditional procurement and delivery models won't make a dent in the scale of the challenge. Relationalism offers a new way for the non-traditional housebuilding sector to collaborate, to drive down cost, but drive up output, quality and environmental performance.

With no real established commercial model or large scale delivery capability, there comes a chance to look afresh at how to build 150,000 homes for people who aren't looking to buy a house with a mortgage. An apt description for what this might look like would be 'a coalition of the willing'. If, as mooted earlier, the answer to meeting need goes outside the confines of current delivery methods and into alternative delivery options, such as MMC, the nature of that market is such that it will require nurturing, collaboration and, most of all, an acceptance that there may be failures as well as successes.

Today, a house built in a factory costs materially more than one built traditionally. However, if you factor in lifecycle costs, snagging costs and the premium to achieve zero carbon, the tables start to turn. However, the best way to close this gap more quickly is to increase volume and increasing volume requires moving away from a price-based assessment, which would preclude the use of MMC, to the collaborative approach that Relationalism fosters.

If councils and housing associations are going to shoulder the burden of delivering the vast majority of the new homes required and, most likely, with limited capacity in the traditional build sector, a substantial proportion of these will need to be delivered by MMC manufacturers. Given that this is an industry that is still very much in its infancy, the traditional procurement processes are unlikely to deliver the step change that is necessary to hit delivery goals.

Another major stumbling block to making this happen is a critical shortage of skills and resources on the client side of the equation. Councils and housing associations have very limited pools of development expertise. Indeed, such that does exist is fully consumed delivering the current numbers of homes they build each year. There is no quick fix for this. Councils in particular have long since lost all of the experts that saw them delivering 200,000 new homes a year in the 1960s and 1970s.

A partnering solution is the only pragmatic solution to moving the needle and doing it in a highly collaborative and supportive way.

Here is an extract from the Construction Playbook (HMG, 2020b):

By adopting the policies in this Playbook, we will:

- *Set clear and appropriate outcome-based specifications* that are designed with the input of industry to ensure we drive continuous improvement and innovation.
- *Favour longer term contracting across portfolios*, where it is appropriate. We will develop long-term plans for key asset types and programmes to drive greater value through public spending.
- *Standardise designs, components and interfaces* as much as is possible.
- *Drive innovation and modern methods of construction*, through standardisation and aggregation of demand, increased client capability and setting clear requirements of suppliers.
- *Create sustainable, win-win contracting arrangements* that incentivise better outcomes, improve risk management and promote the general financial health of the sector.
- *Strengthen financial assessment of suppliers* and prepare for the rare occasions when things go wrong, with the introduction of resolution planning information requirements into critical contracts.
- *Increase the speed of end-to-end project and programme delivery* by investing up front with time and resources to set projects up for success.

The Playbook will, by creating the right environment, enable us to:

- *Improve building and workplace safety* to ensure that we are creating safe facilities and protecting our workforces.
- *Take strides towards our 2050 net-zero commitment* and focus on a whole life carbon approach to fight climate change and deliver greener facilities designed for the future.

- *Promote social value* which will help local communities recover from COVID-19, tackle economic inequality, promote equal opportunities and improve wellbeing.

Groups of councils and/or housing associations need to come together in geographically based clusters to pull together the sort of pipeline of opportunities that will provide a mix of short-, medium- and long-term availability and a mix of small, medium and large sites to provide the chance for a range of manufacturers to engage.

This is where commissioning effectively within a relational framework comes to the fore. It is clear that extending a traditional transactional approach to contracting with new entrants to the market will not enable them to be nurtured, developed and grown. A contract loaded in favour of the client and full of penalties for failure will create a risk-averse response from suppliers. If the goal of the sector as a whole is to deliver a larger number of better homes, it will require all parts of it to collaborate, focus on the need to bring new entrants into the market and encourage them to thrive. Doing this under a relational framework, where the focus is on the collective goal, not the specifics of an individual project, is most likely to achieve the desired outcome of increasing the supply of the right homes in the right places. An enlightened commissioner will keep the focus on the wider objectives and build upon the benefits of Relationalism and not fall into the first procurement pitfall that comes along.

The challenge for MMC manufacturers is that they need to establish a large facility, capable of holding multiple numbers of fully built houses. In doing this they immediately take on a large fixed overhead cost. To meet such an overhead, a reliable and secure pipeline of orders is required. Property is, by its nature, lumpy and unpredictable. This presents challenges to incumbent manufacturers but also presents a bar to entry for others.

By creating partnerships where a steady flow of houses can be delivered and with a client who understands the importance of growing the MMC market, the sector can begin to develop at a faster rate. If each partnership were to offer the kind of pipeline outlined, deal with all of the tedious issues around development such as title issues, planning matters, infrastructure and funding, they can create an ideal environment for MMC manufacturers to thrive.

These partnerships can then take an enlightened approach to selecting their partners. And this is where Relationalism can provide the catalyst to deliver the much needed step change. The entire process of selecting partners to tackle this vital endeavour must be almost nothing to do with cost and everything to do with learning, joint endeavours and shared outcomes. Existing manufacturers can be supported by having access to a steady and robust pipeline. This will allow them to focus on driving down the cost of their product without compromising on quality. New entrants can be given smaller sites and nurtured to help them be successful. Pooling knowledge, sharing best practice, developing new techniques and common specifications will massively help to foster a spirit of collaboration where breaking new ground and making concrete steps to solving the housing crisis are the key objective.

The author's experience of relational partnering over the last decade completely supports this approach. Where both partners are focused on shared goals and objectives the outcomes are always better than where one side feels it has the upper hand over the other and seeks to gain advantage to the detriment of the other. The fleet of foot governance and decision-making processes that we have operated under allow for projects to be evolved and developed quickly and even once up and running for decisions to be taken to change direction without falling foul of rigid contractual frameworks that do the opposite of fostering collaboration, going the extra mile and delivering exceptional outcomes.

The housing crisis is one of the most profound challenges we face as a nation. As is all too evident, the wicked issues that pervade every aspect of children and families' lives brought up in poor quality housing in economically disadvantaged areas last for a lifetime. Starting to move the needle by offering access to high quality and affordable housing is vital. If these houses also happen to be low or zero carbon, then further benefits arise. They will be significantly cheaper to run, thus reducing levels of fuel poverty (*New Statesman*, 2017). Similarly, if they are good news for the occupants, they are great news for the planet, reducing our carbon footprint and delivering benefits on a global level.

Conclusion

Houses are buildings, but they are also homes, and giving everyone access to a decent home can make a profound difference to the lives of individuals, communities and the planet. There is no downside to delivering this goal. It just requires will, innovation and money. If the current cost of housing families in temporary accommodation can, instead, be used to fund new homes, the route to a more equitable and resilient future begins to open up. Relationalism can be the tool to make this happen.

By opening up new housing delivery channels, increasing the capacity of the sector and putting a focus on quality and carbon reduction, profound changes can be made to the nation's housing stock and the stock of those who live in them. This can be achieved by mobilising the public sector and embracing the use of MMC to fundamentally disrupt the current failing housing delivery model and drive material change for the better.

References

HMG (2017) *Fixing Our Broken Housing Market.* MHCLG. https://www.gov.uk/government/publications/fixing-our-broken-housing-market

HMG (2017–2019) *Off-site Manufacture for Construction: Building for Change.* Science and Technology Select Committee. https://publications.parliament.uk/pa/ld201719/ldselect/ldsctech/169/169.pdf

HMG (2020a) *New-build Housing: Construction Defects – Issues and Solutions.* UK Parliament. https://commonslibrary.parliament.uk/research-briefings/cbp-7665/

HMG (2020b) *The Construction Playbook.* Cabinet Office. https://www.gov.uk/government/publications/the-construction-playbook

New Statesman (2017) Zero-carbon homes: Saving money as well as energy. February. https://www.newstatesman.com/microsites/housing/2017/02/zero-carbon-homes-saving-money-well-energy

RIBA (2019) *Modern Methods of Construction: How They Can Help Deliver the Homes This Country Needs.* Royal Institute of British Architects. https://www.architecture.com/knowledge-and-resources/knowledge-landing-page/why-modern-methods-of-construction-are-key

UK Essays (2018) *Modern Methods of Construction (MMC) Benefits.* November. https://www.ukessays.com/essays/construction/drivers-and-barriers-of-modern-methods.php

Case study: Environmental planning in a post-COVID-19 world

Nigel Saunders

Introduction

The current period of global economic recovery from the COVID-19 pandemic, alongside bolstered international efforts to reach net-zero carbon emissions by 2050, presents a hugely relevant opportunity to reconsider the shape and format of relationships between the private, public and third sectors. In the UK meanwhile, a post-Brexit landscape means that the value of partnering must also be considered in the wake of our shifting relationships with Europe.

Perhaps the biggest example of inter-sector success in these times is the development of, and successful procurement of, a COVID-19 vaccine here in the UK.

It has been suggested in some circles that by resisting the pressures to join a complex EU procurement plan for vaccines, Britain – with its exceptional strengths in scientific research and public–private–academic partnerships – progressed much better through the early stages of the COVID-19 vaccination programme. The UK government understood its role in sharing risk with AstraZeneca and other pharmaceutical research companies; accepting that it should carry some of the burden. Whereas the EU took a much more cautious approach to sharing risk and as a consequence has had less favourable terms of access to vaccines. Equally, it may well be shown with the passage of time that earlier on in the pandemic, the UK's government acted too hastily in its procurement of personal protective equipment, at times seemingly not following established competitive processes, or thorough due diligence, in favour of speed in the face of adversity (Anon, 2021; see also Chapter 3).

Arguably, a reason to believe that procurement can change for the better was demonstrated in the 2020 delivery of several temporary Nightingale Hospitals across the UK for the National Health Service (NHS). Here, against the backdrop of cost/quality/time criteria that make up every construction contract, the decision was taken to use a framework-based procurement route named Procure22 in response to the urgent need (for rapid delivery of COVID-19 treatment centres). This form of procurement is based fundamentally upon a partnering ethos centred around mutual trust, understanding and collaboration, to agreed commercial rates. This route enabled an established framework of 'supply chain partners' to be gathered to collectively rise to the challenge of delivering a series of new 'field hospitals' across the UK.

The output requirements were defined by clinicians, to a specified quality, to allow the contractors to devise design solutions to meet those requirements, with price being an open-book process.

This approach significantly enabled the speeding up of contract commencement. The teams were notified at 4pm on Friday 27 March 2020 that four facilities had been approved to proceed. By the Monday, the contractors had commenced delivery following extensive planning work over the weekend. The delivery teams threw themselves into the contracts and appeared to deliver successfully on-time, on-quality, to a price based upon agreed 'cost-plus' rates within a transparent contractual arrangement.

The Manchester project involved over 1,000 people, working 24 hours a day, to complete the 750-bed facility within a Grade II listed building in just 13 days from instruction to proceed. All parties to the contract appeared to benefit from the dynamics of the relationship. Had it not been for the urgency of need, projects like this would ordinarily have followed a much more protracted and potentially more costly procurement route. Overall, the Nightingale projects provide an excellent example of collaboration, across all construction disciplines, local government, the NHS, health specialists, the armed forces, infection prevention and control, designers and supply chains.

All of this helps to set the context for a long-overdue reform of procurement towards a culture of 'partnerships with purpose', between the customer and provider of goods and services. We should be drawing on the learnings to strive towards a contract where the 'why' and the 'outcomes' are defined within a fair and transparent payment arrangement.

As a privately owned architectural business, my practice, Pozzoni Architecture, provides solely design services. The private sector in which we operate depends upon and thrives upon the formation of successful relationships, both within its supply chains and with external organisations including customers, stakeholders and regulators. Strong relationships and aligned values have a fundamental impact upon the success and sustainability of any business. They affect factors such as the ability to grow and deliver repeat business, job creation, the development of people and skills, as well as profitability, reputation enhancement and the quality of outcomes for clients.

While techniques for the formation of partnering relationships vary widely across the private, public and third sectors, the fundamentals remain that for a successful relationship to be maintained, all parties must gain value from the interaction. For relationships to be sustainable, the value gained should neither be short-term nor overly transactional and should be based upon a shared appreciation of the value derived by each party.

Defining 'value' when making decisions to award a contract is at the heart of the public–private **relationalism** debate (see Chapters 8 and 18). Unfortunately, metrics for evaluation are a myriad of tangible and less tangible measures, with price being the most visible and most easily measured metric. Particularly in the context of decision-making accountability, price is relatively simple to account for, whereas 'quality' measures have an inherent subjective element to them. Value has been too often defined, in the construction industry especially, by the 'MEAT' method of assessment. That is, the 'Most Economically Advantageous Tender' as introduced by the European Parliament and enacted by the UK in 2014.

There are recently proposed changes by the UK government which are intended to speed up and simplify procurement processes. The *Transforming Public Procurement* Green Paper (HMG, 2020a) recognised that the MEAT methodology 'can be mistaken as the need to deliver the lowest price when actually there may be scope to deliver greater value through a contract in broader qualitative (including social and environmental) terms'. Instead it defines value as the 'Most Advantageous Tender' (MAT). While seemingly nuanced, this revised focus can allow for broader issues such as suitability, lifecycle, environmental, social value, to have a much greater consideration in assessing tenders. Furthermore, it is encouraging to see government advice that asks commissioning bodies to refer any 'abnormally low bid that is more than 10% lower than the average of all bids' to the Cabinet Office before accepting it.

We have certainly experienced great change in the standard and complexity of procurement in recent years. Long-gone are the days of holding 'standard answers' on file for use across multiple tenders. A new breed of professionals has emerged in the form of the bid-manager and the bid-writer, the former from a related industry, the latter perhaps from a journalistic background. Both are important skill-sets in the armoury of competitive tendering. Their roles are to position and bolden both the narrative and values of any given organisation's proposition.

The professionalisation of bidding has also sown the seeds for the emergence of independent 'framework agreement' organisations, operating as private sector businesses to provide independent, fully managed procurement vehicles for the public and third sectors. The most effective can originate from a private sector entrepreneurial approach, based upon offering a procurement vehicle that is more equitable to both parties. That is, equitable in terms of the effectiveness and efficiency of the tendering process itself, plus delivering the desired outcome for all in the delivered contractual results. Such examples provide procurement options that understand that lowest cost often puts strain on a relationship from the outset, especially where that cost is fixed in nature against an inadequately defined outcome.

As architects, the procurement and tendering process is an essential component of securing work and we want to use our experiences to help facilitate improvements as to how it is done. As an example, the current procurement of new free schools follows a two-stage process, the first stage of which is simple and speedy, to select two bidders for the final second stage. However, from this point on, the second stage requires two bid-teams, at risk, to each commit huge resources to produce an advanced level of design for a new school, fully costed in consultation with the client, before a successful bidder can be selected and awarded the commission. The losing team has to carry the loss. But the reality is bigger than that. The losing team's costs need to be recovered somewhere in the ecosystem of the economy and are therefore 'carried' elsewhere in pricing other work. For tendering to become more effective, we believe there needs to be greater appreciation of the process. If not carefully controlled, the process can become needlessly onerous and expensive to the bidder with costs ultimately impacting the economy and public purse.

As a nation, UK plc is carrying an enormous burden of hidden costs of this nature, which ought to be rationalised and spent more productively in delivering positive outcomes. In a competitive tender process, it is inevitable that there will be winners and losers, but the combined costs of failed bids amount to a huge amount of collateral damage for the private sector and come with little to no additional gain for a public sector that is on the front line of delivering social value outcomes.

For many years, common perceptions of the corporate 'listed' private sector (sometimes rightly justified while at other times simply misinformed) have helped to reinforce the notion that the sole objective of business is to maximise profits. Perhaps this is part of the reason for areas of misunderstanding between public, third and private sectors. Nevertheless, it can be easy to tar all private sector businesses, large and small, with the same brush. Doing so dismisses the myriad of private sector businesses, as well as the increasing number of listed organisations, which operate in a far less lionised manner, whereby profits are recognised as essential, but are purpose-driven and not maximised at the expense of sustainable relationships and compromising values. Times are changing, and with a greater shift towards socially responsible capitalism, profit should not be regarded as a dirty word. Along with purpose, planet and people, profit is an essential ingredient to a sustainable enterprise, without which little will be realised.

In the world of finance, a greater focus on responsible investing over recent years has been articulated in the rise of environmental, social and governance (ESG) factors (see Chapter 10). **Social value** and sustainability assessments increasingly feed into ESG factors that are affected by an organisation's actions and performance. Many industries are now being assessed against ESG to varying degrees. However, there can be a danger of factors like social value becoming only point-scoring lines in a bid process, or focusing on the short-term benefits and not the long-term legacy, which could be perceived as at odds with what ESG increasingly symbolises; encouraging all of us to think wider than our own narrow silos and to 'measure and manage' our impacts on our environment and society.

A move towards increasingly higher standards, better accountability and visibility is helping to mitigate such risks. The rise of 'B Corporations' is developing new ways of operating, to shift the focus of businesses to deliver ESG benefits (PWC, 2020). New 'profit for purpose' businesses are emerging, underpinned by values that address some of the world's most challenging problems: environmental issues, inequality, education, healthcare and more.

Sitting above the more transactional relationships of getting public sector work commissioned and delivered is the hugely important role that the public sector and its constituent parts play in delivering a managed environment in which the private sector can invest and do business. For example, some of the most innovative and efficient local authorities can be founded on a mindset of facilitator and enabler, providing the ecosystem for investors from all sectors to operate and thrive with confidence and support.

Today's context for the debate is also framed by news of ever-stretched resources within the public sector. The private sector too is stretched, particularly in those markets where competition is fierce and consequent margins are thin. So, both sides of the relationship need to support each other's positions, to achieve the outcomes from those relationships, without overreliance on the other. A significant example of this approach can be seen in Manchester, where the culture and ambitions of the city council and the combined authority have aligned with and enabled an entrepreneurial environment to flourish and grow. Indeed, I myself sit on a Greater Manchester Combined Authority (GMCA) working group that is a collective of public, third and private sector bodies, all working together and sharing views towards delivering on GMCA's position as the UK's first Age Friendly city region (GMCA, 2018). And we are making a difference, in partnership together, guiding, enabling and influencing the cross-sector impact across the city-region.

No more so than in our sector, property and construction, is there such a stark need to measure what we deliver with a long-term mindset. Buildings generally are expected to have a life of around 25 years as a minimum, so it seems perverse that scrutiny of a bid should focus exclusively on the design and construction phases only, which often only accounts for a small percentage of a building's full lifecycle cost. Good careful design can pay for itself many times over, but can require a greater investment in the time needed to create that design. Reassuringly, within the government's

Construction Playbook (HMG, 2020b), it has been proposed that projects be assessed against a 'Should Cost Model' which acts as a fair benchmark for the cost of a project over its whole life.

There is, clearly, a need for improvements to the way we work together cross-sector and it is true that there is good, bad and mediocre practice across all sectors. There is also a huge appetite to make change happen, as evidenced by the great work contained within the *Construction Playbook* and the themes running through the government's Green Paper, *Transforming Public Procurement*.

Responsible procurement is a key component of success, placing great emphasis on defining a project's requirements and getting it right from the start – to reduce risk, ambiguity, confusion, and ultimately the potential for delays and claims. The proposed outcome-based approach to procurement as outlined within the *Construction Playbook*, with the focus on whole-life value, performance and cost, rather than scope, is an interesting approach, whereby outcomes are based on wider government strategies, for example, net-zero carbon by 2050, modern methods of construction, use of Building Information Modelling, and so forth. Early supply chain involvement has been proposed by government to help ensure that requirements are realistic and achievable, which is an important part of establishing an appropriate definition of outcome requirements. However, this approach should not become overly onerous on suppliers during the procurement process. 'Soft market testing' is fairly commonplace at the moment but the risk is that some commissioning organisations may see this as an excuse to obtain free advice. Fundamentally, tendering procurement requirements should be proportionate to the size and complexity of a project.

Conclusion

We believe the objective of **relational partnering** is fundamentally straightforward. In terms of construction design and planning we now need to be encouraging parties to adopt and trial the fine recommendations of the *Construction Playbook* and Green Paper (HMG, 2020b). This should not be a subject exclusively between the private sector and the commissioning bodies within the public and third sectors. It has a far wider remit, covering the relationships that need to be in place between all of us, whether that be private–private, private–public, public–third sector, contractor–subcontractor and every other permutation. With concerted efforts to achieve net-zero carbon by 2050, if not sooner, the outcome of better partnering in our industry and elsewhere will be as critical to the long-term social determinants of health as any direct investment into areas such as scientific research and healthcare. If we can all make strides to open up, think differently and adopt emerging best practice, the benefits to public bodies, charitable bodies, companies, society and UK plc will be huge.

Together, we can spend public funds more effectively, deliver faster, to ever-higher quality standards in a sustainable, responsible manner, to the benefit of all.

References

Anon (2021) UK vaccination rollout a rare pandemic success. *Financial Times*, 18 January. https://www.ft.com/content/cdfb7b28-8306-4db2-8dd6-4f85a92b177 8

GMCA (2018) *Greater Manchester's Age-Friendly Strategy*. GMCA. https://www.greatermanchester-ca.gov.uk/media/1166/gm_ageing_strategy.pdf

HMG (2020a) *Green Paper: Transforming Public Procurement*. Cabinet Office. https://www.gov.uk/government/consultations/green-paper-transforming-public-procurement

HMG (2020b) *Construction Playbook: Guidance*. Cabinet Office. https://www.gov.uk/government/publications/the-construction-playbook

PWC (2020) *A Guide to the UK B Corporation Movement: What Is a B Corporation?* PWC. https://www.pwc.co.uk/industries/retail-consumer/insights/b-corp.html

Case study: Central England Co-operative society

Luke Olly and Hannah Gallimore

Introduction

Central England Co-operative is one of the largest independent co-operative retailers in the UK, with gross sales more than £1 billion, over 400 trading outlets, a family of around 8,600 colleagues and more than 330,000 regular trading members.

We trade across 16 counties, from Yorkshire through the Midlands to the East Coast – through more than 250 food stores, 100-plus funeral homes, filling stations, post offices, florists, masonry outlets, a crematorium and a coffin factory.

The business is owned and democratically controlled by its members who can stand for election to the board and who also share in the Society's profits through dividends, community investment and member benefits.

Although independent from other co-operative societies we are part of a wider movement and share the international values of principles of co-operatives. As a movement we channel the power of relationalism and as a business use that power to bring our purpose to life – to create a sustainable society for all. We are committed to a society that is financially, humanly, and environmentally sustainable and inclusive.

Social value through cooperation

On 21 December 1844, 28 working people, the Rochdale Pioneers, opened a co-operative shop. They sold pure food at fair prices using honest weights and measures. They encouraged local people to become members, to take part in controlling the business and to share in the profits. There are now 3 million co-ops around the world with 1.2 billion members. In the UK alone, over 7,000 co-ops contribute £39.7 billion to the economy.[1]

A co-op is a business that is owned and controlled by its members. Members can be customers, employees, residents or suppliers. You can find co-operatives in pretty much every industry, from healthcare to housing, renewable energy to retail, sports to social care. And they are every shape and size from multibillion-pound businesses to small community enterprises.

A co-operative might look like any other business, but they are guided by a core set of values and principles that sets them apart:

- A co-op is owned and controlled by its members and exist for the benefit of the members.
- Co-ops are democratic – every member has a vote and has an equal say in how it is run.
- Every member contributes in some way and has a say in how resources are used, and profits are distributed.
- A co-operative is an independent business, owned and controlled by its members.
- It provides education and training to everyone involved, so they can develop and promote the benefits of cooperation.
- It cooperates and works in solidarity with other co-ops.
- It works to support and sustain the community.

Cooperating on wicked issues

Following on from the exploration of mutuality within the public, private and third sectors covered within the previous volume, *Local authorities and social determinants of health* (Simmons, 2020: 319) we can see that mutuality and in turn cooperation may be defined as 'acting together, in a coordinated way, in social relationships, in the pursuit of shared goals, the enjoyment of joint activity, or simply furthering the relationship' (Argyle, 1991: 15). The co-operative values and principles outlined earlier are designed to build organisations centered on mutual support and cooperation, able to tackle issues in a fair and equitable manner, with the benefits shared among all its members.

This has led to the co-operative model being used in a huge range of contexts, delivering on the ethos of 'stronger together', a sentiment that mutually beneficial partnerships are based upon and one that can be argued the co-operative business model uniquely enables.

Co-operatives look to work in partnership with similar organisations that have values aligned to their own and Central England Co-operative is no different.

The co-operative model has survived and even thrived during the COVID-19 storm, growing as a movement, proving its connection to people and places encourages strength and resilience. Co-operatives cannot claim to be the only business that proactively look to partner with external organisations to help deliver a more sustainable world, but we have led the way since 1844 and continue to do so.

COVID-19 has accelerated, exacerbated, changed and highlighted wicked issues to varying degrees in a hundred different ways. To follow is a snapshot of three Central England Co-operative's projects that address wicked issues our communities are facing. These projects pre-date COVID-19 and have flexed and grown during that time. Taken through a relationalism lens they can be seen to demonstrate how working with organisations with similar values and shared aims delivers solutions that are of greater quality and impact, that can be truly sustainable, financially, humanly and environmentally.

Access to food and food waste

Three WRAP[2] studies published in 2013 and 2016 estimated annual food (Anon 2019) waste (Anon 2020a, Anon 2022b) produced in the UK was around 10 million tonnes, 60 per cent of which could have been avoided. This has a value of over £17 billion a year and is associated with around 20 million tonnes of greenhouse gas emissions.

While retail contributes only a fraction of the total amount of annual food waste (around 240,000 tonnes or 2.5 per cent), society has for many years seen food waste by retailers as an unforgivable sin, and for good reason. While it may have once been viewed as just a cost of doing business, the pictures of edible food filling waste bins at the back of stores when 30 per cent of children live in poverty (Anon, 2021) is no longer acceptable. Central England Co-operative have been looking for solutions to this problem for many years, and better ordering systems and reduce-to-clear processes are key, but food waste still remains. We had trialed back-of-house collections with local charitable partners, but they were unsustainable, convenience stores don't have a lot of waste and daily collections from charity partners takes a lot of resources for small returns.

FareShare is the UK's largest national network of charitable food redistributors, made up of 17 independent organisations getting good quality surplus food to almost 11,000 frontline charities and community groups. We approached FareShare Midlands to support us in delivering a bespoke solution that would deliver significant reductions in food waste while feeding as many people as possible. In 2018, after six months of development with FareShare Midlands and the support of local authority environmental health agencies, Central England Co-operative started rolling out its new food redistribution process.

Uniquely this involved taking all unsold 'best before' products and using our own logistics network that serves our community stores, backhauling them to our chilled distribution centre. This reduces costs and miles and ensures consistency which is essential to ensure food is moved quickly and safely. Products are checked and consolidated and transferred five miles to FareShare's dedicated Central England hub. Here it is sorted and distributed to groups across Central England's trading estate based on their specific needs, daily or weekly, via collection or delivery. This process happens five days a week throughout the year.

With the rollout now complete across our estate we are seeing reductions of 40 per cent in our food waste, enabling us to save on waste disposal costs and offset the costs incurred by FareShare Midlands to deliver the scheme.

This scheme now provides around 1 million meals a year to hostels, holiday clubs, food banks, community centres and many more. The food is predominately healthy fruit and vegetables, a much-needed category, and is consistent in volume and nature, making it possible to support beneficiaries in a predictable, sustainable manner.

Addiction and retail crime

P started taking drugs at 14 and spent £1,000 a week on heroin and crack cocaine. He had over 100 arrests and multiple prison stays on his record. P stole £3,000 worth of retail stock a week to sell on at a fraction of its value to sustain his addiction. P stole from Central England Co-operative, Erdington in Birmingham, among others. He was one of a small cohort addicts responsible for over 50 per cent of shoplifting offences in the North Birmingham policing area.

P is not unusual.

P is now living clean and sober, reconnected to his family. P is newly qualified in health and social care and is supporting others through his volunteer work at Livingstone House Rehabilitation Centre in Small Heath, Birmingham.

Central England have invested heavily in hard security measures such as improved closed-circuit television, training and campaigning. The retail industry is calling loudly for changes in the law to protect key workers who have given their all during the pandemic, who daily uphold the law on age-related sales and who suffer over 450 crimes against them every day costing the retail sector £2.5 billion in the last year.[3]

After reaping the rewards of investment in 2019 and seeing falling crime rates against the national trend in Central England stores, the pandemic has been hard. Fear, frustration, suspicion and falling incomes have led to rocketing levels of abuse and violence in our stores.

PC Stuart Toogood of West Midlands Police was in the early stages of trialling an offender to rehab project in partnership with two Midlands based rehab partners. Looking to disrupt decades of drug use, offending and prison stays, PC Toogood brought together offender management services, rehab experts and the final part of the jigsaw, retailers.

Our values and purpose encourage the positive action needed to deal with the root causes of crime rather than relying on deterrent or punishment.

We have now support more than ten individuals through their residential rehabilitation and beyond. Success is relative, varied and unpredictable, such is the wicked nature of addiction, but this project is life-saving and life-changing for the individuals, our colleagues and the sustainability of our Society.

Relationalism is key to the project – we have a problem, the police have a duty and declining resources, and rehab providers such as Livingstone House have the time, experience, training and commitment to be the solution. The result, a sustainable and valuable improvement in the health and wealth of some of the most vulnerable and hard to reach community members and our Society.

Climate change

The climate emergency is one of the most pervasive and threatening challenges of our time for the health of both our society and the economy that serves it. The UK retail industry contributes approximately 215 MtCO2e through the lifecycle footprint of goods sold annually in the UK, with additional emissions from vehicle fuel sales by retailers of ~50 MtCO2e. This places the sector among the most important contributors to greenhouse gas emissions, contributing approximately 80 per cent more emissions each year than all road transport in the UK (Anon, 2021).

Central England Co-operative recently launched a new target to reduce its carbon footprint by 90 per cent by 2030, from a 2010 baseline. This ambitious target can only be achieved through strong partnerships, and an example of this was the development of a new refrigeration strategy.

Refrigeration gases constitute around 20 per cent of a retailer's carbon footprint (scopes 1 and 2) and the power used by refrigeration systems can be up to 60 per cent of the power consumption of a store. It is therefore a key area for a retailer to decarbonise, particularly as systems can be in use for 10–15 years. A new refrigeration gas was launched in 2018 that Central England Co-operative wanted to use in future refrigeration installations. Due to the nature of the gas, it required new design guidance, additional safety features in cabinets and packs and several components to be redesigned and brought to market. We then needed to get our system designers and installers to understand the requirements of the gas and value engineer the process so that our trading development team could include the new system within the financial models they use when developing new stores.

As the end user of the refrigeration system Central England Co-operative used our position of influence to bring all stakeholders together into a working group. Trials were developed through gaining access to new equipment before it came to market and funding for design guidance was accessed through the gas manufacturer who had an interest in bringing solutions to market. As we made clear our intent to use the new technology, this enabled manufacturers to invest in the research and design of new products, knowing they had a market to sell to. This led to two trial sites being installed in 2019, delivering carbon savings of around 90 per cent on our previous refrigeration systems and this has now become our standard system design.

Conclusion

As demonstrated by these examples, the values represented by the co-operative business model, when they are lived and breathed by its members, enable a co-op business to deliver sustainable social value with integrity. As a trusted partner, we are in a strong position to harness the power of relationalism, build strong, successful partnership and deliver meaningful change.

Customers, colleagues, suppliers and members need to be taken on the journey. Addressing wicked issues such as climate change and food poverty undoubtedly require investment and real change, both of which can pose an uncomfortable challenge to people and business.

A co-op, owned and controlled by its members, guided by shared values and principles, and led by leaders who are passionate about sustainable development and social change, has a strong chance of delivering the level of change society requires on wicked issues.

Notes

[1]   Co-op Economy (2021) Report by Co-operatives UK, p 3. www.uk.coop/get-involved/ awareness-campaigns/co-op-economy#:~:text=The%20Co-op%20Economy%20is%20 the%20nation%E2%80%99s%20only%20comprehensive,resilient%20to%20the%20 economic%20devastation%20caused%20by%20Covid
[2]   WRAP is a climate action NGO working around the globe to tackle the causes if climate crisis, https://wrap.org.uk/about-us
[3]   British Retail Consortium's Crime Survey (2021). https://brc.org.uk/news/operations/ crime-survey-2021/

References

Anon (2019) Food Waste Reduction Roadmap progress report 2019. WRAP. https://wrap.org.uk/resources/report/food-waste-reduction-roadmap-progress-report-2019. Accessed on 29 August 2022.

Anon (2020a) Courtauld Commitment Milestone progress report. https:// wrap.org.uk/resources/report/courtauld-commitment-milestone-progr ess-report Accessed on 29 August 2022.

Anon (2020b).UK progress against Courtauld 2025 targets and UN Sustainable Development Goal 12.3. WRAP. https://wrap.org.uk/resour ces/report/uk-progress-against-courtauld-2025-targets-and-un-sustaina ble-development-goal-123. Accessed on 29 August 2022.

Anon (2021) Child poverty facts and figures. Child Poverty Action Group. https://cpag.org.uk/child-poverty/child-poverty-facts-and-figures#:~:text=%20Child%20poverty%20facts%20and%20figures%20. Accessed on 29 August 2022.

Argyle M. (2014) *Cooperation: The Basis of Sociability*. Routledge.

BRC (2021) Climate action roadmap. British Retail Consortium. https://brc.org.uk/climate-roadmap/. Accessed on 29 August 2022.

Simmons R. (2020) Mutuality in the public, private and third sectors. In Bonner, A. (ed) *Local Authorities and Social Determinants of Health*. Bristol: Policy Press, p 319.

PART VI

Engagement and proposed changes

Richard Smith

The cultural factors that influence the formation of successful inter- and intra-sectoral partnerships cannot be overstated. When it comes to engagement of the partners the commissioning and procurement regime, as a gateway, needs to reflect on a partnering of equals. This should include the role and involvement of the third sector. The Kruger Report makes reference to this as reviewed in Chapter 16.

The post-COVID-19 and post-Brexit effects, whilst taking account of the cost of living crisis, need to be reflected in a change to the approach to contracting products and services. Nowhere is this more important than within procurement. A balance must be struck between over-regulating the sectors and under-regulating them. If innovation is a key driver, then either approach can stifle this through too much prescription or lack of it leading to status quo and the avoidance of challenge.

A key issue to be considered within the context of procurement as a 'gateway' to more effective partnering is a recognition of two distinct activities. Firstly, the role of the specifier and, secondly, the role of the procurement professional, and engagement of contracting parties. Hitherto, these two activities have been regarded as a client function. It is time now to recognise the different and distinctive roles of commissioner and client.

If we are to make a success of this opportunity, the learning of the lessons of the past will be critical. However there is a lack of detailed evidence as to the reasons why some partnerships are successful, while other are disastrous. Academic research has a crucial role in helping to build a new and comprehensive base through its research and its training and educational programmes. All sectors, including the political class, should be 'led by the evidence' in terms of policy creation and guidance.

Future engagement of partners should reflect an environment which has facilitated the building of trust through an open and transparent process. This means a framework that enables full and frank dialogue between all sectors, both specifiers and deliverers. It also includes those having a direct interest in the outcome, including the third sector working within and on behalf of the community. This is the essence of what we mean by **relationalism** and its contribution to **social value** (see Chapter 8).

Reference is made within this book to the establishment of the Centre for Partnering (CfP) which is being developed to introduce the notion of relationalism. This will include a definition of the term, research into the **relational dividends** (see Chapter 1) both from a social and commercial perspective and consideration of the impact this could have on the social determinants of health. The CfP will consider, through its research programme, the impact of relationalism in terms of partnering culture, in a 'commissioning' context.

The compilation of the knowledge base will be key (see Introduction to Part V). This will be drawn, in part, from the experiences gathered through the Exemplar programme (see Case study 17.1). If the future impact of relationalism is to be significant, then this will demand a re-education of the differences between a partnering environment which is based upon current and traditional principles, when compared with a new partnering culture embracing much more flexibility and innovative practices in the legal, financial, social and economic environments. This will include a necessary change to behaviour. A future partnering environment should lead to the inclusion of public, private and third sector participants as equal partners without obstacles being placed in their way, which stifle any one or more of those potential partners offering innovative solutions. This could include a market proposition being initiated and offered to the public sector or a third sector making representations on behalf of it and the local community. An important element in this regard is placing the public sector in a position where it can accept this offer.

Given the need for a change to partnering behaviour in the current economic and political climate, it is timely for the emergence of a new relationalism idea – an idea that focuses more on partnering/contractual outcomes than partnering mechanisms.

Chapter 8, in Part III, reviews the governance framework in which stakeholders understand their contributions and empathetically work together for the public good. As highlighted in the introduction to the book, a **relational partnering** approach should take account of **legal, financial, social, economic, environmental and geopolitical factors**. How do these factors impact the public, private and third sectors?

A legal perspective on client–contractor contracts and related issues on procurement is presented in Chapter 18. This highlights the **process** in establishing **governance**. **Strategic planning** following the COVID-19 crisis includes major infrastructural projects such as the planning of housing and town centres (Case study 17.2) and highways, reviewed by Mike Bresnen in Chapter 19. Strategic planning and economic development have both

Figure VI.1: The types of projects forming part of the Exemplar Initiative and the need for new types of partners to deliver a relational dividend

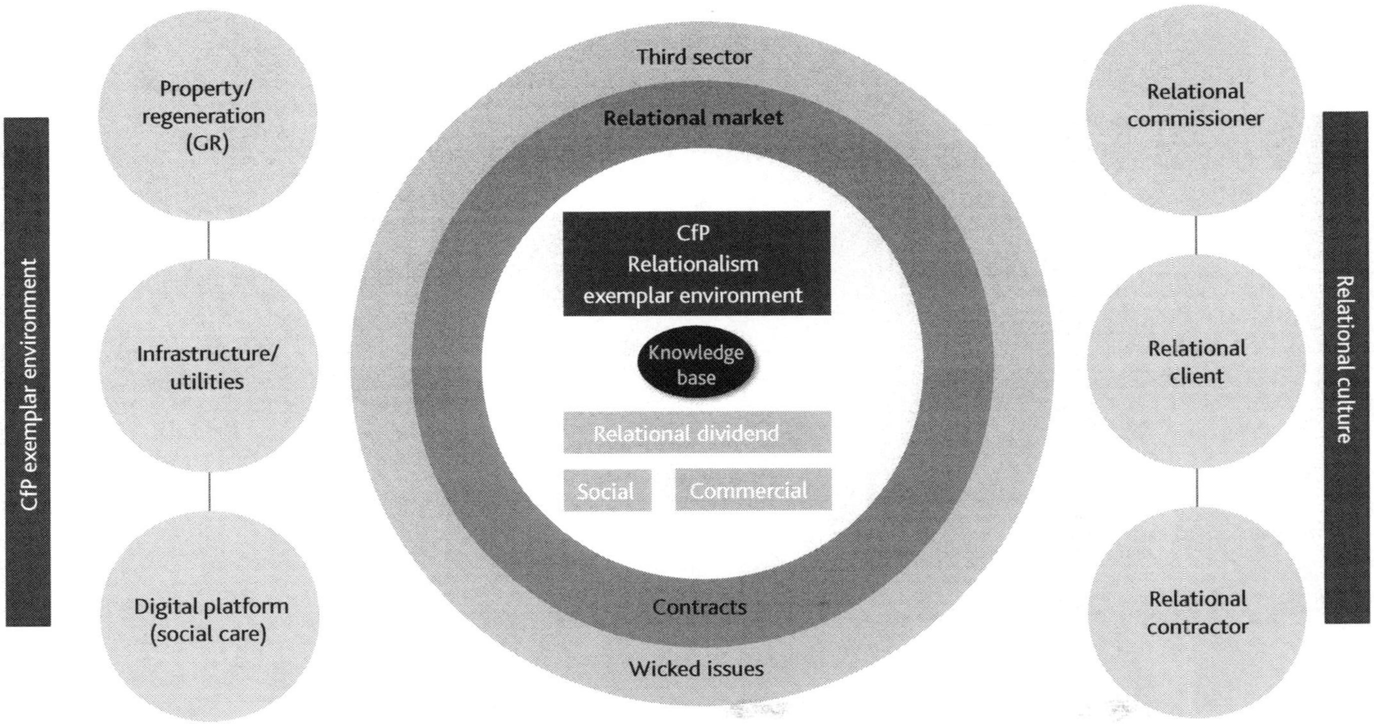

Relational culture

Relational commissioner

Relational client

Relational contractor

Third sector

Relational market

CfP Relationalism exemplar environment

Knowledge base

Relational dividend

Social

Commercial

Contracts

Wicked issues

Property/ regeneration (GR)

Infrastructure/ utilities

Digital platform (social care)

CfP exemplar environment

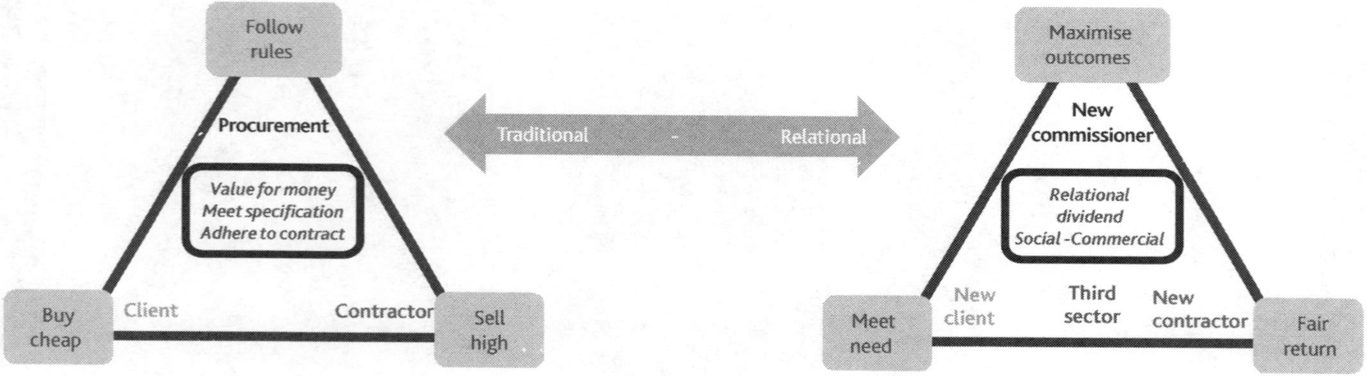

Figure VI.2: The major impact of a relational partnering environment compared with a more traditional approach, with a particular focus on the need for equal partners balancing social and commercial value

regional and national **political** drivers, these sociopolitical levers are discussed in Chapter 20.

Chapter 21, by Nigel Ball, provides an overview of the impact of COVID-19 on the swinging pendulum and citizens' demands as previously discussed in *Local Authorities and Social Determinants of Health* (Bonner, 2018).

In terms of the future evolution of the idea of relationalism, the commissioning role of the CfP will be enhanced through the bringing together of individuals and organisations (some of whom have contributed to this book) within its governance structure and establishment of the alliances between public, private and third sectors. The compilation of a **relationalism knowledge base** will facilitate an educational programme focused on those that commission and/or act in the client/contractor procurement role.

In formulating the ideas that lie behind relationalism it will be important to understand the benefits that arise from its application in terms of balancing social and commercial value. The notion of the relational dividend will be evidenced through the **Exemplar Projects Initiative**, both in terms of generating the additional value that will be possible to create and then significantly giving careful consideration as to how it is ringfenced and spent (Figure VI.1). The opportunity to do this provides the third sector with the option of contributing to the community outcomes that are delivered through the relational dividend.

The application of relationalism to the social determinants of health may give rise to the replacement of **public–private partnerships** with **public–third–private partnerships**. This will demand a change to behaviour. For this to occur, the Centre for Partnering must achieve its overall aim to establish the relationalism accreditation model. Thereafter the Centre for Partnering and its universities will need to educate individuals and organisations from across the partnering sector to network in accredited frameworks so as to achieve partnering outcomes that deliver the relational dividends (Figure VI.2).

References

Bonner, A. (ed) (2018) *Social Determinants of Health: Social Inequality and Wellbeing*. Bristol: Policy Press.

18

Soft and hard measures in optimising wellbeing through procurement, commissioning and partnering

Mark Cook

Introduction

The essential components to enhancing well-being in commissioning and procurement are public authorities, especially National Health Service (NHS) bodies and councils, and these have been responsible for a wide range of services for the public for many decades, through the exercise of a wide range of statutory duties but also powers. The means by which such services have been delivered have however tended to be altered by successive governments restructuring the NHS, whereas councils have tended to have had their statutory functions constrained or broadened on a constantly fluctuating basis. In many ways the delivery of high quality public services has been shaped by the 'make or buy' question that has arisen and been to the fore since the introduction of compulsory competitive tendering (CCT) for a number of local authority services in 1989 that was then succeeded by a 'best value' regime that came into force in 2000.

It would be wishful thinking for any government to take an interest in a wholesale review of NHS and local government functions so that we can have a comprehensively integrated offer in terms of health and social care but also other services. So, we can expect that when changes are made they will continue to be adding layers of adjustments such that the image that can come to mind for the legislation that governs public services is of an Egyptian mummy with plaster casts and adhesive tape all over it.

In the absence of any interest in integrated legislation and central coordination by central government (preferring the easier and expedient approach of meddling and interference), it is arguably down to councils and local NHS bodies to do the best that they can for the communities that they serve and to establish the coordinated and engaged approach that local services require.

Given this, the opportunity to engender the greatest social, economic and environmental wellbeing should perhaps be determined by the ascertainment of need, an understanding of the resources required to meet that need, a programme to work out the best way of attracting the right resources to address that requirement and then a route map for delivering that programme. However, instead what often happens is that a public authority considers the best way of meeting its statutory duties, establishes the budget that is available to meet that duty and then commissions and procures or delivers itself services to meet that duty limited by the budget that it has available and often by deeply entrenched ways of doing things – and therefore without necessarily meeting the need that is there to be met.

This chapter seeks to address this anomaly by considering:

- how a full understanding of social value can unlock better value and meet actual need in public services;
- how creating partnering and collaborative relationships can help to meet the wellbeing of communities – and why a good governance framework is essential to each of the participants in any such relationship but also to the vehicle for that relationship itself;
- what can be done to move from a binary commissioning–contracting framework that yields a decreasing cycle of outcomes to a multistakeholder approach that negotiates an upward rachet of benefits generated through collaboration.

Social value in public procurement: recent developments

Policy-led public procurement has been a global phenomenon for decades, but in the UK was dealt a heavy blow with the introduction of the 'non-commercial considerations' legislation (Part II Local Government Act 1988) which outlawed councils from taking into account prescribed factors at various points in a procurement process, in direct response to the Greater London Council undertaking such measures in its contracting arrangements. This legislation was put in place at the same time as the extension of CCT to a range of services. The factors that were outlawed included:

(a) the terms and conditions of employment by contractors of their workers or the composition of, the arrangements for the promotion, transfer or training of or the other opportunities afforded to, their workforces;

(b) whether the terms on which contractors contract with their sub-contractors constitute, in the case of contracts with individuals, contracts for the provision by them as self-employed persons of their services only;

   (c)   any involvement of the business activities or interests of contractors with irrelevant fields of Government policy;

   (d)   the conduct of contractors or workers in industrial disputes between them or any involvement of the business activities of contractors in industrial disputes between other persons;

   (e)   the country or territory of origin of supplies to, or the location in any country or territory of the business activities or interests of, contractors;

   (f)   any political, industrial or sectarian affiliations or interests of contractors or their directors, partners or employees;

   (g)   financial support or lack of financial support by contractors for any institution to or from which the authority gives or withholds support;

   (h)   use or non-use by contractors of technical or professional services provided by the authority under the Building Act 1984 (Designing Buildings 2021) or the Building (Scotland) Act. (HMG, 2003)

It was this legislation that stopped councils from advancing the kind of policy-led commissioning procurement, that is now advocated so widely and which was identified in the seminal publication *Achieving Community Benefits through Contracts: Law, Policy and Practice* (Macfarlane and Cook, 2000)), as a major barrier to opportunities for training and employment being incorporated into procurement contracts, much more so than EU law which was given much blame by those sceptical of such positive arrangements. The same report identified the *Finnish Buses* case as the route for embedding social characteristics in public procurement (by analogy with its support of environmental characteristics pursued by policy). In essence this case enabled advocates of community benefits in procurement to pursue the following good practice: adopt corporate policy that enables such measures; adopt them within the specification of the contract as being core to the requirement; create a way of evaluating them within the criteria for awarding the contract; and then ensure that they are achieved by robust contract management. The Joseph Rowntree Foundation report also made the most of relaxations introduced at that time by statutory instrument to the non-considerations legislation that allowed targeted training and recruitment requirements to be incorporated in procurement exercises.

Much of first decade of the 21st century saw a galvanising of all those committed to sustainable procurement creating a considerable amount of evidenced good practice. Two highlights of this in the UK were:

• the Scottish government's embracing of community benefits in public procurement in its policy, evidenced by pilots and good practice learning, that was shared nationally; and

- the Sustainable Procurement Task Force, jointly funded by the Department for the Environment, Food and Rural Affairs and HM Treasury and set up under the direction of Sir Neville Simms. The National Action Plan, 'Procuring the Future', delivered its findings and recommendations on 12 June 2006. (HMG,2011b)

Numerous toolkits of good practice were created during this decade that were established not only by local authorities, the prime proponents of such methodologies, but also the NHS on a regional basis (especially the North West Health Authority).

The election of a new UK government in 2010 saw the disruption of such consensual progress with the reorganisation of the NHS and the onset of austerity in public services. But in addition, a very strange thing happened: a private member's bill made it all the way through to being passed as legislation which has had a most catalytic effect on the way that public procurement has been exercised, especially in more recent years, such that what was deemed heresy in the beginning of the century is now arguably regarded as desirable good practice at the heart of HM Treasury thinking, albeit with a centrist slant. The Public Services (Social Value) Act 2012 was initiated by Chris White MP, with the support of what is now Social Enterprise UK, and politicians of all political complexion. It was able to progress forward when the Cabinet Office decided to lend its approval to its current form, which is narrower than originally intended but nevertheless is possibly one of the best examples of statute with a 'nudge' effect (HMG, 2021b).

When procuring services, in short, the 2012 Act requires contracting authorities in England to consider how to:

- improve the economic, social and environmental wellbeing of the area served by it through procurement;
- how to undertake the process of procurement with a view to securing that improvement; and
- consider whether to undertake any consultation on that improvement.

The constitutional importance of this is usually missed as this small but beautiful Act effects a duty on all contracting authorities to consider wellbeing at the heart of their procurement of services in relation to the place they serve. Those three pillars of wellbeing mirror the underpinning of UN Sustainable Development Goals as well as an important power that councils had at the time to promote the economic, social and environmental wellbeing of the areas that they served (a useful power that was swept away in England by the Localism Act 2011 in the belief that the general power of competence that Act brought rendered the wellbeing power superfluous – a fundamental mistake in thinking and a reflection of the still extant failure to grasp the opportunity for wellbeing to be at the heart of council powers, rather than an add-on) HMG (2011a).

In Scotland more comprehensive legislation was passed as led by the Scottish government in the form of the Procurement Reform (Scotland) Act 2014. Part 2 of the 2014 Act sets out a number of duties and requirements that are wider and deeper than anything comparable elsewhere in the UK (HMG, 2014b).

Under the 2014 Act, contracting authorities are required by law ('the sustainable procurement duty') to consider how their procurement activity can be used to improve the economic, social and environmental wellbeing of their area, with a particular focus on reducing inequality, and how they will facilitate the involvement of small and medium enterprises, third sector and supported businesses and promote innovation.

But it goes beyond this, such that:

- Scottish ministers can and do publish guidance on the exercise of the sustainable procurement duty;
- it promotes procurement exercises being limited to supported businesses (which are ones that have high proportions of people with disabilities or who have been unemployed);
- it provides for distinct treatment of contracts for health or social care services, including the issuance of guidance specific to them;
- it requires any contracting authority which has significant procurement expenditure (equal to or greater than £5,000,000) to prepare and review a procurement strategy setting out how the authority intends to carry out regulated procurements and in particular how the authority intends to ensure that its regulated procurements will contribute to the carrying out of its functions and the achievement of its purposes, deliver value for money and be carried out in compliance with its sustainable procurement duty, including:
  - a statement of the authority's general policy on the use of community benefit requirements, consulting and engaging with those affected by its procurements, the payment of a living wage to persons involved in producing, providing or constructing the subject matter of regulated procurements, healthy and safety compliance, the procurement of fairly and ethically traded goods and services;
  - a statement on how contracts for the provision of food will improve the health, wellbeing and education of communities in the authority's area, and promote the highest standards of animal welfare;
  - setting out how prompt payment will be enabled to contractors and subcontractors.

In Wales procurement has tended to be directed by guidance issued by its government, but it has developed its own far-reaching legislation that extends across all public body functions, in the form of the Well-being of Future Generations (Wales) Act 2015 (HMG, 2015). The 2015 Act establishes the office of the Future Generations Commissioner for Wales. She has the general duty:

(a) to promote the sustainable development principle, in particular to—
  (i) act as a guardian of the ability of future generations to meet their needs, and
  (ii) encourage public bodies to take greater account of the long-term impact of the things that they do, and
(b) for that purpose to monitor and assess the extent to which well-being objectives set by public bodies are being met. (HMG, 2015)

Under the 2015 Act each public body must carry out sustainable development, meaning the process of improving the economic, social, environmental and cultural wellbeing of Wales by taking action, in accordance with the sustainable development principle (that is, the body must act in a manner which seeks to ensure that the needs of the present are met without compromising the ability of future generations to meet their own needs), aimed at achieving the wellbeing goals. These goals are set out in an explanatory table in section 4 of the 2015 Act, covering these goals: a prosperous Wales, a resilient Wales, a healthier Wales, a more equal Wales, a Wales of cohesive communities, a Wales of vibrant culture and thriving Welsh language, and a globally responsible Wales (HMG, 2015).

Procurement post-Brexit and the embedding of social value in projects appraisal

In some ways it has been the political turns of events surrounding Brexit rather than Brexit itself that are contributing to the approach now being taken to wellbeing and its place in public services, certainly in England. In particular the election of a UK government mandated with a large majority and winning seats in what has been described as 'Red Wall' areas has resulted in HM Treasury looking for ways to justify much more interventionist approaches to public investment.

A second significant contributor is the COVID-19 pandemic and the application of public funding to keep the economy as afloat as possible, with a range of 'Build Britain Back' measures that are intended to improve local infrastructure and stimulate employment and growth.

A third important event is the hosting of COP26 held in Glasgow in November 2021 which reflected the strong interest taken in measures to tackle the worldwide climate crisis, such that capital investment in the UK both in the public and private spheres is programmed to enable buildings and other assets to achieve net-zero carbon levels faster than the UK government's stated timeline of 2050 (HMG, 2021a).

It is within this landscape that the publication in November 2020 of *Green Book Review 2020: Findings and Response* by HM Treasury is significant (HMG, 2010). Right at the beginning of this document the following explanation is given:

1.2 The Green Book is the government's guidance on options appraisal and applies to all proposals that concern public spending, taxation, changes to regulations, and changes to the use of existing public assets and resources. It is vital for designing interventions that both achieve government policy objectives and deliver social value for money – that is, that maximise the delivery of economic, social and environmental returns for UK society for every pound of public funds spent. It is supported by detailed HM Treasury guidance on developing business cases which reflects its principles, and by departmental guidance that addresses issues specific to their policy concerns.

1.3 The review was set up in response to concerns that the government's appraisal guidance may mitigate against investment in poorer parts of the UK and undermine the Government's aim to 'level up' these areas. This has therefore been the central focus of investigation, but many of the findings and the action that the Government intends to take to address them have a much wider relevance to how appraisal can support decision-makers to deliver their priorities. These changes will therefore turn the Green Book into a vital tool for progressing the Government's priority outcomes and wider public value agenda.

1.4 Given the UK's recent legal requirement to achieve net zero carbon emissions by 2050 and the 25 Year Environment Plan (2018), the review has also revisited the guidance included in the 2018 Green Book on appraising environmental impacts. In addition, the Government has taken the opportunity to refresh guidance on best practice in appraising the impact of interventions on equalities. (HMG, 2010)

Of significance is this assertion:

1.10 One of the fundamental issues that the review has identified is the common failure of those writing appraisals to engage properly with the strategic context in which their proposal sits. Specifically, business cases frequently do not demonstrate the necessary understanding of:

- the proposal's specific contribution to the delivery of the government's intended strategic goals (such as levelling up or net zero); and
- the specific social and economic features of different places and how the intervention may affect them;
- Other strategies, programmes or projects with which the intervention may interact, including in a particular geographical area.

Three highlights of the changes to the Green Book are the recognition that:

- business case preparation must start with a strategic aim that is expressed clearly (that is, policy-led projects are promoted as best practice);
- any such business case can be applied to 'place' at a local or regional level so it makes sense in the context of where people actually live. Furthermore, the benefits to be achieved do not have to all be monetised; and
- environmental impacts over time can be measured with reference to an acknowledgement of the value that society places on health but also the welfare of future generations (in fact a whole chapter of this Review is devoted to appraising environmental impacts). (HMG, 2010)

As the Green Book Review concludes:

1.23 Ultimately, this should promote better decision-making in support of clearly expressed policy objectives, and improved public confidence in that process. And as a result of the changes set out in this report, including more robust analysis of transformational potential, including in areas that have been considered as 'left behind', and improving the analysis of regional and local impacts more generally, the Government would expect future investments to be better aligned with its ambitions to level up the country. (HMG, 2010)

These changes herald an opportunity to embed social value at the heart of the public arena but it remains to be seen to what extent this is truly reflected in the way in which government departments and their ministers make judgements about public expenditure and the achievement of holistic outcomes centred around wellbeing.

Just after the publication of the Review the UK government's Green Paper, *Transforming Public Procurement*, was published, exploring ways in which procurement processes could be simplified and made more flexible in a manner that is consistent with trade treaty obligations and also ensures good practice without unnecessary 'red tape' (HMG,2020).

Chapter 1 of the Green Paper says that the government proposes that the following principles should be 'included in the new legislation'. These principles are:

- Public good – although it is not clear from the paper exactly what is meant by 'public good' and how it interfaces with social value.
- Value for money – although this duplicates obligations many contracting authorities are subject to already – and needs to fit in with Green Book principles.
- Transparency – although it is not clear how the tension between this and the principles of integrity and fair treatment of suppliers, in relation to things like the disclosure of tendered prices and method statements, is to be resolved.
- Integrity – in terms of avoiding conflicts of interest, respecting suppliers' confidential information and running procurements professionally.
- Fair treatment of suppliers – without reducing procurement to a tick-box exercise but also requiring consideration of other duties, for example, those of local authorities under the Care Act 2014 (HMG,2014a).
- Non-discrimination based on nationality – although government procurement guidance PPN 11/20 recommends discrimination based on area for below threshold contracts, which will therefore also discriminate against non-national suppliers who are not within the designated area.

The Green Paper explores the evaluation of contracts with reference to matters that do not necessarily relate to the subject matter of contract, providing that government guidance and directions are adhered to. The risk with public procurement is that it replaces the principles-based approach of the European Commission with a much more directional political stance taken by an incumbent government.

It would be arguably better to adopt the more encompassing approach that both the Scottish and Welsh governments have established, particularly in Wales with regard to future generations and then for all public bodies to make their decisions with reference to a broader canvas.

The principles established in the Green Paper as described here look likely to be implemented following the government's response to the consultation, with the new legislation likely to take effect earliest in 2023.

How good governance creates the framework for success in partnering relationships

A holistic approach to public services commissioning and procurement requires more than a buyer–seller relationship if it is to succeed. Particularly in long-term contracts it is not unusual to make provision for liaison between the authority and the contractor, including joint working groups.

However a number of public bodies, especially local authorities, have established joint ventures which entail creating a vehicle in which both the council and its private sector partner have a share, typically with a reasonably long contract between that authority and the vehicle, and with a framework arrangement established enabling other described contracting authorities to purchase from that joint business. This kind of practice began with the large 'hosting' procurements undertaken in the 1990s to bypass CCT legislation but in recent years has been used by councils to leverage the opportunities from the skilled workforce that they have developed in certain services. Such joint ventures are invariably established after an exhaustive procurement exercise.

Other joint ventures are established for making the most of the resources that each party brings as the basis for a broader collaboration. Typically, these commercial ventures are intended to enable the council or other authority to make better use of their land holdings with a view to achieving policy aims. For example, several councils have established joint ventures with housing associations to enable more affordable housing to be built in their area. Often it has been possible to establish such arrangements without undertaking a procurement exercise for the selection of the joint venture partner. Instead competition has been leveraged down the line in establishing the supply chain for the works (Anon, 2021).

The key components for such joint ventures succeeding are manifold but include:

- The officers and political leadership of both organisations being willing players, with leadership from the top ensuring continuity in approach.
- Creating governance documents that enable equal bargaining power and a robust means of resolving differences, but particularly being clear as to how any joint business plan is to be agreed, profit is to be accounted and allocated, and the joint venture unwound should this be necessary.
- Each side taking time to understand the different drivers of each party, but with an exploration of how a shared culture and set of co-owned values might be developed.

It is equally important for the decision-making operations within a public body to be clearly established in relation to its statutory responsibilities so that a correct approach is taken to the persons it appoints as directors or corporate representatives of any joint vehicle (bearing in mind that conflicts of interest will arise with companies, but less so with limited liability partnerships). It is also important in the case of companies for the shareholder function to be discharged at the appropriate level and in accordance with an apt scheme of delegation. In turn the commissioning activity of the authority must be conducted separately from the shareholding function.

Properly constructed, good governance within a public body alongside good governance within the joint venture entity is important. It should not, however, be forgotten that private businesses are increasingly under scrutiny for their governance by their investors and therefore a successful partnership between the sectors will inevitably entail all parties demonstrating robust accountability structures for them to fully play a role as good team players with each other.

Taking commissioning and contracting beyond a binary relationship

The opposite approach to a commissioning–contracting model is to construct a resource focused approach to meeting public need. This can be realised by seeking to engender the greatest social, economic and environmental wellbeing by the ascertainment of need, an understanding of the resources required to meet that need, a programme to work out the best way of attracting the right resources to address that requirement and then a route map for delivering that programme.

On that basis perhaps procurement and commissioning might be refashioned to place commissioner and contractor on a collaborative footing to deliver better and more honest outcomes. Since the Second World War historically it is the state that has played the role of commissioner. But is this correct in a context where individual users and local communities have often the best grasp of what serves their best interests? It is also often the case that the service deliverer has a better idea of what should be commissioned. Equally many commissioners have a very clear grasp of what good delivery might look like. These questions should therefore be asked:

- Who is the real commissioner: the state, the individual user, the community, the contractor (in so far as the contractor determines how delivery works)?
- Conversely, who is the contractor and how dependent is delivery really on the expertise and input of the commissioner?
- How might procurement be reconfigured to reflect these realities?

And that is where, when it comes to the wellbeing of any place, any of the locally based public bodies, any community stakeholder group and any deliverer of services should perhaps have the right to convene a public need resources conversation, in which all participants assess the need, offer the resources that they have between them and then work out how the optimum resources can be found and used to meet that need, including any gaps to be filled. All this can be done as a way of scoping what is to be procured and who is to be the procurer. It would be interesting to develop pilots of such an exercise just to see where they lead to. With wellbeing at the heart of such an exercise, good collaboration will be paramount, taking into account the considerable learning developed in this connection.[1]

A good model for drawing all these strands is the co-operative – and we are beginning to see signs of the full use of it being introduced to public services especially in North West England, with its roots in Rochdale.

Wellbeing cannot be achieved by 'same as usual' and it is hoped that this chapter offers clues as to how a holistic approach can be manifested fully to achieve the widest benefits possible for all.

Note

[1]   A good organisation to follow on this is 'do-tank' Collaborate: https://collaboratecic.com/

References

Anon (2021) *Collaborate: For Social Change.* https://collaboratecic.com

Designing Buildings (2021) *The Building Act 1984.* https://www.designi ngbuildings.co.uk/wiki/The_Building_Act

HMG (1984) *Building Act 1984.* https://www.legislation.gov.uk/ukpga/ 1984/55

HMG (1988) *Local Government Act.* https://www.legislation.gov.uk/ukpga/ 1988/9/contents

HMG (2003) *Building (Scotland) Act 2003.* https://www.legislation.gov.uk/ asp/2003/8/contents

HMG (2010) *Final Report of the Green Book Review.* HM Treasury. https:// www.gov.uk/government/publications/final-report-of-the-2020-green- book-review

HMG (2011a) *Localism Act 2011.* https://www.legislation.gov.uk/ukpga/ 2011/20/contents/enacted

HMG (2011b) *Procuring the Future: The National Action Plan.* Department for Environment, Food and Rural Affairs. https://www.gov.uk/governm ent/publications/procuring-the-future

HMG (2014a) *Care Act 2014.* https://www.legislation.gov.uk/ukpga/2014/ 23/contents/enacted

HMG (2014b) *Procurement Reform (Scotland) Act 2014.* https://www.legislat ion.gov.uk/asp/2014/12/contents

HMG (2015) *Well-Being of Future Generation (Wales) Act 2015.* https://www. futuregenerations.wales/about-us/future-generations-act/

HMG (2018) *25 Year Environment Plan.* Department for Environment, Food and Rural Affairs. https://www.gov.uk/government/publications/ 25-year-environment-plan

HMG (2020) *Green Paper: Transforming Public Procurement.* Cabinet Office. https://www.gov.uk/government/consultations/green-paper-transforming-public-procurement

HMG (2021a) *COP: UN Climate Change Conference UK 21.* https://www.gov.uk/government/topical-events/cop26 Download on 17 08 2021

HMG (2021b) *Social Value Act: Information and Resources.* https://www.gov.uk/government/publications/social-value-act-information-and-resources/social-value-act-information-and-resources

Macfarlane, R. and Cook, M. (2000) *Achieving Community Benefits through Contracts: Law, Policy and Practice.* Joseph Rowntree Foundation. http://socialeconomyaz.org/wp-content/uploads/2011/06/jr129-community-benefits-contracts1.pdf

19

Relational procurement: translating lessons learned from large infrastructural projects

Mike Bresnen, Sarah-Jane Lennie and Nick Marshall

Introduction

Relational contracting has had a marked influence on contemporary discourse about improving performance within the construction and engineering industries. Experience with delivering large-scale infrastructure projects through a partnering approach provides valuable lessons to be learned about the antecedents, processes, outcomes and possibilities associated with public–private partnering. However, that rich experience has also provided considerable insight into the complexities and challenges of developing and embedding relational contracting in practice and in directing that joint effort to achieve superordinate (project) goals. Added to the wicked problems those efforts attempt to address are the many challenges and tensions associated with translating the rhetoric of partnering into the reality of collaboration on the ground. Drawing upon established research and thinking on partnering in major infrastructure projects, this chapter elaborates on and explores those challenges and tensions and examines how they may unfold in the context of public–private collaboration designed to address wicked social and cultural issues. Particular emphasis is placed upon understanding the organisational cultural antecedents of partnering and how these may evolve as collaborative relationships are established and develop between organisations that straddle the public–private divide.

Relational contracting in the construction industry

The origins of relational contracting in the construction industry can be traced back to the search for a solution to communication and coordination problems that bedevilled construction industry performance in the postwar period. From the 1960s onwards, UK government and industry-led reports highlighted the fragmentation within this project-based industry (between clients, designers, builders) and observed how it had consistently led to delays in project completion, exorbitant costs and problems in meeting client specifications and quality standards (for example, Higgin and Jessop, 1965; Latham, 1994). Competitive tendering, the system of contracting commonly used on infrastructure projects, was seen as a major contributing factor. By driving down tender prices, it created incentives for successful bidders to exploit complexities and uncertainties in the construction process, as well as variations introduced by clients, by pricing the additional work required to recoup the costs of tendering and squeezed margins. The result was what many industry insiders depicted as a 'contracting culture', characterised by adversarial relationships and frequent recourse to the law to settle disputes (Eriksson and Laan, 2007; Challender et al, 2017).

The drive towards relational contracting gained momentum in the 1990s, inspired by a number of influential reports that called for greater trust and cooperation between contractual partners. In the US, the Construction Industry Institute (1991) attributed poor performance to fragmentation and a lack of trust and cooperation between contractual partners, as did the National Economic Development Office in the UK (NEDO, 1991). The scene was thus set for the emergence of partnering in construction, which was to herald a move away from confrontation and a commitment to resolve problems jointly and informally through inter-firm collaboration (Bennett and Jayes, 1995; Barlow et al, 1997). A further major influence was the Latham (1994) report in the UK, which reinforced calls for improved working relationships and greater supply chain integration. The enrolment of key institutional players (such as the Institution of Civil Engineers and the Chartered Institute of Building) helped consolidate and institutionalise the trend towards collaboration (Bresnen and Marshall, 2010). This received a further boost with the publication of the Egan (1998) report, which drew upon lessons learned from the automotive sector in supply chain integration, just in time delivery and lean production.

Early definitions of partnering in construction emphasised the long-term strategic commitment envisaged between clients and builders (for example, Construction Industry Institute, 1991: iv). The intention was to ensure that each organisation achieved its own (business) objectives, while at the same time enabling the achievement of joint project objectives (Bennett and Jayes, 1995: 2). Also emphasised were the performance benefits, in terms of project time, cost and quality. Cost reduction was a key driver and performance indicator in many industry reports. However, scheduling improvements were also important, with earlier involvement in design by building contractors promoting value engineering and ensuring the constructability of engineering and architectural designs (Construction Industry Institute, 1991: 9). Important too were other key performance criteria, notably improved quality due to continuous improvement (of both building products and construction processes); improvements in health and safety; and greater customer focus and client satisfaction (Construction Industry Institute, 1991; NEDO, 1991; Loraine, 1993; Bennett and Jayes, 1995; Bennett et al, 1996). For contractors, greater continuity of work allowed better long-term planning and the more effective use of resources, in turn enabling more investment in training and research.

Early independent evidence of the effects of partnering highlighted its positive impact on measures of project success (for example, Barlow et al, 1997; Larson, 1997). However, these findings need to be tempered with the observation that partnering successes at that time were widely showcased and research was often anecdotal. Exemplars were used to illustrate the benefits of partnering (for example, Weston and Gibson, 1993) and, while there was not much published work highlighting failures, there were some early examples (for example, Angelo, 1998). Consequently, much of that early work was heavily prescriptive (for example, Bennett and Jayes, 1995; Bennett et al, 1996).

Nevertheless, over the past 20 years, partnering has become central to understanding ways of working in the construction industry, infusing both industry practice on the ground and wider discourse around the value of relational contracting within the sector. The claimed benefits of partnering are essentially the same as they were nearly 30 years ago: a reduction in lead and programme time, increase in innovation, sharing of risk, reward, resources and knowledge, and reduction in costs and disputes (Beach et al, 2005; Bygballe et al, 2010; Challender et al, 2017). Relational and cultural benefits are recognised too: open and clear communication, inclusivity and equality, organisational flexibility, the ability to learn and to solve problems, and increased commitment. Additional intangible benefits accrue from suppliers who, no longer pressured on price but motivated by further work prospects, are more open and honest about the limitations of products and more willing to add value to customers' businesses.

At the same time, examining experiences of partnering in the UK through interviews with key players within the industry, Challender et al (2017) note the failure of partnering to yield expected benefits in some instances and significant industry scepticism about the approach, with trust not necessarily translating into behaviour on the ground. They point out that key 'soft' human factors (motivation, team building, trust and respect) are still important influences on project success. Consequently, individual behaviour, rather than the choice of a partnering arrangement per se, is the important factor (Challender et al, 2017: 549). Sundquist et al (2018: 365) describe this as the 'actor bond' and a number of other studies make a similar point (Anvuur and Kumaraswamy, 2007; Hameed and Abbott, 2017; Evans et al, 2020).

While the principles of collaboration that partnering encapsulates have received widespread recognition and buy in across the sector, debates still continue therefore about how partnering functions within the construction industry (Anvuur and Kumaraswamy, 2007; Bygballe et al, 2010; Gottlieb and Haugbölle, 2013; Hosseini et al, 2016). In particular, attention has shifted more towards understanding practical manifestations of partnering and how it is embedded in particular project and organisational circumstances and contexts (Gottlieb and Haugbölle, 2013; Sundquist et al, 2018; Bygballe and Swärd, 2019). Partnering's emergent relational properties also makes a focus on situated behaviour and lived experiences just as fruitful, if not more so, than the search for an objective definition and success criteria (Bresnen, 2009; Bygballe et al, 2010).

Complexities and challenges of partnering

Despite the presumed and demonstrated benefits of partnering, there have remained a number of real tensions and dilemmas in the way in which it has reflected and shaped industry practice. These revolve around definitional issues, cultural change expectations, and scope of application (international, sector). Many of these tensions and dilemmas feed through into a consideration of the possibilities for public–private partnering and so are central to the concerns of this volume (and explored further in the next section). However, they also suggest partnering itself is a wicked problem, given the many paradoxes that emerge and that need to be resolved for it to work effectively (Alderman and Ivory, 2007; Bresnen, 2007).

First, there is the question of definition. Given the emphasis on long-term cooperation, partnering sits rather uneasily with shorter-term projects or programmes of work, which are more common in project-based industries such as construction. Early distinctions drawn between project-based alliances and longer-term (programme-based) partnering (for example, Loraine, 1993) merely highlighted, rather than resolved, this tension between the (expected) longer-term benefits of partnering and its mobilisation as a short-term collaborative solution. Indeed, debates continue about the feasibility of project-based partnering (Sundquist et al, 2018). Yet, for the most part, the approach to partnering within industry is still to apply it to single projects, at the possible expense of long-term benefits (Beach et al, 2005; Anvuur and Kumaraswamy, 2007; Bygballe et al, 2010; Hosseini et al, 2016; Challender et al, 2017; Sundquist et al, 2018).

Practitioners have often taken an understandably pragmatic view of the measures needed to develop a more collaborative approach (for example, Loraine, 1993; Sundquist et al, 2018). Such measures might include a risk/ reward contractual formula (so-called gainshare/painshare arrangements), the use of facilitators, partnering charters and workshops, team building exercises, performance management and improvement programmes and dispute resolution mechanisms (Bresnen and Marshall, 2000a, 2000b).

However, the selection of particular practices, tools and techniques is often dependent on client preferences and the needs of the organisation, its context, culture and existing supplier relationships (Beach et al, 2005; Gottlieb and Haugbölle, 2013). This not only thwarts attempts at developing a coherent and consistent approach that has universal applicability, it also creates problems in developing a clear definition or template against which partnering can be assessed. Partnering as originally envisaged reflected a set of values and principles around improved collaboration, rather than a carefully crafted programme of action with universally applicable tools and techniques. It is not surprising, therefore, that partnering takes many different forms, with the use of particular mechanisms varying enormously between projects and clients (Hosseini et al, 2016). The inevitable outcome is a somewhat piecemeal and selective approach to the choice of methods for building collaboration (Bresnen and Marshall, 2000b).

Another consequence is the tendency towards an instrumentalist view of how to develop partnering and an 'engineering' logic that pervades some approaches – perhaps reflecting wider orientations within the sector (Bresnen and Marshall, 2000a, 2010). Many commentators have stressed the importance of using the full range of tools and techniques available to actively build collaboration – including on short-term, one-off projects (for example, NEDO, 1991; Loraine, 1993; Bennett and Jayes, 1995). Yet, on such projects, there is not only the problem of moving swiftly through a learning curve to develop trust and collaboration, there is also the lack of incentive associated with follow on work opportunities (Anvuur and Kumaraswamy, 2007; Gottlieb and Haugbölle, 2013; Sundquist et al, 2018).

Early analysis suggested that this generated a tension between those who argued for a more informal, *developmental* approach to relational contracting and those who took a more formal, *instrumental* perspective (Bresnen and Marshall, 2000a, 2002). Indeed, over the last 25 years, the diffusion of partnering has continued to be associated with a duality in approach. While some emphasise the soft power of collaborative discourse, based upon concepts of cooperation and trust (Eriksson and Laan, 2007; Evans et al, 2020), others emphasise the search for practical tools, techniques, systems and metrics to engineer change (Graca and Camarinha-Matos, 2016; Habibi et al, 2019).

Second, and connected with these points, are questions around cultural change expectations. Partnering specifically, and the shift to relational contracting more generally, was intended to signify a move away from confrontation and 'adversarialism' towards greater collaboration and cooperation. Evidence over the last 20 years does suggest that the rhetoric of partnering at least is now a feature of industry discourse (Bygballe and Swärd, 2019). Nevertheless, the question remains of whether this shift in behaviours marks a deeper change in attitudes and values; or, instead, whether it reflects market conditions and a more superficial alignment with the principles and practices of an approach that, after all, helps contractors gain more work.

A further, related question about cultural change concerns the extent to which external advocacy of a collaborative approach mirrors and shapes each participants' own organisational cultural values and practices in ways that are internally consistent, as well as mutually reinforcing. Much of the work on partnering has focused, quite naturally, on relationships between clients and contractors; and, in some cases, between contractors and their subcontractors (Beach et al, 2005; Bygballe et al, 2010; Sundquist et al, 2018). Rather less attention, however, has been given to delving more deeply into the organisational correlates of relational contracting – that is, internal structural and cultural capabilities. Work in this area continues to emphasise the importance of internal leadership and championing of a collaborative approach and the need for cultural adaptation (Nifa and Ahmed, 2010). Moreover, considerable emphasis has also been placed on the importance of behavioural change at the individual and group level (Evans et al, 2020). However, we still know little about how these internal capabilities feed into cultural transformation at the *interstices* between organisations and, in turn, whether this signifies a more profound change of culture within the industry (Crespin-Mazet et al, 2015; Sundquist et al, 2018).

More generally, the question still remains of how well partnering manages to overcome some of the tensions and challenges associated with each party's attempts to reconcile their own and others' commercial and other interests (Bresnen, 2007). For clients (buyers), there is a paradox in the desire for greater collaboration based on a negotiated agreement, while forgoing the benefits of competition in procurement. For contractors (suppliers), there are potential gains in securing future work, but at the cost of taking on greater risk and potentially reduced margins – particularly in buyer's markets. Whether sharing risks and rewards based on performance improvement initiatives are sufficient to resolve these tensions and paradoxes is something that can only really be assessed with reference to the terms and conditions of exchange and each party's satisfaction with the resultant outcomes.

Third, there is the further question of the scope of application of partnering across both international contexts and (industrial) sectors. After a spike of initial interest in the US, UK and Australia, partnering quickly became more internationally widespread (for example, Chan et al, 2003, 2008; Eriksson and Laan, 2007; Hosseini et al, 2016; Evans et al, 2020). However, not only has that diffusion been somewhat concentrated in specific contexts (notably the Far East and Scandinavia), but the spread of interest and application has still not yet been matched with a full enough systematic investigation of the impact of international cultural and/or institutional differences (Phua, 2006). Consequently, relational contracting not only takes many forms internationally, it is also inevitably shaped by fundamentally different institutional norms and practices associated with differences in political institutions, legal frameworks, market conditions, social conditions and technological capabilities (cf Whitley, 1999).

With regard to sector, the principal question surrounding partnering has been its relevance and application to public sector infrastructure projects, as well as its positioning in debates related to PPP (Public–Private Partnering) and PFI (Public Finance Initiative). Given the importance of these issues to the current volume, these are turned to next.

The public–private dimension of partnering in construction

While it emerged principally from developments in the private sector, initial thinking around prospects for partnering was that it could apply equally to public sector projects (Loraine, 1993; Loraine and Williams, 1997). Indeed, a number of early contributors emphasised the value that partnering could bring to procurement across the public sector and examples were presented of early success stories (for example, Weston and Gibson, 1993). However, the importance of compulsory competitive tendering for projects, combined with the development of new forms of contract in the late 1990s in the UK that effectively proscribed non-competitive approaches to tendering (Pinch and Patterson, 2000) meant a much slower and more constrained uptake (Reeves et al, 2017).

However, over the 20 years, an easing of such restrictions in the UK, combined with the extension of public–private partnering through PFI and PPP have opened up the possibilities for public sector clients to pursue more collaborative contracting approaches (Corner, 2005; Carrillo et al, 2008).

PFI and PPP were driven by the UK government's objectives of achieving good Value for Money (VfM), benefiting from private sector expertise, and reducing government exposure to risk through partnering with the private sector (Corner, 2005; Li et al, 2005; Nisar, 2007; Henjewele et al, 2011). Typically, in a PFI contract, the agent will bear the risk of any increased costs but be incentivised by including allowance for risk in pricing the contract (Nisar, 2007; Carrillo et al, 2008). Risk is also contracted in for the whole life of the project, leading to an increase in construction standards (and cost) in the initial build phase, but longer-term financial benefits due to a reduction in maintenance costs (Nisar, 2007). Therefore, PPP enables a long-standing relationship where risk allocation drives quality construction, which, over time, sees cost benefits to both parties (Corner, 2005; Nisar, 2007).

However, this cost driven approach to what is, essentially, a collaborative partnership, soon came into question as cost savings were not universally realised. Bidding costs were also higher than under traditional procurement routes, with projects often delayed due to increased lead times as a result of complex negotiations (Li et al, 2005; Nisar, 2007; Carrillo et al, 2008).

Consequently, the strong emphasis on cost as the driving factor, combined with a penalty/reward regimen that stressed penalties meant that the emphasis on relational factors in the 'partnership' was low (Smyth and Edkins, 2007). Moreover, research also suggests that inconsistent VfM returns and increased times delays were contributed to by changes in client requirements as projects progressed (Henjewele et al, 2011). This may all reflect the poor relationship management reported within PFI and PPP projects in the UK, where there has been more emphasis on contractual compliance and rather less emphasis on the development of trust and other relational attributes between private and public partners (Smyth and Edkins, 2007).

Consequently, partnering and collaboration in the context of public sector infrastructure projects has seen a disconnect between the rhetoric of partnerships as reflected in PPP and the reality of arrangements driven more by financial and accounting imperatives and reflecting more traditional, adversarial modes of contracting. At the same time, the drive to improve collaboration in public sector infrastructure projects still has momentum. Most recently, thinking in the construction and engineering industries has crystallised around 'Project 13', an initiative designed to spread the tenets of collaboration further among major clients, including those in the public sector (Institute of Civil Engineers, 2017, 2018). The development of stronger relational bonds between clients and contractors on major projects is expected ultimately to lead to more integrated working across supply chains (Browne, 2018).

Nevertheless, while such collaboration is increasingly commonplace, public sector organisations have less experience to draw upon in pursuing a collaborative approach and face particular challenges and constraints associated with their public sector status. Moreover, considerable adverse publicity over the last decade concerning PPP and PFI, culminating in the recent Carillion collapse, has inevitably created greater caution in approach (Hajikazemi et al, 2020). Indeed, the UK government has since discontinued PFI, and its successor PF2, for future infrastructure projects. Wider research in the public management field also continues to question the precepts of public–private partnering at the level of public policy, as well as in the context of major public sector infrastructure projects (Sherratt et al, 2020). Nevertheless, while a recent National Audit Office report on learning from major programmes scarcely mentions their relational character (NAO, 2020), the UK government's recently announced national infrastructure strategy promises 'to move away from a confrontational approach, towards stronger relationship and contract management which will deliver continuous improvement over time' (HM Treasury, 2020: 86).

Notwithstanding this wider public policy debate and the ambivalence surrounding public–private partnerships it reveals, research into the micro-processes of public–private partnering still remains scarce and we know comparatively little about manifestations of partnering in public sector projects. This is particularly the case when we direct attention away from large-scale infrastructure projects and towards smaller scale, more local initiatives. Consequently, there is an important gap to be filled in understanding the correlates of relational contracting in this context, bearing in mind what we know more widely about how partnering works in the private domain. Filling this gap in understanding is important, since it provides not only further insights into collaboration in such relatively underexplored organisational and institutional conditions, but also helps inform that wider public policy and management debate. This is particularly important in a context in which public services globally are becoming more 'corporatised' and expected to operate in more commercial or 'business like' ways (Andrews et al, 2020). Consequently, there is considerable value in efforts to blend or bridge what we know about private sector management practice with the institutional imperatives associated with delivering public sector projects.

Implications for public–private partnership, wicked problems and health issues

A useful starting point for considering relational contracting in the context of public–private partnerships is to draw together a model that can act as a framework for understanding the lessons learned from partnering in the construction industry. That will also highlight some of the key tensions and dilemmas that mark out achieving successful partnering not only as the resolution of a wicked problem in itself, but also something of a social accomplishment, given the latent (market) factors that continue to encourage non-collaborative behaviour.

The framework presented in Figure 19.1 is an attempt to capture some of the key parameters shaping elements of the discussion so far.

The model is centred around the progression of a partnering relationship from early stage collaboration, through tendering and contracting processes, to project delivery and outcomes. It is important to highlight the importance of the wider institutional and socioeconomic context in helping shape collaborative antecedent conditions (for example, legal context, competitive conditions, cultural factors, organisational capabilities) and the contracting and collaborative mechanisms available and used. However, the model also drills down to emphasise not only the structural and cultural conditions shaping the formation of partnering relationships on the ground, but also the factors driving and mediating the relationship (contracting and collaborative mechanisms) and the range of potential outcomes (including continuity in the relationship).

As with private sector partnering, there are three principal points of tension for partnering between public and private organisations. First, the

Figure 19.1: Summary model of public–private commissioning and contracting

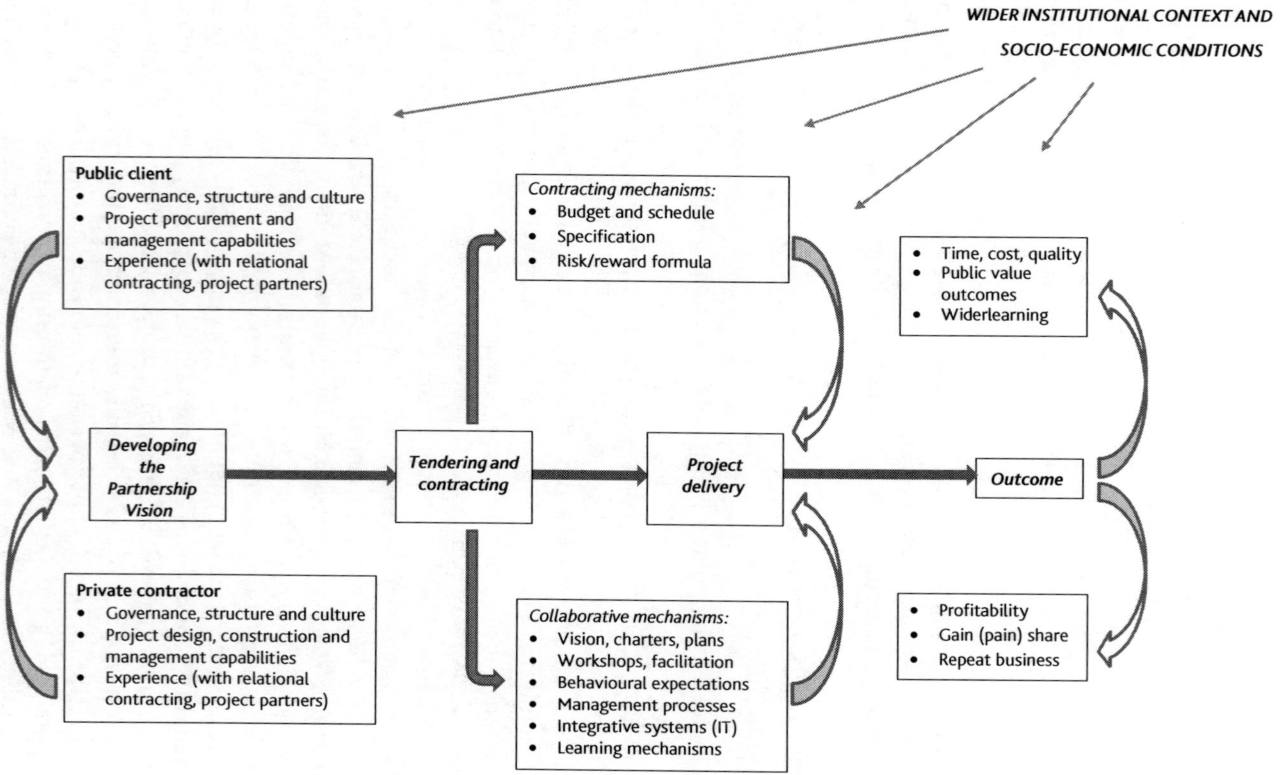

WIDER INSTITUTIONAL CONTEXT AND SOCIO-ECONOMIC CONDITIONS

Public client
- Governance, structure and culture
- Project procurement and management capabilities
- Experience (with relational contracting, project partners)

Developing the Partnership Vision

Tendering and contracting

Contracting mechanisms:
- Budget and schedule
- Specification
- Risk/reward formula

Project delivery

- Time, cost, quality
- Public value outcomes
- Wider learning

Outcome

- Profitability
- Gain (pain) share
- Repeat business

Private contractor
- Governance, structure and culture
- Project design, construction and management capabilities
- Experience (with relational contracting, project partners)

Collaborative mechanisms:
- Vision, charters, plans
- Workshops, facilitation
- Behavioural expectations
- Management processes
- Integrative systems (IT)
- Learning mechanisms

cultural predispositions and compatibilities shaping behaviour on the ground (which are likely to be shaped significantly by private and public sector differences that may hinder cultural alignment). Second, the commercial relationship that underpins the terms and conditions of exchange and its relationship with other wider outcomes (which will be shaped particularly by the importance to the relationship of achieving VfM in public services delivery). Third, the mediation of collaboration through non-contractual mechanisms and behavioural change (which is where, on the other hand, one might observe significant differences in the experiences and capabilities of organisations and individuals to achieve effective relational contracting).

The other significant points to emphasise from this modelling are, first, the importance of seeing relational approaches to contracting as a multilevelled phenomenon – shaped by institutional level forces (for example, policy and legal context), but also significantly impacted by relational conditions at the meso-(project) level, by capabilities at the organisational level and by behaviours at the individual and team levels. Second, relational contracting also has a dynamic quality to it, where the attributes and effects of collaboration not only produce cycles of positive or negative reinforcement, but also are directly conditioned through the ongoing evaluation of past actions and assessment of future finite possibilities (Crespin-Mazet et al, 2015).

Conclusion

This chapter has focused on the lessons learned from experiences of relational contracting in the construction sector. It has charted the development of partnering over the last 30 years, particularly in the private sector and drawn out from that a number of pointers for continuing research on public–private collaboration. The chapter has presented achieving collaboration through partnering as something of a wicked problem, insofar as it presents a number of challenges, tensions and dilemmas that are far from resolved within the construction industry context – despite a plethora of interest and the widespread diffusion of partnering practice. In particular, it has emphasised not only the challenges of recognising, reconciling and managing these tensions and dilemmas (Bresnen, 2007), but also the importance of conceptualising forms of collaboration such as partnering as a complex, multilayered and dynamic construct.

As such, relational contracting in practice defies easy definition, is situated in practice and shaped by context, and is characterised as much by its emergent properties as by its conscious design. Moreover, confrontational relationships, competing interests and adversarial cultures are still being referred to in industry discourse and policy debates, showing their persistence decades after partnering first appeared. This suggests that partnering, in all its variety, is not a one-off relational shift, but something that has to be continually recreated and renewed, both to be sustained in existing inter-organisational contexts and as it spreads into new ones. The project of developing more effective public–private partnerships for the achievement of public service provision that generate social value, can therefore only benefit from the lessons learned from such experiences.

References

Alderman, N. and Ivory, C. (2007) Partnering in major contracts: Paradox and metaphor. *International Journal of Project Management*, 25: 386–393.

Andrews, R., Ferry, L., Skelcher, C. and Wegorowski, P. (2020) Corporatization in the public sector: Explaining the growth of local government companies. *Public Administration Review*, 80(3): 482–493.

Angelo, W.J. (1998) Partnering goes awry on Connecticut bridge job. *ENR*, 240(18): 17.

Anvuur, A. and Kumaraswamy, M. (2007) Conceptual model of partnering and alliancing. *Journal of Construction Management and Engineering*, 133(3): 225–234.

Barlow, J., Cohen, M., Jashapara, A. and Simpson, Y. (1997) *Towards Positive Partnering*. Bristol: Policy Press.

Beach, R., Webster, M. and Campbell, K.M. (2005) An evaluation of partnership development in the construction industry. *International Journal of Project Management*, 23(8): 611–621.

Bennett, J. and Jayes, S. (1995) *Trusting the Team: The Best Practice Guide to Partnering in Construction*. Reading: Centre for Strategic Studies in Construction/Reading Construction Forum.

Bennett, J., Ingram, I. and Jayes, S. (1996) *Partnering for Construction*. Reading: Centre for Strategic Studies in Construction.

Bresnen, M. (2007) Deconstructing partnering in project-based organisation: Seven pillars, seven paradoxes and seven deadly sins. *International Journal of Project Management*, 25(4): 365–374.

Bresnen, M. (2009) Living the dream? Understanding partnering as emergent practice. *Construction Management and Economics*, 27(10): 923–933.

Bresnen, M. and Marshall, N. (2000a) Partnering in construction: A critical review of issues, problems and dilemmas. *Construction Management and Economics*, 18(2): 229–237.

Bresnen, M. and Marshall, N. (2000b) Building partnerships: Case studies of client-contractor collaboration in the UK construction industry. *Construction Management and Economics*, 18(7): 819–832.

Bresnen, M. and Marshall, N. (2002) The engineering or evolution of co-operation? A tale of two partnering projects. *International Journal of Project Management*, 20(7): 497–505.

Bresnen, M. and Marshall, N. (2010) Projects and partnerships: Institutional processes and emergent practices. In P. Morris, J. Pinto and J. Söderlund (eds) *OUP Handbook of Project Management*, Oxford: Oxford University Press, pp 154–174.

Browne, D. (2018) Project 13 blueprint to end stranglehold of short termist construction. *Highways Magazine*, 4 May. Available at: https://www.highwaysmagazine.co.uk/Project-13-blueprint-to-end-stranglehold-of-short-termist-construction/4068 (accessed 25 November 2020).

Bygballe, L.E. and Swärd, A. (2019) Collaborative project delivery models and the role of routines in institutionalizing partnering. *Project Management Journal*, 50(2): 161–176.

Bygballe, L.E., Jahre, M. and Swärd, A. (2010) Partnering relationships in construction: A literature review. *Journal of Purchasing and Supply Management*, 16: 239–253.

Carrillo, P., Robinson, H., Foale, P., Anumba, C. and Bouchlaghem, D. (2008) Participation, barriers, and opportunities in PFI: The United Kingdom experience. *Journal of Management in Engineering*, 24(3): 138–145.

Challender, J., France, C. and Baban, H. (2017) So why is UK construction partnering not working the way it was intended? Proceedings, International Research Conference 2017: Shaping tomorrow's built environment, University of Salford, 11–12 September, pp 544–551.

Chan, A.P.C., Chan, D.W.M. and Ho, K.S.K. (2003) An empirical study of the benefits of construction partnering in Hong Kong. *Construction Management and Economics*, 21(5): 523–533.

Chan, A.P.C., Chan, D.W., Fan, L.C., Lam, P.T. and Yeung, J.F. (2008) Achieving partnering success through an incentive agreement: Lessons learned from an underground railway extension project in Hong Kong. *Journal of Management in Engineering*, 24(3): 128–137.

Construction Industry Institute (1991) *In Search of Partnering Excellence. CII Special Publication*. Austin: University of Texas.

Corner, D. (2005) The United Kingdom private finance initiative: The challenge of allocating risk. In G. Hodge and C. Greve (eds.) (2005) *The Challenge of Public–Private Partnerships: Learning from International Experience*, Cheltenham: Edward Elgar Publishing, pp 44–61.

Crespin-Mazet, F., Havenvid, M.I. and Linné, Å. (2015) Antecedents of project partnering in the construction industry: The impact of relationship history. *Industrial Marketing Management*, 50: 4–15.

Egan, J. (1998) *Rethinking Construction*. London: Department of the Environment, Transport and the Regions.

Eriksson, P.-E. and Laan, A. (2007) Procurement effects on trust and control in client-contractor relationships. *Engineering, Construction and Architectural Management*, 14(4): 387–389.

Evans, M., Farrell, P., Elbeltagi, E., Mashali, A. and Elhendawi, A. (2020) Influence of partnering agreements associated with BIM adoption on stakeholder's behaviour in construction mega-projects. *International Journal of BIM and Engineering Science*, 3(1): 1–17.

Gottlieb, S. and Haugbölle, K. (2013) Contradictions and collaboration: Partnering in-between systems of production, values and interests. *Construction Management and Economics*, 31(2): 119–134.

Graca, P. and Camarinha-Matos, L.M. (2016) Performance indicators for collaborative business ecosystems: Literature review and trends. *Technological Forecasting and Social Change*, 116: 237–255.

Habibi, M., Kermanshachi, S. and Rouhanizadeh, B. (2019) Identifying and measuring engineering, procurement, and construction (EPC) key performance indicators and management strategies. *Infrastructures*, 4(14).

Hajikazemi, S., Aaltonen, K., Ahola, T., Aarseth, W. and Andersen, B. (2020) Normalising deviance in construction project organizations: A case study on the collapse of Carillion. *Construction Management and Economics*, 38(12): 1122–1138.

Hameed, W. and Abbott, C. (2017) Critical review of the success factors of strategic alliances in the UK. *Construction Innovation*, 4: 53–65.

Henjewele, C., Sun, M. and Fewings, P. (2011) Critical parameters influencing value for money variations in PFI projects in the healthcare and transport sectors. *Construction Management and Economics*, 29(8): 825–839.

Higgin, J. and Jessop, N. (1965) *Communications in the Building Industry*. London: Tavistock.

HM Treasury (2020) *National Infrastructure Strategy: Fairer, Faster, Greener*. London: HM Treasury.

Hosseini, A., Wondimu, P.A., Bellini, A., Tune, H., Haugseth, N., Andersen, B. and Laedre, O. (2016) Project partnering in Norwegian construction industry. *Energy Procedia*, 96: 241–252.

Institute of Civil Engineers (2017) *From Transactions to Enterprises: A New Approach to Delivering High Performing Infrastructure*. London: Institution of Civil Engineers.

Institute of Civil Engineers (2018) Project 13. Available at: https://www.p13.org.uk/library/ (accessed 25 November 2020).

Larson, E. (1997) Partnering on construction projects: A study of the relationship between partnering activities and project success. *IEEE Transactions on Engineering Management*, 44(2): 188–195.

Latham, M. (1994) *Constructing the Team*. London: HMSO.

Li, B., Akintoye, A., Edwards, P.J. and Hardcastle, C. (2005) Critical success factors for PPP/PFI projects in the UK construction industry. *Construction Management and Economics*, 23(5): 459–471.

Loraine, R.K. (1993) *Partnering in the Public Sector*. London: Business Round Table.

Loraine, R.K. and Williams, I. (1997) *Partnering in the Public Sector.* Loughborough: European Construction Institute.

NAO (2020) *Lessons Learned from Major Programmes.* London: National Audit Office.

NEDO (1991) *Partnering: Contracting without Conflict.* London: HMSO.

Nifa, F.A.A. and Ahmed, V. (2010) The role of organizational culture in construction partnering to produce innovation. Proceedings of 26th Annual ARCOM Conference, 6–8 September, 725–734.

Nisar, T.M. (2007) Value for money drivers in public private partnership schemes. *International Journal of Public Sector Management*, 20(2): 147–156.

Phua, F.T.T. (2006) When is construction partnering likely to happen? An empirical examination of the role of institutional norms. *Construction Management and Economics*, 24(6): 615–624.

Pinch, P.L. and Patterson, A. (2000) Public sector restructuring and regional development: The impact of compulsory competitive tendering in the UK. *Regional Studies*, 34(3): 265–275.

Reeves, E., Palcic, D., Flannery, D. and Geddes, R.R. (2017) The determinants of tendering periods for PPP procurement in the UK: An empirical analysis. *Applied Economics*, 49(11): 1071–1082.

Sherratt, F., Sherratt, S. and Ivory, C. (2020) Challenging complacency in construction management research: The case of PPPs. *Construction Management and Economics*, 38(12): 1086–1100.

Smyth, H. and Edkins, A. (2007) Relationship management in the management of PFI/PP projects in the UK. *International Journal of Project Management*, 25(3): 232–240.

Sundquist, V., Hulthen, K. and Gadde, L.E. (2018) From project partnering towards strategic supplier partnering. *Engineering, Construction and Architectural Management*, 25(3): 358–373.

Weston, D. and Gibson, G. (1993) Partnering project performance in US Army Corps of Engineers. *Journal of Management in Construction*, 9(4): 331–344.

Whitley, R. (1999) *Divergent Capitalisms: The Social Structuring and Change of Business Systems.* Oxford: Oxford University Press.

20

The impact of 'the lost decade' on developing a relational culture in public–private partnering

Michael Burton

Introduction

The years 2010–2020 that economists often dub 'the lost decade' has been among the most volatile in modern British history. They included the Great Recession at the beginning, austerity economics and the convulsions of Brexit in mid-term and COVID-19 at the end. Each of these events were seismic on their own and yet were interwoven, creating a convulsion in the body politic unparalleled in postwar Britain. The resulting shift in public policy was to envisage a more interventionist role for the state and the need for a less confrontational, more **relational culture** between private and public providers, together harnessed to delivering social value for communities dislocated by recession, austerity and the pandemic.

The widening inequalities gap

The thread that ran through these years and which set the political priorities for the following decade was Britain's widening socioeconomic inequality. The recession and its devastating impact on the public finances led to austerity and a stagnation in living standards for the lower paid, generating a resentment that found its expression in the vote for Brexit in the 2016 EU referendum. The pandemic then laid bare the socioeconomic inequalities that had been exacerbated by the recession and the negative impact of austerity on public services which the government from 2017 onwards felt compelled to address. One consequence was the reorientation of traditional political allegiances with an ostensibly right-wing Conservative government, elected in 2019 through the support of working-class pro-Brexit voters in England's industrial North and Midlands, henceforth committed to removing regional economic inequalities and addressing social **wicked issues** through state intervention and public spending supported by private sector investment.

While therefore austerity through spending cuts in the first half of the decade signalled a downgrading of the state's role, Brexit and the pandemic signalled the opposite through an unprecedented rise both in public spending and in the high profile role of key state services like the National Health Service (NHS) and local government in tackling COVID-19. The new political landscape marked a step change away from the traditional left–right divide as well as heralding a more pragmatic era in the relationship between public and private providers. This was accelerated by the pandemic, with private hospitals drafted in to help the NHS, local government involved in test and trace, and private providers called on to deliver vital protective equipment for the public sector. The highly successful vaccination programme, a collaboration between state funding and private scientific expertise, was described by the World Economic Forum as driven by a 'public-private alliance' and was 'a moment of great pride, and one made possible only by an unprecedented degree of collaboration between the public and private sectors' (Seriot et al, 2021).

By 2021 therefore, as Britain was emerging gradually from the pandemic, the stage was set for a more interventionist role for the state backed by private investment, a more pragmatic relationship between public and private partners operating under a less onerous procurement regime and a relentless focus on reducing the nation's regional inequalities. This strategy had to be carried out at the same time as the government embarked on its long programme of reducing the huge deficit in the public finances caused by tackling the pandemic. If austerity was out of favour, efficiency was not. The government's planned reforms to the procurement regime summed up how it saw the state's huge buying power reorientated to achieving these socioeconomic goals while also harnessing private sector efficiencies. The December 2020 Green Paper on transforming public procurement stated that:

> The huge power of some £290 billion of public money spent through public procurement every year in the UK must support Government priorities: to boost growth and productivity, help our communities recover from the COVID-19 pandemic, and tackle climate change.
> … Linking the elements of social value through into procurement is critical to ensuring the social, economic and environmental benefits are delivered through the contract. (HMG, 2020)

Procurement was no longer a case of just finding the cheapest price to deliver a contract: it was about the client and contractor together efficiently delivering social outcomes with bureaucratic obstacles removed. But as the Green Paper recognised, 'there will need to be a shift in the behaviour of commercial teams'. The new procurement regime implied a change of attitude between public and private to a more relational, rather than purely contractual, culture.

The background to 'the lost decade'

The events that were to lead to a more corporatist role for the state and a more relational public–private partnering culture focused on delivering social value had their origins in the previous decade. Fifteen years without a recession convinced politicians in Britain by the mid-2000s that the era of 'boom and bust' was over and the public to believe that rising living standards would eventually eradicate poverty and solve ingrained socioeconomic challenges putting an end to the wicked issues that had challenged public policy for many decades. In 2008 that assumption was shattered by the fiscal crash and the consequent wider Great Recession which shredded the public finances. By 2010 the deficit, the amount the government had to borrow just to cover its outgoings was an unsustainable 10 per cent of Gross Domestic Product (GDP) (Burton, 2016). How politicians addressed this budget hole through spending cuts, what the long-term negative impact of what became known by economists as the Great Recession had on the standard of living of lower income groups, why the political expression of this discontent found its outlet through the EU referendum in 2016 plus the general election of 2019 and in what manner politicians responded, is the theme of this chapter. It covers a turbulent ten years in British politics dubbed 'the lost decade' by economists because of the stagnation in household incomes (Pope, 2018). These years were bookended by the recession and the pandemic; the common thread throughout was the recognition of the social determinants of health, that those households adversely hit by the recession were the same ones worst affected by COVID-19 (Burton, 2022).

Technically the Great Recession in the UK ended around 2011 when the economy began to recover but having shrunk by more than 6 per cent between the first quarter of 2008 and the second quarter of 2009, the UK economy then took five years to get back to the size it was before the recession. So-called fiscal consolidation, or austerity as it was termed, being the government response to the deficit in the public finances, added further deflation to an already weakened economy. In particular austerity was partly blamed for delaying recovery from the recession and for persuading its victims to vote for the populist far right and Brexit. It led to Conservative politicians from 2016 firstly rejecting the austerity they had hitherto supported, then to turn it on its head and develop 'Red Toryism' with big spending pledges for those same parts of the country which had been worst hit by spending cuts. COVID-19 then only further emphasised the division between the 'haves' and the 'have nots'.

The Great Recession runs through the UK's political and socioeconomic history of the last decade. We will never entirely know its devastating impact on household, let alone the public, finances. The Institute for Fiscal Studies later estimated in 2018 that the economy was £300 billion smaller than it would have been had there been no recession and GDP growth had continued its pre-2008 trajectory. It put the cost per person as £5,900. The extra income from tax revenues would have funded the NHS and social care budgets and made austerity irrelevant (Cribb and Johnson, 2018).

Data from the Office for National Statistics for 2018/2019 showed that real mean disposable income was no higher in 2018/2019 than in 2007/2008 while for the typical household it was just 6 per cent higher. The income of the poorest fifth of the population was no higher in 2018/2019 than in 2004/2005. As the think tank the Resolution Foundation commented:

> Real income growth of 6% over a 14 year-period is an unprecedently poor economic performance for working-age households. If we look at 10-year growth rates over time, the 5% growth of the last decade for the non-retired population compares to an average of around 30% pre-crisis. That is a lot of lost growth. (IFS, 2010)

The recession's negative impact on poorer areas of the UK reinvigorated the debate about how the public and private sectors could together address the shortfall in resources and tackle long-term wicked issues, especially following COVID-19, and so reduce socioeconomic inequalities. In rejecting austerity as a solution to eliminating the deficit caused by the pandemic the Boris Johnson administration from 2019 set out to use the private sector to deliver social value as part of a renewed focus on infrastructure spending targeted at those areas most affected by previous austerity cuts.

The rise and decline of austerity

The Conservatives had hoped to win the general election outright in 2010 but without winning an overall majority were instead forced to join with the Liberal Democrats to create the first coalition government since 1945. Both parties were nonetheless committed to reducing the deficit and total borrowing. Labour's original plans had envisaged a mix of 70 per cent cuts to 30 per cent tax rises. In 2010 the balance now looked more like 74 per cent to 26 per cent, which was more than the Conservative government targets after the previous 1990s recession which aimed for a 50 per cent to 50 per cent mix between cuts and tax rises (IFS, 2010). Inevitably the 2010 spending cuts fell mainly on those in receipt of welfare like housing benefit and other state aid. The housing benefit bill paid to low income tenants had soared over the previous decade but this was largely due to a dearth of social housing exacerbated by the sale of council-run housing and the lack of a replacement.

There were big cuts in local government, especially in specific grants which had been created to target poorer areas on top of general local government funding. The cuts in specific grants especially hit struggling former industrial metropolitan areas in the North, North West and the Midlands. In areas of high welfare dependency cuts in benefits did not only hit individual households but also took millions of pounds out of the local economy as invariably welfare grants were spent in local shops. These areas were then doubly hit by the withdrawal of private sector funding for regeneration and housing projects as the recession made such schemes no longer viable.

The NHS was spared actual cuts in its budget but as health inflation averaged 4 per cent a year and its increase in spending around 1 per cent, in practice this meant year-on-year reductions, ending the years of above inflation budget rises awarded by the Labour government. One notable, but often ignored, reform was the transfer of public health responsibilities from the NHS to local government in 2013. Ministers recognised that health was determined by social and environmental factors like housing, employment, pollution, diet and exercise and that the focus should be on prevention not just medical treatment. In effect the transfer was a return to local government's original remit to improve health by improving environmental conditions. Unfortunately once transferred to cash-strapped local government and out of the relatively protected NHS public health funding was then cut by the government.

The government's austerity plans were predicated on the economy improving and, as GDP increased, the deficit declining and eventually the private sector returning to normal activity, a virtuous circle. The classic economic model proposed by the famous economist Keynes was that public spending should replace private spending during recessions and then be rebalanced as the private sector recovered. Critics of austerity argued that the Coalition government had misjudged the timing, that it had brought in spending cuts too early believing the economy was on the mend when the modest growth in 2010/2011 was actually down to public sector infrastructure spending in the last year of the Labour government. The critics therefore argued that austerity helped the recession to last much longer than it needed to. Defenders of austerity pointed out that the plans were completely overturned by the crisis in the eurozone and low growth in the European Union, the UK's biggest export partner, and rises in oil prices and other commodities that increased inflation and reduced consumer spending. Real household disposable income fell by 2.3 per cent in 2011, a postwar record, while growth forecasts were reduced. Less tax revenues meant higher borrowing and higher public spending and in turn austerity being continued further into the future.

Despite ambitious plans laid out in 2010 the Coalition government's key fiscal targets were missed. Its Emergency Budget in June 2010 had predicted the deficit would be 1.1 per cent of GDP by 2014/2015 thanks to its austerity programme. In fact it was still at 4.9 per cent that year. The Budget also forecast total spending would be down to 67.4 per cent of GDP in 2015/2016. The actual figure was 80 per cent. Yet despite the impact of austerity on the poor the Conservatives managed to win their first overall majority in the 2015 general election since 1992, forming their own government for the first time since 1997 thanks to the collapse of the Liberal Democrats and a weak Labour opposition. Soon afterwards the Conservative government abandoned some of its more ruthless planned spending cuts. Austerity was not quite dead and buried but it was certainly no longer the flavour of the times though it would be three years before a future Prime Minister officially read the last rites (Anon, 2018).

As the Institute for Fiscal Studies later said in September 2018 in its commentary on recovering from the financial crisis:

> We should never stop reminding ourselves just what an astonishing decade we have just lived through, and continue to live through. The UK economy has broken record after record, and not generally in a good way: record low earnings growth, record low interest rates, record low productivity growth, record public borrowing followed by record cuts in public spending. (IFS, 2018: ix)

The Great Recession was unlike its predecessors for two prime reasons. One was that employment remained relatively robust, mystifying economists who assumed that in a recession jobs are cut. The second reason was that the Great Recession had a long tail: wages remained stagnant or low paid, below pre-2008 levels in real terms. Economists began to refer to these years as the lost decade because many of the lower paid were worse off than ten years previously. These two issues, robust employment levels but low wages, were of course connected. Productivity growth was 0.3 per cent a year after 2008 whereas during the previous decade it had been 2.3 per cent annually. There were jobs but they were low paid, unskilled or semi-skilled. Employers found it easier to hire poorly paid labour than invest in training or technology. In some cases they found it even easier to hire cheap but comparatively well-educated European immigrants rather than take on the costs of training local labour.

Britain's economy in 2015 appeared to be on the mend but underneath remained persistent inequalities that fuelled populist resentment against the so-called 'elite' of big business, politics, the media and the City. Actually the UK's big regional capitals were a success story. The problem was not with Manchester, Leeds or Newcastle, which had successfully reinvented themselves as cities competing on a global stage, but with the smaller towns and cities. Spending cuts had fallen disproportionately on the former industrial areas of the North and the Midlands and in pockets of deprivation in the South such as ailing seaside resorts or rural counties. The long-standing regional divide was exacerbated by the recession with low-paid jobs in retail, call centres and logistics replacing well-paid manufacturing work. The geographic divide was reflected in an income divide between the very wealthy and the rest with low- to middle-income households experiencing weak growth in pay in the decade after the fiscal crash. A substantial number of households were on the breadline or just about managing with little prospect of improving their lot because without training the only jobs on offer were low paid. The Resolution Foundation, a think tank studying low pay, produced the first of its audits on 'low to middle earners' in 2009 and found they were too poor to benefit from the opportunities provided by the private sector but not so poor that they qualified for welfare.

These income and regional differences were often blamed on globalism, which created winners and losers. The former were skilled, educated workers based in the booming financial centre of London or the science powerhouses of Cambridge and Oxford. The losers were those workers, mainly in manufacturing, who saw their livelihoods decimated by competition from cheap labour overseas. Multinationals had no local roots; they went to the areas of the world where labour was cheapest so they could in turn sell their goods cheaply.

Power had moved away from labour to capital. Low interest rates benefited those who owed assets. The global rich flocked to London to buy up investment properties while young people struggled to buy their first home at inflated prices and rents soared. The bankers were back with their bonuses even as the poor struggled with stagnant wages. There was a dearth of social housing because councils could no longer build homes as they had done in previous decades, meaning the housing benefit bill, paid by the taxpayer to landlords, rocketed. As in so many aspects of public spending, cuts in one area turned up as new costs in another.

The EU referendum, the 'left behind' and 'levelling up'

A rash pledge by Prime Minister David Cameron to hold an in-out referendum on remaining in the EU in June 2016 became a lightning-rod for discontent. Those who felt financially unstable, resentful of globalism, disgusted at the excesses of the very rich, convinced there was an establishment doing very well at their expense, used the vote to make their views known by voting to leave the EU even though their grievances had very little to do with EU membership. There were plenty of people without any of these concerns who still voted to leave but the political, financial and media establishment, shocked at the 52–48 majority to leave, focused on the former industrial areas of the Midlands and the North and deprived areas in other parts of the UK where the leave vote had been highest. As it happened most of these areas were Labour strongholds.

The new Prime Minister, Theresa May, who was elected by her party after Cameron's resignation in June 2016, recognised the link between the vote to leave the EU and deprivation. Austerity, in name at least, vanished from the government's lexicon. She began to refer to 'the left behind' and the 'just about managing', an appeal to those who were not welfare dependents but most likely in work on low wages and who, as it happened, had also been hard hit by the recession and by cuts in local government services. Her language initially was even quite anti-big business, picking up the populist revolt against the global elite and multinationals. The collapse of contractor Carillion in 2018 gave further impetus to public disillusionment at the idea that the private sector was the only answer to providing public services. Eventually, as she was sucked into Brexit negotiations, May's spotlight on reducing inequality and helping the just about managing dimmed to the point of extinction.

It was therefore left to her successor Boris Johnson to rediscover their party's commitment to helping the 'left behind' households. There were sound political reasons for doing so: most of the ex-industrial areas adversely affected by the recession and the years of stagnant incomes were traditional Labour voting areas and dubbed the 'Red Wall'. With Labour in disarray over Brexit the pro-Brexit 'Red Wall' was ripe for conversion to the new 'blue collar Toryism' with its call to 'get Brexit done' and in the December 2019 general election duly handed Johnson an 80-seat majority in the House of Commons, cementing him into power for five years. In the North East, North West, Yorkshire and Humberside and Wales and the Midlands the Conservatives gained 50 seats from Labour.

Austerity was now well and truly banished. The mantra by the new government was 'levelling up' to the more prosperous regions of the UK those areas in the North, Midlands, parts of Wales, and pockets in the otherwise economically dynamic South which had previously been dubbed 'the left behind'. Whatever their name these households had been worst hit by the long tail of the recession, were trapped in low-paid jobs with lack of opportunities, had worse health outcomes and were most affected by the wicked issues. Furthermore, there was now a political imperative since the new Conservative MPs in the former 'Red Wall' areas had their eyes on the next election.

However 'levelling up', which in reality had been a soundbite to win the 2019 general election, proved difficult to define as a government policy, let alone deliver. The pandemic laid bare health inequalities which were founded on long-standing socioeconomic inequalities, the wicked issues that had for decades been a challenge for policymakers and governments and were not going to be solved with a soundbite. A government decision in November 2021 to abandon part of the hugely expensive HS2 high speed rail link to Leeds drew accusations from MPs, including Tory MPs representing former 'Red Wall' seats, that ministers' commitment to levelling up was superficial. Concerned that the centrepiece of his strategy was unravelling, Prime Minister Boris Johnson in September 2021 appointed the experienced politician Michael Gove to take charge, making him Secretary of State for Levelling Up, Housing and Communities.

Conclusion

The pandemic marked the end of 'the lost decade' as well as a new era in the role of the state which acquired huge powers, both authoritarian in imposing lockdowns, and interventionist in its purchasing of medical supplies and vaccines. In rejecting austerity as a solution to eliminating the deficit caused by COVID-19 the Boris Johnson administration set out to stimulate public–private partnerships to deliver social value as part of a renewed focus on infrastructure spending targeted at those areas most affected by previous austerity cuts. The challenge for both public and private partners was how to adapt to the more flexible culture implied by the new priorities.

The 2020 Green Paper on the procurement regime stated that its 'proposals provide significantly more flexibility; with this will come greater discretion for contracting authorities on how they conduct procurements as the rules will not be as prescriptive' (HMG, 2020). It was a green light for a more relational culture between public and private, focused not just on profits or contracts but on delivering social value outcomes.

References

Anon (2018) Theresa May's speech to the 2018 Conservative Party Conference. *PoliticsHome*, 3 October. Available at: https://www.politicsh ome.com/news/article/read-in-full-theresa-mays-speech-to-the-2018-conservative-party-conference (accessed 24 August 2021).

Burton, M. (2016) *The Politics of Austerity: A Recent History*. London: Palgrave Macmillan.

Burton, M. (2022) *From Broke to Brexit: Britain's Lost Decade*. London: Palgrave Macmillan.

Cribb, J. and Johnson, P. (2018) *10 Years On: Have We Recovered from the Financial Crisis?* Institute for Fiscal Studies, September. Available at: https://ifs.org.uk/publications/13302 (accessed 24 August 2021).

HMG (2020) *Green Paper: Transforming Public Procurement*. Cabinet Office. Available at: https://www.gov.uk/government/consultations/green-paper-transforming-public-procurement (accessed 24 August 2021).

IFS (2010) *Emergency Budget 2010 Report.* Institute for Fiscal Studies, June. Available at: https://ifs.org.uk/tools_and_resources/budget/330 (accessed 24 August 2021).

Pope, T. (2018) *The Lost Decade: Spring Statement 2018.* Institute for Fiscal Studies, 14 March.

Seriot, P., Hatchett, R. and Berkley, S. (2021) Public-private alliance drive historic vaccination programme. *World Economic Forum*, 10 March. Available at: https://www.weforum.org/agenda/2021/03/public-private-alliance-drives-historic-vaccination-programme/ (accessed 24 August 2021).

When the politically impossible becomes the politically inevitable: has the moment arrived for the wholesale adoption of relationism?

Nigel Ball

Introduction

What is relationism? In its broadest sense, it can be understood as the assumption that positive relationships will lead to positive outcomes. Enhancing the quality of relationships between people and organisations is increasingly favoured as a way to improve the delivery of public services and thus social outcomes. Yet much of the institutional machinery built by industrialised societies in the modern era has focused on ensuring that individuals cannot cosy up with each other to take advantage of others (think of arm's-length legal principles or procurement rules, for example). Still, it seems unlikely that a move towards relationism is inspired by a sense that modern standards of probity have gone too far. More likely, those serving the public are striving to find new types of relationship that avoid past dangers while unlocking some of the benefits that positive relationships must surely bring.

What might these new types of relationship look like? And is there evidence that that they will lead to better outcomes? And if these new types of relationship are to have a future in delivering services to the public and improving social outcomes, what might enable their widespread adoption – an electorally endorsed wholesale reform, or continued experimental, incremental adjustments?

This chapter will attempt to describe some of the emerging **relational tools** that leaders and practitioners working in different sectors have made use of, before examining how widespread these practices might become.

Unpacking relationism

What sort of tools and practices count as 'relational'? What many of the examples seem to have in common is a focus on maintaining and enhancing the quality of personal and organisational relationships, by increasing the pro-social behaviour of people who work together in a place, policy domain or system. This pro-social environment might be characterised by certain attitudes, for example:

- *Inclination to trust.* People might assume that associates have an intrinsic motivation to do a good job, which counterbalances extrinsic motivators related to personal gain. This might lead them to trust in others to do the right thing, rather than treat them with scepticism or suspicion.
- *Concern for long-term reputation.* People might understand that reputational incentives act as a motivator, leading to a long-term and widespread desire not to look bad to one's peers.
- *Valuing of transparency.* People might actively seek to build a culture of open and transparent communication, to undergird mutual scrutiny and support.

These informal attitudes might find their way into the formal mechanisms that govern relationships in a place, policy domain or system. There may be an emphasis on different types of contracts or written agreements, with fewer inducements and restrictions. There may be new forums and governance bodies that aim to take advantage of the pro-social culture to cultivate aligned working.

This shows that the relational behaviours of individuals can translate into relational mechanisms for organisations. After all, relationships between respective organisations are fundamentally made up of many individuals holding relationships with many other individuals who are professional peers: a criss-crossing web of interpersonal associations. Much attention is given to how bilateral relationships between two organisations operate, but most organisations also share multiple relationships across a complex network. I will consider both types in turn under the heading of 'inter-organisational relationships'.

Organisations can also hold a relationship with individuals who are not part of another organisation and are not peers. Most obviously these are the relationships with their clients, service users or customers, but public organisations also need to consider their relationship with citizens, due to the public accountability demanded by spending taxpayers' money. I will consider these types under the heading of 'extra-organisational relationships'.

Enhancing inter-organisational relationships

Improving bilateral relationships

We live in the era of outsourcing. The UK government spends £284 billion per year with external suppliers (Institute for Government, 2018), which is equivalent to over a fifth of all public spending (Brien, 2021). Many large organisations, both companies and charities, have grown considerably on a diet of government contracts. The biggest suppliers, who receive over £100 million a year in revenue from the government, are designated 'strategic suppliers' in recognition of their importance in delivering government services. According to the Institute for Government, between 2013 and 2017, strategic suppliers went from receiving an eighth of all central government procurement to a fifth (Davies et al, 2018).

However, this growth has not been universally good for either the companies or the government. The problems were brought dramatically to the fore by the collapse of one of the strategic suppliers, Carillion, in January 2018. Other strategic suppliers have survived moments teetering on the brink, such as Serco in 2014 and Interserve in 2019. Most analysis attributes these issues to a mix of poor procurement practice from the government, and poor corporate governance within the organisations. I will examine each in turn.

The weaknesses in procurement practice are now well-established. Often the initial decision to outsource is insufficiently justified. Engagement with the market of potential suppliers is poor or absent. An excessive focus on low cost leads to a deterioration in quality and transfers unsustainable risks to companies (often sardonically called the 'race to the bottom'). And poor contract management enables, or even encourages, suppliers to do the minimum after winning the contract (Davies et al, 2018).

In 2019 the UK government published the *Outsourcing Playbook* (updated in 2020 and renamed the *Sourcing Playbook*) (Cabinet Office, 2020a). This provides a thorough set of guidance attempting to overcome these issues. But could reform could go further, and does 'relationism' have something to offer?

Part of the problem, well established in economic theory (for example, Williamson, 1975), is that when there are small numbers of buyers and suppliers in a market, the buyer and supplier become co-dependent. Neither can easily exit the relationship, even if it is harmful for one or both of them, due to a lack of alternative buyers or suppliers. This problem is not unique to public sector contracting, and lessons could be learnt from attempts to solve it in the private sector. Nobel prize-winner Oliver Hart and colleagues describe a 2005 contract between two large corporations whereby although the supplier performed all the requirements of the contract, the buyer felt more could be done to cut costs and improve quality. Gradually trust and confidence was eroded, but the buyer could not easily switch supplier and the supplier could not afford to forego the contract. It had become a 'lose-lose' situation (Frydlinger et al, 2019). Hart proposes that a **relational contract** can alleviate these challenges.

A relational contract is useful when both buyer and seller understand the end goal, but face uncertainty about the means of achieving it, or what the costs will be. Such uncertainty makes drafting a conventional contract, specifying a service and the price to be paid for it, difficult. A relational contract instead focuses on describing how the parties should align their goals, share ongoing risks, and continually interact and negotiate with each other as they learn about delivery or as external circumstances evolve. It attempts to mingle the trust and informality inherent in positive relationships with the legal protections of a contract. Achieving long-term social outcomes is a good example of when a relational contract might be useful. Neither the government (as buyer) nor a supplier can predict exactly what will need to be done for each service user, for how long, or what that might cost. The arrival of external shocks, like COVID-19, adds to the uncertainty.

Relational contracts have a major drawback: they are unlikely to offer the same recourse as a conventional contract if things go wrong. They rely on trust and reputation as their principal mechanism of enforceability. It takes time (and money) to build the required level of trust. Even then, in dire circumstances, one party may be tempted to take advantage of the other if breaching trust (and potentially damaging their reputation) is a less costly option – imagine the case of looming bankruptcy for a supplier, or a political scandal hitting the government. Still, a group of US academics has explored the use of relational contracts in the public sector, looking at large-scale military procurement (Brown et al, 2013), and they deserve more experimentation (Ball, 2020a).

Even if formal relational contracts do not become common, contract tender and award processes could also make use of a relational approach. Currently, the emphasis is on open competition, lowest cost is favoured, and minimising the risk of challenge to the decision is paramount.[1] The government is revising procurement rules in the light of Brexit, as it is no longer bound by EU regulations (Cabinet Office, 2020b). But the rules already give latitude for procuring authorities to do things differently. Instead of open competition, it is already possible to award via negotiation with a closed group of suppliers (Villeneuve-Smith and Blake, 2016). Instead of favouring lowest cost, the evaluation of bids could focus more on quality and how actors will work together. With reform to the rules, past record could be taken into account more explicitly (Sloan, 2019). And with training and the establishment of communities of practice, procurement professionals might feel more empowered to stand behind unconventional award decisions.

But public sector procurement professionals do not bear all the responsibility for the failures of outsourcing; after all, suppliers still bid for an won these contracts. The collapse of Carillion followed that of fashion retailer BHS and foreshadowed that of holiday company Thomas Cook, and together these failures have led to a slew of inquiries into corporate governance practices (Kingman, 2018).

Perhaps the response to these corporate disasters may set the scene for a more relational approach on the supplier side. These failures stand in sharp contrast to a growing movement that promotes business as a force for good. The concept of shareholder primacy – that profit-seeking is a company's sole purpose – is being challenged by proponents of 'stakeholder capitalism' who argue that a company's relationships with its customers, suppliers, employees and community are just as important (Taylor, 2020). Companies have co-opted this pro-social message. In August 2019, the US Business Roundtable, representing chief executive officers of major US companies, redefined the purpose of a company to reflect this shift in thinking (Business Roundtable, 2019). In November 2019, the British Academy followed suit in their *Principles for Purposeful Business* (British Academy, 2019). Neither are these ideas brand new: they have a rich pedigree dating back to 19th-century British industrialists like Titus Salt. They are also well developed intellectually, such as in a seminal 2011 article in the Harvard Business Review by Michael Porter and Mark Kramer, which describes the 'Shared Value' concept, which they define as follows: 'policies and operating practices that enhance the competitiveness of a company while simultaneously advancing the economic and social conditions in the communities in which it operates' (Porter and Kramer, 2011).

Why might this move towards socially responsible business practice be important for more **relational procurement** and contracting approaches? Perhaps it improves the chances of goal alignment between buyer and supplier. Businesses who are explicitly aiming at broader goals than just profit seeking – and demonstrating that through their behaviour – might be more easily trusted by public bodies whose principal goal is the public interest. That trust could support relational approaches (with all the potential benefits and risks those bring).

Improving networks of relationships

Relational contracting and procurement approaches might have potential when it comes to improving bilateral relationships between organisations, but that is not enough. The steady growth in outsourcing and departmentalism has led to a public service delivery system that is characterised by a complex set of inter-organisational relationships between manifold national and local agencies – be they public, private or civil society. For example, reducing rough sleeping might require the action of housing authorities, homelessness charities, the police, emergency healthcare, long-term healthcare, and perhaps many more – as well as the consent, agency and participation of those affected. Each of these actors is working to a different set of incentives and professional norms.

My closing chapter of the previous volume in this series, *Local Authorities and the Social Determinants of Health*, asked 'how might these actors interact with each other so as to create masterful theatre rather than depressing farce?' (Ball, 2020b). The quality of the relationships between these actors can be the difference between success and failure. To address the fragmented system where vulnerable and costly-to-help people are shunted around from one agency to another, forward-thinking leaders are working out how to collaborate and make services more joined-up.

But an array of research shows that an appetite for collaboration is not enough on its own to make complex networks work better. There need to be individuals and organisations who instigate and manage the collaboration. Leaders who wish to do this must nurture 'the ability to see the larger system. ... [This] enables collaborating organisations to jointly develop solutions not evident to any of them individually' (Senge et al, 2015). Large and complex networks need a separate organisation dedicated to the task of coordinating the other actors, variously described as a 'backbone' (Kania and Kramer, 2011), an 'ecosystem orchestrator' (Ebrahim, 2019) or a 'network administrative organisation' (Provan and Kenis, 2008).

What counts as an ecosystem orchestrator? Do Mayoral Combined Authorities fit the description? Greater Manchester Combined Authority, which has the most devolved powers of any in the country, expresses an aspiration to perform some of the functions demanded of one. The 'Greater Manchester Model of public service delivery' involves 'organising resources – people and budgets – around neighbourhoods of 30,000–50,000 residents, rather than around themes or policy areas as is traditionally done' (Greater Manchester Combined Authority, 2019). What about the National Health Service's (NHS) new Integrated Care Systems? A November 2020 publication from NHS England sets out requirements for 'stronger partnerships in local places' and '[p]rovider organisations being asked to step forward in formal collaborative arrangements' (NHS England, 2018). Perhaps individual local authorities can continue to take up the mantle, much as Wigan famously did (as described in *Local Authorities and the Social Determinants of Health*; Arden et al, 2020). Essex County Council manages the Essex Partners, a loose coming together of the myriad public agencies, voluntary organisations and companies operating within the footprint of 'Greater Essex'. The Bishop of Chelmsford, a member of the board, has reflected on the challenge of understanding how such a grouping should operate: 'is it like the United Nations – and so we are still locked inside our own organisational identity – or is it more like a national football team, where all club loyalties are put to one side?' (Morris, 2020).

Enhancing extra-organisational relationships

So far I have discussed organisation-to-organisation relationships, but relationships between organisations and individuals need consideration as well: with both the users whom an organisation serves, and with the citizens to whom any organisation receiving public money should ultimately be accountable.

The importance of public organisations' relationships with their service users can scarcely be overstated, but it is beyond the scope of this chapter.[2] Users of public services are, of course, citizens too. But we wear the identities differently. We all rely on public services, but not to an equal degree and not uniformly over time. Yet we are all, always, citizens. And to be a citizen means accepting a reciprocal relationship with others, even people we will never meet. Rights are typically paired with responsibilities because we understand that a sense of two-way obligation is what binds societies together (Collier, 2018: 44). Today, this core 'social contract' is seen through the lens of the nation-state and we tend to identify ourselves as citizens of a country. But we might also consider ourselves citizens of our neighbourhood.

The COVID-19 pandemic showed how people look out for their neighbours, with a widely reported boom in volunteering and mutual aid. According to the UK government, 21 per cent of people in England formally volunteered at the beginning of the pandemic, and 47 per cent of people informally volunteered during the pandemic's first wave in 2020 (Office for Civil Society, 2020). These are striking numbers, but may have been boosted by the government's employment support scheme temporarily creating a large corps of people whose income was maintained while they were unable to work in their usual jobs. One big way of helping to give volunteering greater political attention would be to quantify its economic value. Andy Haldane, the Bank of England's Chief Economist, advocates for its inclusion in the National Accounts (Haldane, 2019).

However, increasing volunteering is just one way to unlock people's appetite to fulfil their responsibilities and reciprocal obligations in society. It suffers from two limitations. One is that people have limited time, and ever more tantalising choices about how spend it. The other is that dedicating time for free in one's own community is not enough to affect matters of public policy that stretch beyond it – which is most of them. Citizens' sense of reciprocal obligation cannot be fully exploited if they cannot be actively included in actions beyond their immediate sphere of influence.

Of course, this is what our democratic structures are for. But they are imperfect, and public (or publicly funded) organisations can take active steps to close the so-called 'democratic deficit' that can leave citizens feeling powerless and therefore apathetic or hostile.

What holds back relationism?

So far, I have demonstrated that there is ample good practice to draw on when it comes to relationism in public service delivery. So why are such practices not more common? Part of the answer may be that they remain experimental. But the persistence of the status quo can also be explained by analysing the governing orthodoxy that has prevailed over public service delivery over the past three decades: ever-increasing centralisation and control.

The modern welfare state was founded in the 1940s with the promise of the state looking after its citizens, slaying Beveridge's 'five great evils' (Beveridge, 1942). Reforms under Thatcher in the 1980s left their legacy on the welfare state in the form of the purchaser–provider split and outsourcing (Hood, 1991), and further reforms picked up by New Labour from 1997 to 2010, such as 'choice and voice' and targets. This replaced a monolithic public service delivery system with a complex and fragmented one. But it has not led to a reduction in central control as one might expect. Despite the sprawling organisations and dispersed delivery networks of public services, the centre hoards power via a dizzying array of tools: rules, inspections, inducements, commands, targets, competition – even censure (Ball, 2020c). Power is further concentrated in the 'centre of the centre', with the Treasury acting as gatekeeper to billions of pounds of spending in other departments: measured by the proportion of revenue raised centrally rather than locally, Britain is the most centralised country in the G7 (Booth, 2015). Ensuring that delivery at the local level does not fall foul of this torrent of considerations is part of the reason why innovation is so difficult in public agencies.

The moral philosopher Onora O'Neill wrote about the dangers of this approach two decades ago, in the BBC Reith lectures:

> Our new culture of accountability, which is promoted as the way to reduce untrustworthiness and to secure ever more perfect control of institutional and professional performance, [is] taking us in the wrong direction. … We are imposing ever more stringent forms of control. We are requiring those in the public sector and the professions to account in excessive and sometimes irrelevant detail to regulators and inspectors, auditors and examiners. The very demands of accountability often make it harder for them to serve in the public sector. (O'Neill, 2002)

If O'Neill is right, perhaps reversing centralisation is a prerequisite to enabling an 'era of relationism'. Is it likely to happen? The Conservative government that came to power in 2019 under Boris Johnson suggested that it might pick up the mantle of devolution from successive predecessor governments. Yet a White Paper on the matter promised in early 2020 had been delayed four times by January 2021 (Hill, 2020). It was then repurposed to focus instead on the much broader and less well-defined goal of 'levelling up', eventually appearing in that guise in February 2022.

The government's centralised handling of the COVID-19 pandemic did not offer many indications of a taste for devolution either, even for those elements of crisis response that were thought at the time to be better handled at the local level. The centrally run test and trace system was compared unfavourably with Germany's decentralised system, which was run by local public health authorities. An attempt at what the Prime Minister called a 'whack-a-mole' approach to local lockdowns during the so-called second wave in autumn 2020 failed partly because it was not decided in consultation with the places concerned. A show-down with the Mayor of Manchester in October 2020 showed the government's unwillingness to listen to local leaders. The battles with local authorities over the closing and opening of schools over the holiday season in 2020–2021 further reinforced that impression.

The Johnson government made much of the political catchphrase of 'levelling up' Britain's regions without clearly setting out where it meant the levelling to take place. One of Britain's leading psephologists suggested that the 'Red Wall' of former Labour-held seats that went Conservative in 2019 would be the main target – because the government would have an existential need to shore up its new coalition of voters in the North (Kanagasooriam, 2019). A succession of announcements of billions of pounds in funding nominally targeted at 'levelling up', such as the Towns Fund, Levelling Up Fund and Shared Prosperity Fund were not strategically co-ordinated. But the incoherence perhaps mattered less than the fact that the government made places compete to win a slice of this funding against centrally-decided criteria, thus maintaining decision-making power on how the money was to be spent. Local leaders understand what their areas need and can think of ways to draw connections between different initiatives, but only if they have the powers to shape implementation. A government that continues to hoard power centrally undermines these efforts.

Compounding the centralisation problem is the spectre of more austerity. Like governments around the world, the British government unleashed unprecedented fiscal stimulus to support the economy through COVID-19. Government fiscal announcements and continued economic turmoil since the end of the pandemic's worst periods have left ambiguity as to whether the government might re-introduce austerity to 'balance the books' following post-COVID-19 public debt. Certainly society's worse-off look to be bearing the brunt of harsh fiscal decisions and a turbulent economic environment. During 2020, still at the height of the pandemic, the government announced a new public sector pay freeze, and declined to fund free school meals for poor children in the holidays or to extend the boost to Universal Credit, the main benefit for low-income families. The *Financial Times* reported on 'austerity by stealth' (Giles and Bounds, 2020). 'National insurance' tax rises announced in 2021 hit the low-paid hardest, as did much higher inflation beginning in 2022.

This scenario shows how regressive fiscal decisions, and a difficult macro-economic environment , can compound the challenges for local governments, who deal at the frontline with the increased social needs that ensue. That further strains already squeezed local government capacity, closing off opportunities for them to develop the skills and person-capacity to implement meaningful reform or even learn through experimentation. This lack of capacity then undermines a devolution agenda through a vicious cycle. Local agencies lack the powers that would create the imperative to increase their capacity; yet their lack of capacity undermines the confidence needed to offer them more powers (Collier and Kay, 2020: 139).

Might the COVID-19 crisis beget a new era of reform?

These structural features of the British state indicate that widespread adoption of relational approaches like those I have described are unlikely without wholesale reform. I argue three things are needed for that, in sequence. The first is a strong intellectual foundation for the approach. The second is adoption of the ideas by the main political parties who are likely to have a chance at governing in the coming decades. The third is the consent of voters, which is most likely to occur by them electing a party that has backed this philosophy. I will discuss each in turn.

A strong intellectual foundation for the new approach

History might suggest that fringe ideas can be made mainstream by a crisis. Milton Friedman is generally recognised as one of the main architects of the philosophy of shareholder primacy and the 'greed is good' capitalism that has prevailed at the end of the 20th century and start of the 21st. Near the start of that era, he famously said:

> Only a crisis – actual or perceived – produces real change. When that crisis occurs, the actions that are taken depend on the ideas that are lying around. That, I believe, is our basic function: to develop alternatives to existing policies, to keep them alive and available until the politically impossible becomes the politically inevitable. (Friedman, 1982: ix)

Indeed, the alternatives he and his acolytes had promoted a decade earlier were politically adopted by Reagan's Republican Party in the US and Thatcher's Conservative Party in the UK, after a troubled decade in the 1970s. The Britain that Thatcher created in the 1980s, driven by these ideas, is the Britain we live in today. Might the pattern Friedman identified occur again, in light of the COVID-19 crisis? And if so, what are the 'ideas that are lying around' this time?

One can certainly observe a marked shift away from an individualistic and rights-based narrative towards a more communitarian and responsibility-based one, among some prominent thinkers. I have mentioned Hilary Cottam and Andy Haldane already. Alongside them are others like Paul Collier and John Kay who tell us 'greed is dead' (Collier and Kay, 2020), and Colin Mayer who tells us business must be led by purpose (Mayer, 2020). Other economists like Mariana Mazzucato, Kate Raworth and Joseph Stiglitz are increasingly well known and offer new theories that depart considerably from those of the status quo.

There is no perfect consensus, but certain themes recur: the dangers of economic inequality, particularly inequality within nation-states. The limitations of gross domestic product as a measure of human flourishing. The destructiveness of greed and individualism as a governing philosophy. The importance of reciprocity. Taken together, these concepts expand the role of businesses, governments and communities beyond protecting the rights of the individuals towards articulating a common destiny and promoting mutual responsibility. This is fertile intellectual ground for relationism and localism. Within such a narrative, the changes necessary to unlock the benefits of local – and relational – approaches have a chance to move beyond the fringes and into the mainstream.

Adoption of the ideas by the main political parties

In the midst of the COVID-19 crisis, when getting through it consumed almost all political attention, it was difficult to discern a coherent governing philosophy in any of the main British political parties. The governing Conservative Party offered some clues via its policy decisions, though as noted earlier, these did not appear to follow a consistent narrative. This could be regarded as a symptom of the inevitably chaotic nature of governing through a pandemic. But the Conservative Party also offers a cautionary tale: all political parties are broad coalitions, but not all the political ideas they try to incorporate can prevail.

Much of today's Conservative Party takes its intellectual cue from Thatcherism, and Thatcher famously declared in 1987 'there is no such thing as society' (Thatcher, 1987). This sounds like a bad starting point for adopting relationism, and certainly, her premiership is perhaps remembered most for the rampant individualism she appeared to unleash. However, in the same interview, Thatcher goes on to say: 'It's our duty to look after ourselves and then, also to look after our neighbour. … There's no such thing as entitlement, unless someone has first met an obligation.' Her point, which in her own words was 'distorted beyond recognition' (Thatcher, 1993), was about the importance of reciprocity – which as we have seen is a fundamental prerequisite of relationism.

While many will find these comments inconsistent with the thrust of Thatcher's economic policies, the clarification is important, as it shows that the importance of local community and a duty to others have been enduring values of Conservative thought. Indeed, David Cameron, when he became leader of the opposition in 2007 and Prime Minister in 2010, tried to make a governing orthodoxy out of this idea: 'Big Society' was an attempt to politically mainstream the idea that small-scale community groups, bound together by personal relationships, could drive forward meaningful public service reform (Cameron, 2009). Danny Kruger, one of the architects of this narrative as a speechwriter to David Cameron during his time as leader of the opposition, is now an MP and ministerial advisor. Kruger attributes the eventual failure of Big Society to its association with austerity. He claims that the ideas were misinterpreted as an effort to get communities and volunteers to step forward into the void left by the retreating state. In a 2020 report on civil society commissioned by the Prime Minister, he rehearses these ideas once again, setting out 'a vision for a more local, more human, less bureaucratic, less centralised society in which people are supported and empowered to play an active role in their neighbourhoods' (Kruger, 2020).

The consent of voters to implement the ideas

The Labour Party, at time of writing the main opposition party, could legitimately lay claim to a similar set of **relational principles**. But their failure to prevail in the Conservative Party, despite an enduring presence in that party's mix of ideas, perhaps demonstrates that there are deeper, cultural reasons for their non-adoption which can be instructive for any political movement seeking to gain the consent of voters for a new governing philosophy. The individualistic and entitled economic structures of our society are deeply entrenched. These condition us to look out for ourselves first and foremost, and to expect predefined individual rights to be upheld with minimal regard to the corollary obligations (Collier and Kay, 2020: 34). While volunteering may be thriving by some measures, it is more commonly practised by wealthier people (Payne, 2017), potentially excluding lower-income groups from its reciprocal benefits. The sense of solidarity that once typified traditional 'working-class' communities, embodied in co-operative movements and labour unions, has sharply declined in the past decades; many once-proud communities are now characterised as 'left behind' and beset by social problems (Collier, 2018: 8).

The idea of being more relational, whether as citizens or as organisations delivering public services, cuts sharply against this culture. This makes it likely that any attempts to mainstream these ideas politically could continue to fail – unless the COVID-19 crisis genuinely does lead to a watershed moment where a new political consensus can emerge.

Conclusion

In my chapter for the previous volume, *Local Authorities and the Social Determinants of Health*, I observed that approaches to public service reform come in and out of fashion – but that actual change is both more incremental and less linear, often beset by backward steps and dead ends (Ball, 2020b). We do not yet know what the post-COVID-19 world holds. Central government may double down on its grip, further weakening delivery agencies and closing down the space for trying relational approaches. Alternatively, local agencies may find ways to snatch away powers and start doing things their own way (Davies et al, 2020).

In the absence of a coherent narrative that is adopted politically and consented to by citizens, reform towards a more relational approach will continue to be incremental, often marginal, and sometimes in spite of considerable barriers. But it will not be impossible, with much good practice to draw on already. Perhaps this government or the next one will seize the post-COVID-19 political moment to drive an electorally endorsed culture change through the heart of government. Only then might a more radical, faster and deeper shift towards relationism take place.

Acknowledgements

The first part of this chapter, discussing the tools of relationism, draws considerably on the research of the Government Outcomes Lab at the Blavatnik School of Government. I am grateful to several colleagues for insights on particular topics: Ruairi MacDonald (procurement); Gwyn Bevan (contracting theory); Mara Airoldi, Michael Gibson and Stéphane Saussier (relational contracting); Ian Taylor (responsible business); Jo Blundell, Franziska Rosenbach, Tanyah Hameed and Clare FitzGerald (collaboration); Eleanor Carter (network governance); and Leigh Crowley and Ruth Dixon (user voice).

Notes

[1] These issues are frequently discussed by the Procurement of Government Outcomes peer learning group hosted by the Government Outcomes Lab at Oxford University, chaired by Professor Anne Davies.

[2] For readers interested in this topic, I highly recommend Hilary Cottam's 2018 book *Radical Help* which is an inspiring manifesto for how to improve public organisations' poor relationships with their service users.

References

Arden, K., Cunliffe, K. and Cook, P.A. (2020) Cultural change and the evolution of community governance: A north-west England perspective. In A. Bonner (ed) *Local Authorities and the Social Determinants of Health*. Bristol: Policy Press, pp 149–172.

Ball, N. (2020a) *Reflecting on the Social Outcomes Conference 2020.* Government Outcomes Lab. https://golab.bsg.ox.ac.uk/community/blogs/reflecting-social-outcomes-conference-2020/

Ball, N. (2020b) Steadying the swinging pendulum: How might we accommodate competing approaches to public service delivery? In A. Bonner (ed) *Local Authorities and the Social Determinants of Health.* Bristol: Policy Press, pp 401–420.

Ball, N. (2020c) *The Missing Link between Trust and Accountability.* Government Outcomes Lab. https://golab.bsg.ox.ac.uk/community/blogs/missing-link-between-trust-and-accountability/

Beveridge, W. (1942) *Social Insurance and Allied Services.* https://www.parliament.uk/about/living-heritage/transformingsociety/livinglearning/coll-9-health1/coll-9-health/

Booth, P. (2015) *Federal Britain: The Case for Decentralisation.* https://iea.org.uk/publications/research/federal-britain-the-case-for-decentralisation

Brien, P. (2021) *Public Spending: A Brief Introduction.* https://commonslibrary.parliament.uk/research-briefings/cbp-8046/

British Academy (2019) *Principles for Purposeful Business.* https://www.thebritishacademy.ac.uk/publications/future-of-the-corporation-principles-for-purposeful-business/

Brown, T., Potoski, M. and Slyke, D. (2013) *Complex Contracting: Government Purchasing in the Wake of the U.S. Coast Guard's Deepwater Program.* Cambridge: Cambridge University Press.

Business Roundtable (2019) Business Roundtable redefines the purpose of a corporation to promote 'an economy that serves all Americans'. Business Roundtable – Opportunity Agenda. https://opportunity.businessroundtable.org/ourcommitment/

Cabinet Office (2020a) *Green Paper: Transforming Public Procurement.* GOV. UK. https://www.gov.uk/government/consultations/green-paper-transforming-public-procurement

Cabinet Office (2020b) *Updated Outsourcing Playbook.* GOV.UK. https://www.gov.uk/government/news/updated-outsourcing-playbook

Cameron, D. (2009). David Cameron: The Big Society. http://conservative-speeches.sayit.mysociety.org/speech/601246

Collier, P. (2018) *The Future of Capitalism: Facing the New Anxieties.* London: Penguin.

Collier, P. and Kay, J. (2020) *Greed Is Dead: Politics after Individualism.* London: Penguin.

Davies, N., Chan, O., Cheung, A., Freeguard, G. and Norris, E. (2018) Government Procurement. https://www.instituteforgovernment.org.uk/publications/government-procurement

Davies, T., Kili, T. and Pollock, R. (2020) Four scenarios for local government to manage uncertainty. Apolitical. https://apolitical.co/solution-articles/en/four-scenarios-for-local-government-to-manage-uncertainty

Ebrahim, A. (2019) *Measuring Social Change: Performance and Accountability in a Complex World*. Stanford: Stanford University Press.

Friedman, M. (1982). *Capitalism and Freedom*. Chicago: University of Chicago Press.

Frydlinger, D., Hart, O. and Vitasek, K. (2019) A new approach to contracts. *Harvard Business Review*. https://hbr.org/2019/09/a-new-approach-to-contracts

Giles, C. and Bounds, A. (2020) England's councils face austerity by stealth. *Financial Times*, 9 December. https://www.ft.com/content/98699aef-e6be-44a0-a5bf-302755485744

Greater Manchester Combined Authority (2019) Greater Manchester model. Greater Manchester Combined Authority. https://www.greatermanchester-ca.gov.uk/what-we-do/greater-manchester-strategy/

Haldane, A.G. (2019) The third sector and the fourth industrial revolution. Speech at the Pro Bono Economics 10th Anniversary Lecture.

Hill, J. (2020) How the devolution white paper went missing in action. Local Government Chronicle (LGC). https://www.lgcplus.com/politics/lgc-briefing/how-the-devolution-white-paper-went-missing-in-action-30-09-2020/

Hood, C. (1991) A public management for all seasons? *Public Administration*, 69(1): 3–19.

Institute for Government (2018) Summary: Government procurement: The scale and nature of contracting in the UK. Institute for Government, 11 December. https://www.instituteforgovernment.org.uk/summary-government-procurement-scale-nature-contracting-uk

Kanagasooriam, J. (2019) How the Labour party's 'red wall' turned blue. *Financial Times*, 14 December. https://www.ft.com/content/3b80b2de-1dc2-11ea-81f0-0c253907d3e0

Kania, J. and Kramer, M.R. (2011) *Collective Impact (SSIR)*. https://ssir.org/articles/entry/collective_impact

Kingman, J. (2018) *Independent Review of the Financial Reporting Council (FRC)*. GOV.UK. https://www.gov.uk/government/publications/financial-reporting-council-review-2018

Kruger, D. (2020) *Levelling Up Our Communities*. https://www.dannykruger.org.uk/new-social-covenant

Mayer, C. (2020) *The Future of the Corporation and the Economics of Purpose* (SSRN Scholarly Paper ID 3731539). Social Science Research Network. https://doi.org/10.2139/ssrn.3731539

Morris, R. (2020) *Essex Partnership*. https://www.essexfuture.org.uk/boards-networks/essex-partners/bishop-roger-morris-epb-message/

NHS England (2018) *NHS England: What Are Integrated Care Systems?* https://www.england.nhs.uk/integratedcare/what-is-integrated-care/

O'Neill, O. (2002) Reith 2002: *A Question of Trust – Onora O'Neill.* https://www.open.edu/openlearn/ou-on-the-bbc-reith-2002-question-trust-onora-oneill

Office for Civil Society (2020) *A Look at Volunteering during the Response to COVID-19.* GOV.UK. https://www.gov.uk/government/publications/a-look-at-volunteering-during-the-response-to-covid-19/a-look-at-volunteering-during-the-response-to-covid-19

Payne, C. (2017) *Changes in the Value and Division of Unpaid Volunteering in the UK.* Office for National Statistics. https://www.ons.gov.uk/economy/nationalaccounts/satelliteaccounts/articles/changesinthevalueanddivisionofunpaidcareworkintheuk/2015

Porter, M.E. and Kramer, M.R. (2011) Creating shared value. *Harvard Business Review,* 1 January. https://hbr.org/2011/01/the-big-idea-creating-shared-value

Provan, K.G. and Kenis, P. (2008) Modes of network governance: Structure, management, and effectiveness. *Journal of Public Administration Research and Theory,* 18(2): 229–252.

Senge, P., Hamilton, H. and Kania, J. (2015) *The Dawn of System Leadership (SSIR).* https://ssir.org/articles/entry/the_dawn_of_system_leadership

Sloan, L. (2019) Market Design in Complex Social Services. Presentation at the Social Outcomes Conference 2019, Oxford.

Taylor, I. (2020) *Responsible Business: A Challenging Opportunity.* Government Outcomes Lab. https://golab.bsg.ox.ac.uk/our-projects/responsible-business-challenging-opportunity/

Thatcher, M. (1987) Interview for *Woman's Own* ('no such thing as society'). Margaret Thatcher Foundation, interview. https://www.margaretthatcher.org/document/106689

Thatcher, M. (1993) *The Downing Street Years.* London: HarperPress.

Villeneuve-Smith, F. and Blake, J. (2016) The art of the possible in public procurement. E3M.

Williamson, O.E. (1975) *Markets and Hierarchies: Analysis and Antitrust Implications.* http://archive.org/details/oliver-williamson-markets-and-hierarchies

Conclusion

Adrian Bonner

The six parts of this book have focused on global concerns relating to the **wicked issues** of the COVID-19 pandemic and the climate change crisis. Lessons learned from international, national and local approaches to these wicked issues provide an insight into the linked issues of social and health inequalities, individual and family poverty, loss of employment, domestic abuse, housing and homelessness, and other adverse determinants of health. In 2023 the world is at a tipping point in relation to the control of the COVID-19 pandemic and the threats to human life and the environment resulting from climate change, and the threat of global conflict emerging from the invasion of Ukraine by Russia. At the time of writing more than 4 million refugees have left Ukraine, and the number of deaths is in excess of 7,000 (Anon, 2022c).

Globalism and the increasing connectedness of communities around the world have contributed to the spread of the COVID-19 virus and its variants as a result of large-scale movements of people travelling between countries. From a socioeconomic perspective the major impact of lockdown measures, in the various countries, has had a severe economic impact on the viability of a large number of businesses with consequences for employment and the financial security of individuals and families. During the pandemic the aviation related industries were at particular risk during lockdown and the closing of national borders. Paradoxically, the significant drop in passengers using the global airlines, intended to reduce the spread of the virus and its mutations, reduced atmospheric emissions leading to clearer skies, which, in addition to other new experiences of people coping with lockdown, have increased the relationship between people and their awareness of the natural world, providing a political opportunity to progress the climate change strategy being developed, by a relational approach being promoted globally. However, local political divisions on reducing car use and energy generation are not without problems as noted in Chapter 6.

Although the number of deaths, worldwide, resulting from COVID-19 has not, to date, reached the levels of previous pandemics (see Introduction), the impact on individuals, families and local economies is considerable, leading to reflections on pre-COVID-19 lifestyles, community governance, and promoting questions relating to existing political, economic and behavioural arrangements. In reflecting on 'Building Back Better, Fairer' (Marmot et al, 2020), what system changes are needed?

Part I of this book addresses wicked issues, which should be differentiated from **tame problems** (see Chapter 1), and how navigating identified wicked issues requires alternative leadership approaches, best developed within the concept of **relationalism** (see Chapter 2). From a UK perspective, this country experienced one of the highest mortalities in comparison with other countries, and together with the US has recorded significantly more deaths than other Western democracies. In the UK, poor resilience due to a decade of austerity budgeting (Chapter 20), prior to COVID-19, left people at the lower end of the social gradient, and the elderly, at particular risk of infection and dying as a result of the virus. In Chapter 3, a critical analysis of the unpreparedness of the UK health system focuses on delays in healthcare systems integration, problems in procuring personal protective equipment, ventilators, implementing an effective test and trace system and lack of integration between health and social care. The overriding message of the chapter is the inadequacy of strategic leadership and poor communications by central government.

Regional and geopolitical factors have been important vulnerability of people and communities to the harms caused by COVID-19, and approaches to dealing with the pandemic. The chapters in Part II highlight specific examples in the North East of England (Chapter 5) and a London borough (Chapter 6). The impact on children in deprived communities as experienced in the UK is exemplified in Chapter 4, in the Bronx, New York (Case study 7.1), and increased cases of domestic abuse at in South Africa (Case study 7.2).

It is evident that reductions in community wealth, the stage of development of health systems and culture are playing an important role in the pandemic. In considering what system changes are needed to address current and future pandemics and other global wicked issues there is a need to consider public governance, local authority responses to housing and homelessness, and social care. Addressing social and health inequalities, and reviewing sustainability from local, national and global perspectives are considered in Part III. This section provides a public sector perspective and begins to identify the cultural changes needed for future system changes, including housing and homelessness, and social care.

Relationalism and wicked issues

One of the central themes running through this book is the need to consider wicked issues from the perspective of relationalism. The importance of building and maintaining relationships between countries, between people, and within communities, should be promoted by an understanding of a relational approach within and between public, private and third sectors.

The outcomes of enhanced relationships within communities can be seen within the large range of community actions in the third sector. In Part IV, the increased benefits to **social value** is exemplified by the provision of food banks, volunteering and the activities of both large and small charities. The Kruger Report (Kruger, 2020: 22) promotes the need for *social value purpose* and proposed that the government should legislate that the whole purpose of public spending is to deliver value for society. In promoting the concept of *purpose* in public spending, social value should encourage a more collaborative and trusting model of service design and commissioning'. Several of the chapters of this book critically evaluate the concepts of public value leading to social value. Liddle (Chapter 8) and Cook (a lawyer, who helped formulate the Social Value Act, 2016: Chapter 18) make the case that a technical approach to measuring social value should not overshadow the qualitative aspects of social value, a concern expressed by Ritel and Webber (see Introduction). Furthermore, across the public, private and third sectors, the values–based ethos of an organisation should guide strategic planning and organisational development.

The generation of social value is much less obvious in the private sector, however case studies in Part V provide examples of where this occurs in housing and homelessness (Case study 17.2), environmental planning (Case study 17.3) and co-operative retailing (Case study 17.4).

In learning from the major health, social and economic challenges to local, national and global communities since January 2020, there is a need to consider the resilience of health care systems, adult social care, public health, education and the wider economy, demographic profiles and international travel. A framework for assessing preparedness for future pandemics and global crises (for example, climate change) has been proposed by the King's Fund (see Introduction, Figure I.2, and Anon 2021a).

Relationalism at a global level, requires political cooperation across all countries to stop future pandemics. This quintessential aspect of COVID-19 (see Introduction) contrasts with other global issues such as climate change. Goldwin has commented that there are ten top emitters of greenhouse gases, however a consensus of only three countries, the US, China and India, along with the European Union, is pivotal in stabilising and hopefully reversing the buildup of carbon dioxide in the atmosphere. '[N]ine countries have the capacity to generate nuclear war ... a small number of countries are systemically important in finance and could bring about global financial collapse' (Goldwin, 2021). In the case of pandemics, they can arise from any global environment and have been linked to the major environmental destabilisations linked to rapid increases in species extinction rates and impacts on human sustainability (UNSDG, 2020). Increased habitat destruction has been reported to increase the transfer of diseases like COVID-19 from animals to humans. Climate change could further exacerbate this (Zimmer, 2019; Khetan, 2020; Lorentzen et al, 2020).

Wicked issues and politics

Beyond the political rhetoric of 'Building Back Better' there is a widespread acknowledgement that the COVID-19 pandemic presents an opportunity for radical reform and the end of individualism. The promotion of Thatcher's comments that 'there's no such thing as society … it is our duty to look after ourselves' and Ronald Regan's statement that 'government is not the solution to our problem; government is the problem' (Anon, 2021b) are now viewed as contributing social health inequalities. In 2021, the collaboration of government and communities were key issues on the agendas of politicians and commentators. In the early phases of the COVID-19 pandemic, community activity and neighbourliness supplemented the work of local authorities to address a common threat which increased the visibility of the elderly, the lonely, and families suffering financial hardship due to the closing down of the economy (see Chapter 14). At this time (10 May 2022), trust in politicians and political systems has come under scrutiny, and significantly affected the outcomes of the May 2022 local elections, causing shock waves across the governing UK Conservative Party (Anon, 2022d). During 2020–2022 there has been a deterioration of democracy and human rights in over 80 countries related to COVID-19 measures. Governments have used that emergency to restrict opposition and dissenting voices and employed authoritarian control. In his commentary on the changing nature of national and local government, Goldwin discusses 'rescue politics' as politicians focus on normalising societies and taking account of long-standing issues underpinning Black Lives Matter protests, levelling up communities and divided societies (Goldwin, 2021).

Business as usual?

The rapid expansion of globalism involving interconnected supply chains of commodities, such as food and consumer goods and international travel, has highlighted the interconnections and interdependency of countries across the globe. Manufacturing and international trade was significantly slowed during the financial crash of 2008. Although manufacturing and international trade has been reduced by a fifth during the pandemic, supply chains are being restructured to diversify sources and single points of failure risks addressed. It has been estimated that up to 25 per cent of global supply chains and 50 per cent of pharmaceutical products could be restructured by 2025 (Anon, 2020a). The resilience of global business is a reflection of the adaptability of the business world to the challenges of the pandemic. Competition gave way to cooperation, in which the 'strategic interests' of governments led to political decisions as to which businesses should live or die. Lifelines to prevent the wholesale collapse of businesses has led to a change in the power balance of businesses and government. During the pandemic, procurement rules were largely ignored and due process in funding public services was neglected. In the UK, the National Audit Office reported that £17 billion in pandemic contracts were awarded without competitive tendering and that a 'VIP lane' was created through which friends and family of government ministers were ten times more likely to be awarded government contracts (Anon, 2020c, 2020b). A UK Research and Innovation funded evaluation of procurement during COVID-19 is being undertaken by Simmons (see Chapter 1 and the forthcoming volume in this series).

The increase in the number of billionaires during 2020–2021 (Anon, 2021c), reflected in the rise of sales of high-end goods, including luxury cars and boats, indicates that, for some, business has been booming. However, some sectors such as health and leisure, the arts and entertainment have been particularly devastated by the predicted and less predicted consequences of lockdown.

COVID-19 and the social determinants of health

Clearly there have been winners and losers in the pandemic. During COVID-19 the government, aware of the public health threats of people sleeping on the streets, allocated £3.2 million in funding and guidance, via the Everyone In strategy, aimed at finding accommodation for every rough sleeper during the first lockdown (HMG, 2021). A further investment of £1.5 million was allocated to address homelessness over the next two years, but this is not available to support people with no recourse to public funding (Goldin, 2021).

Clearly homelessness is a wicked issue, and is beyond solutions which can be provided solely by local or central government. Being homeless, in most cases, is usually not the result of a recent catastrophic event, the trajectory into homelessness frequently begins in the early years (see Bonner, 2008, 2018, 2020; Skelton et al, 2009). Risk factors leading to becoming homeless have been critically studied by van den Bree (van den Bree et al, 2009) and reported to be driven by socioeconomic factors which can be visualised by the social gradient described by Marmot (Marmot, 2010; Marmot et al, 2020), and linked to geopolitical factors (Bambra et al, 2018). The impact of lockdown on childhood adversity will be evident in future years (see the section on 'The progression of COVID-19' in the Introduction, and Chapter 4).

The Kruger Report (Kruger, 2020; see Chapter 16) recommends **strength-based approaches** to promoting resilience in communities:

> Society should be viewed as being composed of assets not liabilities. 'If people left behind are not problems to be solved but opportunities to be realised; the principle of self-sufficiency, people have a capacity with the right help to effect positive changes in their lives and the lives of others should be at the heart of our social system'. (Kruger, 2020)

Identifying the needs of 'people left behind' is important in addressing the disproportionate impact on Black, Asian and minority groups (Chapter 4 and Case study 7.1). Other vulnerable groups include the homeless (Chapter 11 and Case study 16.1), trafficked people (Case studies 7.3 and 16.3) and people subjected to domestic abuse (Case study 7.2 and Chapter 17).

Part VI of this book provides reflections from members of the Centre for Partnering (CfP), from legal (Chapter 18), procurement (Chapter 19), political (Chapter 20) and government policy (Chapter 21) perspectives. Experiences and literature reviews presented in this book underpinning monthly CfP working groups. This work is undertaken in the CfP governance structure shown in the Appendix. Key questions from CfP discussions and conclusions drawn in the six parts of this book have been formulated as follows:

- What is relationalism?
- How does relationalism make a difference to partnering?
- How does relationalism impact on the social, economic, environmental, legal, and financial outcomes?
- How does relationalism make a difference to our understanding of the social determinants of health framework to understand and navigate wicked issues?
- What are the essential cultural changes that are necessary to enhance the roles of public, private and third sectors in terms of their delivery of social value?

Responses to these questions can be informed by the lessons learnt in addressing the COVID-19 pandemic and the climate change crisis. In both of these wicked issues a linear technical approach is insufficient to deal with these real-world challenges. In the case of climate change there are three competing perspectives: profligate consumption (related to production patterns, contributing to the build-up of carbon dioxide in the atmosphere); population growth in certain regions of the world (placing local and global ecosystems under pressure and dangerously out of control); and the price of natural resources (important in both controlling the demand and footing the bill for environmental protection). From a relationalism perspective the lessons being learned from the climate change crisis highlight the importance of **relational values**, between countries, between people and the natural environment. **Relational autonomy** should be promoted in order to empower people to make decisions in the interest of the wider system; and **social justice solidarity**, the acknowledgement that not everyone is equally situated. These are some of the softer relational issues which were part of the global discussions in COP26, a pivotal conference held in Glasgow November 2021, sponsored by the United Nations (HMG, 2021).

At the beginning of 2021, there was increased hope of collaboration between the US and China working more relationally and addressing the urgent issues of the climate change crisis. There was hope that the political changes in the US and increased recognition by China of the urgency for a climate change strategy would drive the development of green economic strategies, supported by public and' private sectors. However the invasion of Ukraine by Russia is beginning to unravel these developing relationships and is causing perturbations in the global economy.

Levelling up or levelling down?

The cost of Brexit, COVID-19 and climate change strategy, relational autonomy and social justice solidarity, as noted here, reflect the need to address the gaps between those who have more resources than others, and between developed and developing countries. Two 'levelling up' agendas have been identified in this book. In Parts II and III the inequalities between the regions in the UK, and within countries such as the US and South Africa, have been described. A second levelling up agenda between the third sector, public and private sectors is reviewed from the perspective of the Kruger Report in Part IV. The availability and the validity of evidence in addressing both COVID-19 and climate change is paramount to navigating these wicked issues. This book is intended to reframe the questions needed to bring about system change, and increase public, social and environment values.

'Boris Johnson's green agenda has been plunged into chaos amid fears that the costs of reaching net zero could cripple working class families' (Malnick, 2021). The poorest households will be hit hardest with the implementation to strip our domestic gas boilers and switching to electric or hydrogen cars. Currently there is concern about rising inflation and the cost of living. In the UK it has been estimated that 25 per cent of people in some regions of the UK will be in destitution by 2023 (Anon, 2022a).

The tension between the financial deficit in the UK resulting from the response to the COVID-19 pandemic, ambitious targets for the UK to reach **net zero** and the unforeseen costs of the UK leaving the EU are reflected in the rising political tensions between the Prime Minister's Office and the Treasury. Three months prior to COP26 global climate conference, chaired by Boris Johnson, a COP26 adviser commented: 'I don't think ministers knew what they were getting into when they set targets for the conference, such as securing commitments from attendees that will limit the rise in global temperatures to no more than 1.5c' (Malnick, 2021).

The cost of the UK leaving the EU (Springford, 2021), health and economic costs of responding to COVID-19 (Ben, 2021), and the need to lead large-scale change in the UK economy (for example, electrification of transport, decarbonising domestic and business energy utilisation, and so on) (Morales and Mathis, 2021), all impact on national and local resources. This immense drain on public finances requires new innovative relational responses. Careful planning, with respect to the needs of the various sectors of society, is required to avoid even greater social and health inequalities. While community wealth, required to support health and care systems, is important, personal and community capacity underpin health and wellbeing. However, the interconnection and interdependence of the various domains of the rainbow model of **social determinants of health** suggest the need for a route map to balancing the various needs of people and communities and the socioeconomic environment in which they co-exist, and, hopefully influence a 'fairer society', via just and democratic processes.

In a post-Brexit world in which COVID-19 is now endemic, with an international global strategy to address the climate crisis, it remains to be seen what impact there will be on people, their health and wellbeing and their aspirations for a new world order. However, the destablisation of the world order by the invasion of Ukraine by Russia, and lack of opposition to this aggressive action by China, will hopefully not derail global consensus on limiting and reducing global temperatures. The combined influences of migration of large numbers of people due to climate change and conflict in war zones are already exacerbating the global migratory patterns which will have a knock-on effect on housing and homelessness in European countries including the UK. The large number of refugees from Ukraine, mainly into European countries (Anon, 2022b), and the socioeconomic impact on global supply chains, along with the increased costs of oil and food, will further exacerbate the deprivation of people already impacted by the wicked issues which have been the main focus of this volume. The socioeconomic driver of change in the UK, Europe and other countries will be the focus of the fourth volume in this social determinants of health series.

Drivers of change into the next phase of UK and global history will be the focus of the next volume in this series.

References

Anon (2020a) Risk, resilience and rebalancing in global value chains. McKinsey Global Institute, 6 August.

Anon (2020b) The magnifying glass: How COVID revealed the truth about our world. *The Guardian*, 11 December

Anon (2020c) 'Watchdog' criticises government over awarding £17bn COVID contracts. *Financial Times*, 18 November.

Anon (2021a) Assessing England's Response to COVID-19: A Framework. The Kings Fund, 2021. https://www.kingsfund.org.uk/publications/assessing-englands-response-covid-19-framework

Anon (2021b) The Coronavirus is rewriting our imagination. *New Yorker*, 1 May.

Anon (2021c) The billionaire boom: How the super-rich soaked up COVID cash. *Financial Times*. https://www.ft.com/content/747a76dd-f018-4d0d-a9f3-4069bf2f5a93

Anon (2022a) Destitution levels are rising across the country – and terribly worrying in certain regions. Press release. National Institute of Economic and Social Research. https://www.niesr.ac.uk/news/niesr-press-release-destitution-levels-are-rising-across-country-and-terribly-worrying-certain-regions-niesr-research-shows

Anon (2022b) How the Ukrainian refugee crisis will change Europe. *The Economist*. https://www.economist.com/europe/2022/03/25/how-the-ukrainian-refugee-crisis-will-change-europe?gclid=EAIaIQobChMIy8jWi6XV9wIVROrtCh3ZMAjWEAAYASAAEgKo6fD_BwE&gclsrc=aw.ds

Anon (2022c) Number of civilian casualties in Ukraine during Russia's invasion verified by OHCHR. Statista, 9 May. https://www.statista.com/statistics/1293492/ukraine-war-casualties/

Anon (2022d) UK elections 2022: A really simple guide. BBC News. https://www.bbc.co.uk/news/uk-politics-60304595

Ben, K. (2021) How much is COVID costing the UK and how much will we pay? BBC News, 22 June. https://www.bbc.co.uk/news/business-52663523

Bonner A. (2006) *Social Exclusion and the Way Out: An Individual and Community Response to Human Social Dysfunction*. Chichester: John Wiley.

Bonner A. (ed) (2018) *Social Determinants of Health: An Interdisciplinary Approach to Social Inequality and Wellbeing Social*. Bristol: Policy Press.

Bonner A. (ed) (2020) *Local Authorities and Social Determinants of Health*. Bristol: Policy Press.

Goldin, I. (2021) *Rescue: From Global Crisis to a Better World*. London: Sceptre.

HMG (2021) Coronavirus: Support for rough sleeper (England). House of Commons Library, 14 January. https://commonslibrary.parliament.uk/research-briefings/cbp-9057/

Kruger, D. (2020) *Levelling Up Our Communities: Proposals for a New Social Covenant. A New Deal with Faith Communities*. A report commissioned by the Prime Minister. https://www.dannykruger.org.uk/files/2020-09/Levelling%20Up%20Our%20Communities-Danny%20Kruger.pdf

Malnick, E. (2021) Boris Johnson's push for net zero plunged into chaos. *The Telegraph*, 7 August.

Marmot, M. (2010) *The Pandemic, Socioeconomic and Health Inequalities in England*. London: Institute of Health Equity.

Marmot, M., Allen, J., Goldblatt, P., Herd, E. and Morrison, J. (2020) Build back fairer: The COVID-19. https://www.health.org.uk/sites/default/files/2020-12/Build-back-fairer--Exec-summary.pdf

Morales, A. and Mathis, W. (2021) UK's $904 billion climate push to bring bigger economic boost. Bloomberg Green, 23 April. https://www.bloomb erg.com/news/articles/2021-04-23/u-k-says-benefit-of-climate-targ ets-outweigh-904-billion-cost#:~:text=The%20U.K.%20estimated%20t hat%20delivering,environment%20will%20be%20far%20greater

Springford, J. (2021) The cost of Brexit: February 2021. Centre for European Reform, Insight, 13 April.

van den Bree, B.M., Shelton, K., Bonner, A., Moss, S., Thomas, H. and Taylor, P. (2009) A longitudinal population-base study of factors in adolescence predicting homelessness in young adulthood. *Journal of Adolescent Health*, 45(6): 571–578.

The Centre for Partnering

The Centre for Partnering (CfP) collaborators are based in the universities of Cardiff (Business School), Manchester Metropolitan (Business School, PERU), Stirling (Social Science), Northumbria (Newcastle Business School) and Oxford (Blavatnik). CfP promotes discussion within Working Groups within the university network and with public, private and third sector representatives, on a monthly basis. CfP aims to facilitate collaborative research, develop products (for example, assessment tools) and influence policy (disseminated via its advisory group). These activities are framed within a constitution and Memorandums of Understanding between CfP and each university.

In addition to the five universities, the fuse network (The Centre for Translational Research in Public Health) has become a partner in these activities.

The ideal of partnering, promoted by CfP, is to generate additional value by combining each partner's contributions in a positive sum equation. CfP's purpose is to explore the idea that relationships are a necessary precondition of successful contractual partnerships. CfP's programme of activities is focused on research activities related to procurement and investment in infrastructure. It aims to consider appropriate risk and reward outcomes that provide mutual community benefits related to health and social care, the environment, transport and retail sectors in particular.

CfP promotes the development of joint research grant applications by collaborating universities, and the promotion of organisational links with professional groups including the Society of Local Authority Chief Executives, Association of the Directors of Public Health, the Chartered Institute of Public Finance and Accounting, and other groups including the National Audit Office, National Council of Voluntary Organisation and the Department for Work and Pensions. The purpose of CfP is to promote the value of partnering through a relational framework between public, private and third sectors. CfP has facilitated a successful UK Research and Innovation (UKRI) bid of £450,000 which will enable the network to explore procurement during COVID-19.

Recommendations for system change

In order for future recommendations to be more robust and sustainable it is necessary to reflect on the different perspectives of the public, private and third sectors and their cumulative contributions regionally across the UK. The Regionalism Group of the CfP focuses primarily on the North East of England and the government's levelling up agenda. The Third Sector Group promotes discussion on the levelling up of this sector with the public and private sectors, to increase public and social value.

New data from the CfP facilitated UKRI funded COVID-19 research will add to the evidence base being developed by CfP.

The recommendations being generated from CfP take account of issues raised by the contributors to this book and members of the CfP in discussion and research groups. The governance of the CfP is shown in Figures A.1 and A.2.

The five pillars representing the organisation governance of CfP are shown in Figure A.1. The organisational relationship of CfP Working Groups, Research and Policy activities is presented in Figure A.2.

The conceptual basis of the development of CfP is based on the following statement based on MoUs and partnership agreements with collaborating organisations.

The Centre for Partnering promotes:

- The formalisation and adoption of a set of behaviours that create the bedrock of a form of contract that breaks the mould of power-based transactional relationships. Instead, it focuses on optimising behaviours to achieve shared objectives in a more effective and rewarding way'.
- A better way to bring organisations together to deliver long-term benefits to all.
- True partnering, not a transactional contract run over a longer period.
- The use of academic evidence from behavioural economics to public administration to organisational science, with respect to social determinants of health.
- Relationships based upon honesty, reciprocity, mutual trust and respect.
- The breaking down of the barriers and behaviours typically associated with 'partnering' or outsourcing contracts (transactional – client/contractor – power based). (Centre for Partnering Group, https://www.centreforpar tnering.org)

Figure A.1: The five aims of the Centre for Partnering

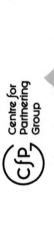

CfP
Centre for
Partnering
Group

1 Purpose

The Purpose of the Centre for Partnering (CfP) is to promote the value of 'partnering' through a 'relational' framework between different sectors. The CfP promotes the idea of partnering that generates additional value by combining each partner's contributons in a positive sum equation, CfP's role will be to explore the idea that relationships are a necessary condition of successful contractual partnerships.

2 Programme

CfP's programme of activities is focused around a series of research projects. Our USP is developing 'connectivity' between the university memebers and the private, public and third sectors. This will improve the quality of research and its impact on community outcomes given the joint participation of each type of organisation in the research programme.

3 Partners

CfP is built on a partnership between five universities.

Key to CfP's approache is develop partnering relations with private, public and this sectors.

In order to ensure cultural compatibility of future partnering organisations the CfP is developing a selection process for private, public and third sectors based on a range of criteria.

4 Product

The CfP Group will develop capacity building tools to support organisations design and deliver new partnering policies and strategies. We will provide self-assessments toolkits, training and capacity building, deep dive reviews, independent research, consultancy and strategic advice. CfP support and services will be based on the 'impact factors' that affect successful partnering outcomes.

5 Policy

Realising CfP's vision of a more effective partnering culture requires CfP to influence policy and practice. To do so CfP will generage a policy and influencing capacity and will work to disseminate its research through bespoke communications and events. The CfP will develop its 'Advisory Group' of influential individuals with experience and expertise to support the CfP agenda promoting a promote the value of 'partnering' through a 'relational' framework.

Figure A.2: Evolution of the Centre for Partnering and relationalism (2018–2022)

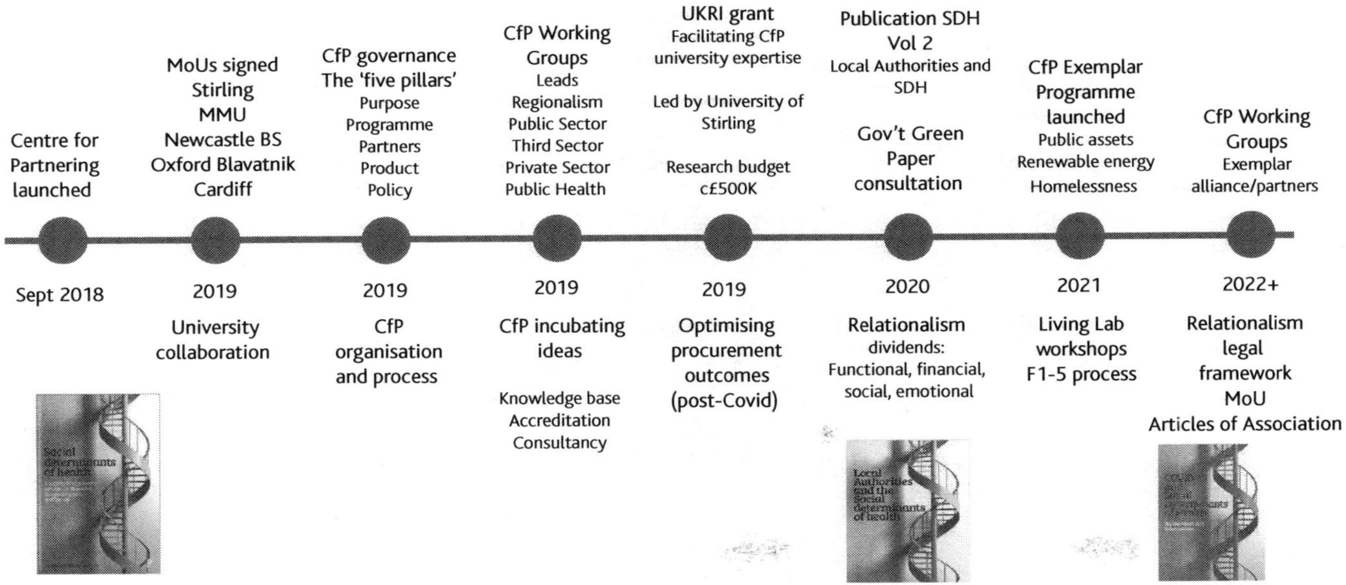
Centre for Partnering launched
Sept 2018
Social determinants of health
MoUs signed
Stirling
MMU
Newcastle BS
Oxford Blavatnik
Cardiff
2019
University collaboration
CfP governance
The 'five pillars'
Purpose
Programme
Partners
Product
Policy
2019
CfP organisation and process
CfP Working Groups
Leads
Regionalism
Public Sector
Third Sector
Private Sector
Public Health
2019
CfP incubating ideas
Knowledge base
Accreditation
Consultancy
UKRI grant
Facilitating CfP university expertise
Led by University of Stirling
Research budget c£500K
2019
Optimising procurement outcomes (post-Covid)
Publication SDH Vol 2
Local Authorities and SDH
Gov't Green Paper consultation
2020
Relationalism dividends:
Functional, financial, social, emotional
Local Authorities and the Social determinants of health
CfP Exemplar Programme launched
Public assets
Renewable energy
Homelessness
2021
Living Lab workshops
F1-5 process
CfP Working Groups
Exemplar alliance/partners
2022+
Relationalism legal framework
MoU
Articles of Association

Figure A.3: The Centre for Partnering: a 'facilitating' organisation

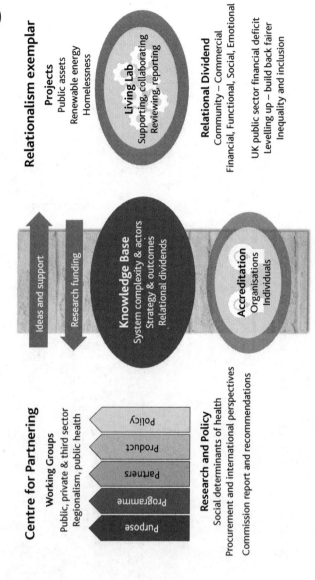

© CfP 2021

Index

References to figures appear in *italic* type;
those in **bold** type refer to tables and boxes.

A

Aberdeen 204–205
abuse 75
 see also domestic abuse
Access to Work programme 233, 234
active travel 107–109
adaptation 26
addiction 329–330
Addison Act 1919 211
adult social care 171, 177, *178*, 182, 190,
 212, 236, 292
adult social care funding 184
'Advancing Assets Programme' 163
affordable housing 216–219
 see also social housing
agency 42
Agostinho, D. 251
aid programmes *see* international
 aid programmes
Aids/HIV 3, 128
air quality 107–109
Alaimo, K. 245
Alarcon de Morris, A. 148
alcohol 125, 127–128, 129
Alderman, N. 354
Aljazeera 134, 136
All Party Parliamentary Group on Faith
 and Society 262
Allas, T. 7
Alma Ata (1978) 143
Anderson, I. 83, 211
Andrews, M.A. 134
Andrews, R. 359
anti-colonialism 45
Anti-Slavery International 137
Anti-Trafficking and Modern Slavery
 (ATMS) unit, Salvation Army 295,
 297–299, 300
 nationalities of potential victims *298*
Anvuur, A. 354, 355
Archer, M. 43
Arden, K. 83
Argyle, M. 327
Argyris, C. 25, 27
Armitage, R. 74
Artiga, S. 115
Asda 255
Asian Americans 117
Association of Chairs 264
asylum-seekers 286

austerity 60, 63, 367, 369–372, 373, 384
aviation industry 392

B

'B Corporations' 323
Baer, P. 75
Baginsky, M. 75
Ball, N. 379, 381, 383, 388
Bambra, C. 1, 58, 72, 88, 396
Bangalore Food Bank 252
Banks, J. 74
Barnardo's 282
Bayliss, F. 18, 46
Beach, R. 353, 354, 355, 356
Beaumont, P. 11
Beddington Zero Energy Development
 (BedZED) 104
Beer, T. 118
Bellis, A. 222
Ben, K. 398
Bennett, J. 352
Benyon, H. 88
Bernstein, L. 49
best practice partnership models 272–273
Better Care Fund 177
Betteridge-Moes, M. 137
Beveridge, W. 383
Beyond Rational Management (Quinn) 26
Bhopal, S.S. 72, 73
Bichard, M. 31
Biden, J. 119
Big Society 162, 163, 247, 387
bilateral relationships 377–380
Black Americans 114, 116–117, 118
Black Death 3
Black, G.S. 49
Black Lives Matter 118–119
Blair administration 216
Blair, T. 283
Blakeley, T. 144
Blood, I. 223
Blunders of Our Government, The (King and
 Crewe) 59
Boast, A. 72
Bolton, P. 197
Bonham, C. 242
Bonner, A. 1, 2, 83, 87, 165, 284
Booth, P. 383
Booth, W. 282, 286–287
Bosman, K. 114
Boswell, K. 259

boundary spanners 271
bounded rationality 21
Bourdieu, P. 42, 50–51
Bovaird, T. 34
Bradbury, A. 258, 263
Breeze, S. 270, 279–280
Bresnen, M. 352, 354, 355, 356, 361
Bretherton, L. 286
Brexit 60, 366, 367
  see also EU referendum
Brien, P. 378
Briggs, J. 43
British Academy 380
British Household Panel Survey 263
Brooks, R. 118
Broughton, J. 219–220
Brown, G. 98
Brown, T. 379
Browne, D. 358
Buchanan, L. 118
buildings 106–107
  see also construction industry; housing
Bump, P. 117
Burns, H. 285, 286
Burton, M. 368
business development 48–50
business rate retention 171–173
Business Roundtable 380
Bygballe, L.E. 355

C

Cahn, M. 26
Calvert, J. 56, 61
Cameron, D. 162, 247, 372, 387
Cameron, K. 30
Campbell, D.J.T. 222
capital 42, 372
capital receipts 174
carbon emissions 195–199, 203, 394
  Central England Co-operative 330
  from housing 204, 221
  from transport 203–204
  see also zero-carbon strategy,
    Sutton Council
Cardow, A. 145
care homes 41, 216, 292–294
care leavers 236
Care Quality Commission (CQC) 292
Carillion 373, 378
Casey, L. 223
Central England Co-operative 326–331
centralisation 61–63, 383–384
Centre for Local Economic Strategies
  147
Centre for Partnering 43, 51, 334, 397,
  402–406
  Exemplar Projects Initiative xxviii, 307,
    309–311, *335*, 337
Challender, J. 353

charges, income from see sales, fees and
    charges income
charities 258–265, 282
  social determinant of health 259,
    260, 261
  volunteering 260–265
  see also Salvation Army, The (TSA);
    third sector
Charity Commission 261, 263
Chasteauneuf, T. 284, 302
Chauraisa, M. 134
Chester, T. 284
Cheung, S.-O. 48
child labour 137
child marriage 137
child trafficking 137
Child Trafficking Advocates 297
childhood adversity 8, 166
childhood poverty 74, 328
children/children and young people
    (CYP)
  health and wellbeing 70–78
    call to action 76–77
    before COVID-19 pandemic 70–71
    impact of COVID-19 pandemic 72–75
    intergenerational justice 75–76
  human trafficking 296
  impact of domestic abuse on 269
  impact of lockdown on 8
  Marmot Reports 18
  online exploitation 136
  violence against women and children
    (VAW/C) 125–127
    third sector collaboration 127–130
children's social care 177, *178*
China 195, 394, 398
Chinese Communist Party (CCP) 48
Christian church 284
Christian institutions 282–283
  see also Salvation Army, The (TSA)
Christian Mission 282
Circle of Concerned African Women
    Theologians 129
Citizen Advice 224
citizen engagement 161, 167
Civil Contingencies Act 2004 92
Clark, D. 118
Clarke, J. 25
Clarke, T. 71
Clean Air Zones (CAZs) 203
clean energy technologies 204–205
climate change 1, 3, 10, 84, 394
  Central England Co-operative 330–331
  competing stories 28
  COP26 10, 45–46, 244, 397
  early concern about 192–193
  historical perspectives on carbon
    emissions 195–199
  and housing 314

key risk areas from 199–200
  flooding 200–201
  heatwaves 201
Kyoto Protocol 193–194
and local authorities 104–105, 109,
  111, 152
and relationalism 45–46
  role of local authorities 202–205
United Nations Framework Convention
  on Climate Change (UNFCCC) 193
  Convention of the Parties 194
United Nations Paris
  Agreement 194, 195
United Nations Sustainable Development
  Goals (SDGs) 194
Climate Change Act 2008 199
Climate Change Committee 199,
  200, 201
climate emergency 100–101, 104, 110,
  111, 202
climate emergency declarations 203
clinical bioethics 46
Cloutier, C. 30–31
clumsy institutions 28
co-operatives 326–327
co-production 34, 275–276
Coalition government 221, 369–371
Cobb, E. 293
Coe, R. 74
Cohen, R.I.S. 73
Colebatch, H. 23, 25, 30
collaboration 151, 245–247, 248, 285,
  352, 381
  frame for examples 249–255
  see also partnering; partnership working
collaborative citizens 246
Collaborative Newcastle **95–96**
Collective Preferences model 159
collectivism 45
Collier, P. 382, 385, 386, 387
Collins, K. 119
combined added value (CAV) 33
Combined Authorities, England and
  North East region 89
commercial income 174, 184
commercial property purchases 175
Commission on Social Determinant of
  Health 143
commissioning 162–163, 164, 166–
  167, 316
  domestic abuse services 273–279
  and good governance 346–348
  relational 285
  resource focused approach 348–349
  wellbeing in 338–339
common good 161
communication 49
communities 145–148
community asset transfer 163

community resilience 396
Community Right to Bid 163
Community Services Unit (CSU),
  Salvation Army 299
community support 299–301
competitive tendering 352
compulsory competitive tendering
  (CCT) 338, 339, 347, 357–358
conceptual work 30, 31
congruence 27, 29
Conklin, H. 17
conservatism 23
Conservative administrations 211–212,
  219, 369, 371, 383
Conservative Party 386–387
construction industry 319–325
  public-private partnering (PPP) 357–361
  relational contracting 351–354
  see also housing
Construction Industry Institute 352, 353
Construction Playbook (HMG,
  2920b) 315–316, 324
contexts 25
contracting culture 352
contracting, relational see
  relational contracting
Coordinated Community Response
  (CCR) 272
COP26 10, 45–46, 244, 397
Core Cities 90
Corner, D. 357
Cosens, M. 233, 236
cost of living 398
council housing 219–220
council tax 171, 186–187
Coventry 204
COVID-19 funding 184
COVID-19 pandemic xxvii, 2, 392
  deaths 3, 6, 8, 41, 56, 91, 134, 392
  and domestic abuse 269–270
  and human trafficking 135–138,
    294–299
  impact of local governments 109–110
  impact on children's health and
    wellbeing 72–75
  impact on North-East region 91–92
  impact on volunteering and
    charities 263–265
  Nepal and India 133–135
  modern slavery and human
    trafficking 135–138
  New Zealand 143–148
  older people and care homes 292–294
  progression 3–10
  and relational marketing 49
  South Africa 125–130
  UK government response 7–8, 42,
    56–57
  assessment framework 9

United States 114–120
volunteering 382
and wicked issues 1
COVID-19 vaccine *see* vaccinations
COVID OneView 163
Cowper, A. 63
Crampton, P. 144
creation 47
Crespin-Mazet, F. 356
Crewe, I. 56, 59, 60
Cribb, J. 369
Crick, B. 58
crime 329–330
crises 17
critical problems 23
Cromar, C. 204
cross-cultural psychologists 45
cultural change 355–356
cultural innovation 26
cultural perspective 45
cultural relationalism 48
Cultural Theory 28
Curran, D. 311

D

Dahlgren, G. 1, 18, 50, 165, 166
Daly, S. 259
Darling-Hammond, S. 117
Dartnell, E. 125, 126, 127, 128
Davies, N. 11
Davies, T. 378, 388
Davy, B. 25
Dawadi, S. 136
Dawson, C. 263
De Leeuw, E. 58
deaths from COVID-19 3, *6*, 8, 41, 56, 91, 134, 392
debt servicing costs *176*
decarbonisation 221, 330
Decent Homes initiative 220
Delmon, J. 246
Deori, U. 135
Department for Education (DfE) 235
Department for Levelling Up, Housing and Communities (DLUHC) 170–171, 184, 186, 187, 190, 217, 222
Department of Health and Social Care (DHSC) 186, 292
Department of Work and Pensions (DWP) 230–231, 232, 233, 235, 236
deprivation levels and gross rates payable per capita *173*
Derissen, S. 23
destitution 398
Development Asset Framework 276
devolution 83, 89–90, 144, 163
devolved administrations 61
'Dilemmas in a general theory of planning' (Rittel and Webber) 21

direction-finding instruments 21
Disability Employment Advisors (DEAs) 231–232, 234
disabled people 231, 232, 233, 237, 296
disruptive innovation 253–255
dissonance reduction 27
District Managers Discretionary Fund 231
Doan, M. 46
domestic abuse 268
partnership working 270–273
prevalence 269–270
Domestic Abuse Act 2021 269, 280
domestic abuse services 273–279
domestic homicides 272
domestic workers 296
double-loop learning 27, 35
drug addiction 329–330
Dublin *288*
Durham County Council 92, **94–95**
Dyer, J. 33

E

Ebrahim, A. 381
economic development 90, 187–188
education 75
educational institutions 136–137
see also schools
Egan, J. 352
Egypt 255
El-Erian, M. 8
Ellis-Petersen, H. 137
Emirbayer, M. 42, 44
emotion 271
emotional value 33
employment rate 237
see also unemployment
employment support 230–234
and local government 234–237
UK Shared Prosperity Fund (UKSPF) 237–239
EnergieSprong 106, 204
energy 106–107
England
assessment of COVID-19 response *9*
deaths from COVID-19 8
English Health and Care Act 2022 66
environmental planning 319–325
environmental, social and governance (ESG) factors 322–323
environmental value 192
Equality Now 136
Erikson, E. 45
Eriksson, P.-E. 352, 355
Essex Partners 381
EU referendum 372–374
see also Brexit
European Social Fund (ESF) 237
European Union (EU) 160, 188, 319, 370
Evans, M. 356

'Everyone In' 182, 186, 190, 222,
    223–225, 289, 396
evidence-based policymaking (EBPM) 22
Exemplar Projects Initiative xxviii, 307,
    309–311, *335*, 337
exploration 24–25
extra-organisational relationships 381–382
extreme weather impact 200–201
Eyban, R. 45

F

Fair Start Scotland 233
faith-based organisations (FBOs) 47–48,
    128–130, 138, 262, 277, 283
    see also Christian institutions; Salvation
    Army, The (TSA)
Fallaize, R. 166
Fareshare 252, 254–255, 328
Farrell, C. 83
federal taxes *103*
Feeding America 250
fees, income from *see* sales, fees and
    charges income
Fernández Campbell, A. 117
Ferris, E. 283
Fiddian-Qasmiyeh, E. 283
financial sustainability, LAs 170–191
    central government action 184–187
    change in service demand *178*
    change in service spend *180*
    changes in components of spending
        power *172*
    commercial property purchases *175*
    cost pressures *183*, *185*
    before COVID-19 pandemic 170–176
    debt servicing costs as share of spending
        power *176*
    effect of COVID-19 pandemic
        on 182–184
    effect of funding reductions 177–182
    effect on economic
        development 187–188
    levels of deprivation and gross rates
        payable per capita *173*
    social care as share of service spend *181*
    year on year price changes *179*
Financial Times 384
financial value 33
Fineman, S. 271
Finnish Buses case 340
Fisayo, T. 8
Fiske, A.S.P. 45, 49
Fitzpatrick, S. 220
Flexible New Deal 231
flooding 200–201
Foley, L. 136
folk society 44
Food Bank Regional Network
    (FBRN) 255

food banks 245, 247, 250, 251, 253,
    254
food delivery service 299
food deserts 248
food hubs 242–243
food insecurity 245
    collaboration 246–247, 248
    frame for examples of collaboration and
        innovation *250*
    innovation 246–247, 248–249
        disruptive 253–255
        incremental 249–251
        institutional 252–253
food waste 328–329
Francis-Devine, B. 74
free schools 322
Friedman, M. 385
Friends of the Earth 104
Frydlinger, D. 378
Fuchs, T. 30, 43
functional value 33
fundraising 263
furlough scheme 7
future shocks and stressors 10–11

G

Gamble, A. 58
Garvie, D. 224
Gaskell, J. 59
Gauthier, D. 44
gender-based violence 125–126, 128
    see also violence against women and
        children (VAW/C)
general election 2019 60–61, 87, 156,
    384
Gennrich, D. 129
geographic variations 83
George, S. 107
George Steven Community Hub 299
Germany 254
Giles, C. 384
Girls Not Brides 137
Glasby, J. 271
globalism 372, 392, 395
Gonzalez, D. 116
goodness 44
GoodWeave International 136
Gorges, R. 115
Goth, U.S. 260, 261, 262
Gottlieb, S. 354
Gough, J. 136
Gould, C. 127
Gove, M. 374
governance 151, 158, 346–348
government funding 102, 171, 184–187
    effect of funding reductions 177–182
government grants 184, 186, 221
Graca, P. 355
Great Recession 368–369, 371

Greater Manchester 187–188, 223, 236, 323, 381
   geographical boundaries *189*
Greater Manchester Working Well project 234
Green Book Review 2020 (HMG, 2010) 344–345
Green Homes Grants Local Authority Delivery Scheme (LAD) 107
Green New Deal for London 105
greenhouse gas emissions *see* carbon emissions
Greenwood, J. 27
Gregorian, D. 118
Griffith Laboratories 252
Grint, K. 22–23, 24, 31
Gronroos, C. 49
Guardian 108, 134
Gundersen, C. 251
Gurung, T. 295

H

habitus 43
Hadebe, N. 129
Hajikazemi, S. 358
Haldane, A. 382
Hamel, L. 116, 117
Hammond, K. 22
Han, J. 260
harm reduction 287
Harris, J. 283
Harrison, D. 125, 127
Hart, O. 378
Hartley, J. 33
Hatch, W. 48
hate crimes 117
Head, B.W. 270, 271
health and social care 90–91
Health and Social Care Act (2012) 84
health and social care futures 92–97
health and wellbeing
   children and young people (CYP) 70–78
      call to action 76–77
      before COVID-19 pandemic 70–71
      impact of COVID-19 pandemic 72–75
      intergenerational justice 75–76
   in New Zealand 143–148
   and public and social value 164–165
   see also social determinant of health
health inequalities 57–58, 114–115, 144, 259, 260, 399
health insurance 115, 137
health lifestyle theory 42–43
health policy 59
health services 75
healthcare 222
heatwaves 201
Henrickson, M. 143
hierarchy of needs 245

Higgins-Dunn, N. 114
Hill Group 290
Hill, J. 383
HIV *see* Aids/HIV
HMT Green Book 155
Ho, D.Y.F.G. 45
Home Office 273, 286
Home Office Single Competent Authority 297
homelessness 177, *178*, 190, 220, 221–225, 396
   Malachi Project 290, *291*
   Night-Time Accommodation Project 291
Homelessness Reduction Act 2020 289
Homelessness Services Unit (HSU), Salvation Army 287–288, 290
   user satisfaction surveys **289**, **290**
homes 106–107
Homes England 221
Hong Kong 254
Hood, C. 64
Hoppe, R. 28
Horton, R. 59
Hosseini, A. 355
Houchen, B. 167
house prices 217, 312, *313*
housebuilding 216
   see also construction industry
household income 369, 372
housing 152, 204, 210–226
   affordability 216–219
   housing associations 220–221, 314–315, 347
   local authorities 219–220
   new homes, 1969–2020 *213–215*
   private sector 212–216
   sector-based analysis 211–212
   see also homelessness
Housing Act 1974 220
housing delivery 312–317
Housing Delivery Test 216
'Housing First' 222–223, 225
Housing (NI) Order (1988) 289
housing tenure **219**
Housing (Wales) Act 2014 289
HS2 high speed rail 374
Hudson, B. 245
human trafficking 135–139, 294–299
Hunter, D.J. 66
Huxham, C. 29

I

Ill Fares the Land (Judt) 68
immigrants 371
   see also migrant workers
income inequality 144, 372, 396
Incredible Edible 253–254
incremental innovation 249–250

Independent Panel for Pandemic
    Preparedness and Response
    (IPPPR) 57, 74
India
    Bangalore Food Bank 252
    carbon emissions 195, 394
    COVID-19 pandemic 133–135
    modern slavery and human
        trafficking 135–139
Indian Health Service 115
indigenous approach 45
indigenous people 147
inequalities see health inequalities
inequalities gap 366–368
infection rates 7–8, 115
inflation 398
infrastructure spending 155
innovation 166
    cultural 26
    food insecurity 246–247, 248–249
        disruptive innovation 253–255
        incremental innovation 249–251
        institutional innovation 252–253
    in local governance 163–164
innovation initiatives 161–162
Inside Housing 221
Institute for Fiscal Studies 369, 371
Institute for Government 378
Institute for Health Metric Evaluation 8
Institute for Public Policy Research
    (IPPR) 102
Institute of Civil Engineers 358
Institute of Employment Studies 285
Institute of Fundraising 258
institutional innovation 252–253
institutional logics 25–26
institutional pluralism 28
institutional work 26
integrated care systems 93
Intensive Personalised Employment
    Support 233
inter-contextuality 25
inter-organisational relationships 377–381
intergenerational justice 75–76
international aid programmes 18, 44–45,
    245
International Energy Agency 195, 203
International Monetary Fund 160
Isba, R. 75
Islam 47

J

James, M. 260, 262
Japan 48
Jenrick, R. 216
Jessop, B. 27
Jeung, R. 117
Job Entry Targeted Support (JETS) 232
Jobcentre Plus 231–232, 236

Jobcentre Plus Work Coaches 232
Johnson, B. 87, 88, 241, 373, 374, 383, 398
Joint Learning Initiative (JLI) 295
joint ventures 347
Jones, B. 64
Joseph, J. 44
Joseph Rowntree Foundation 282–283,
    302, 340
Judt, T. 68

K

Kaiser Family Foundation (KFF) 115, 116
Kanagasooriam, J. 384
Kania, J. 381
Kearns, N. 270, 271
Kelly, G. 34
Kemp, R. 27
Kendon, M. 201
Keohane, N. 212
Key Cities 90
Keynes, M. 370
khichdi 252
Kickbusch, I. 59
'Kickstart' scheme 236
King, A. 59, 62, 66, 67
Kingman, J. 379
Kingston Council 205
knowledge
    competing/complementary forms of **25**
    legitimate 25
Kruger Report 47, 241, 243, 282, 283,
    284, 302, 387, 394, 396
Kunonga, E. 83, 87
Kyoto Protocol 193–194

L

Labour governments 211–212, 219, 220,
    231, 370, 383
Labour Party 87, 387
Lado, A. 49
Lasswell, H. 21, 22, 58
Latham, M. 352
Lawrence, T. 26, 30
learning 26
    see also double-loop learning; single-
        loop learning
Leathard, A. 246
Lee, Y.J. 260
Lefafa, N. 126
LeFevbre, R. 45
legitimate knowledges 25
Lehtonen, A. 46
Leicester City Council 204
Lejano, R. 27, 34
LePan, N. 3
'levelling up' 286
'levelling up' agenda 83, 87–98, 238, 241,
    285, 373–374, 384, 398
    devolution 89–90

health and social care futures 92–97
impact of COVID-19 91–92
NHS long-term plan 90
quangos 90
social determinant of health 156
and third sector 311
'Levelling Up' Index 163
levels of deprivation and gross rates payable
    per capita *173*
Li, B. 357
Liddle, J. 158, 159, 192
life expectancy 58, 114
Link Cafe, Merton 277, 278–279
listening 31
Livability 282
lived experiences 275–276
Liverpool 204, 223
Llyod George, D. 211
local authorities 102
  carbon emissions 203
  and central government 66
  climate emergency declarations
    203
  health inequalities 84
  housing 219–220
  see also local government
*Local Authorities and Social Determinant of
    Health* (Bonner) xxvii, 2, 5, 49, 83,
    87, 241, 284, 285, 380–381, 388
Local Enterprise Partnerships (LEPs) 187
local governance, New Zealand 145–148
local government
  austerity 63
  central government funding 102,
    151–152, 171
  and centralisation 62
  climate change 104–105, 109, 152, 194,
    200, 202–203
    Clean Air Zones (CAZs) and transport
      initiatives 203–204
    clean energy technologies 204–205
    extreme weather impact 200–201
    housing related emissions 204
  employment support 234–237
  financial sustainability 170–191
    central government action 184–187
    change in service demand *178*
    change in service spend *180*
    changes in components of spending
      power *172*
    commercial property purchases *175*
    cost pressures *183, 185*
    before COVID-19 pandemic
      170–176
    debt servicing costs as share of spending
      power *176*
    effect of COVID-19 pandemic
      on 182–184
    effect of funding reductions 177–182

effect on economic
    development 187–188
  levels of deprivation and gross rates
    payable per capita *173*
  social care as share of service spend *181*
  year on year price changes *179*
innovation in 163–164
New Zealand 143
  and NHS 91, 92
    Collaborative Newcastle **95–96**
    Durham County Council **94–95**
  The Salvation Army 289–291
  social care demand *178*
  social care spending *180*
  spending cuts 370
  see also Sutton Borough Council
Local Government Act 1929 202
Local Government Act 1988 339–340
Local Government Act 2002, New
    Zealand 145–146
Local Government Association 108,
    109, 203
Local Growth Fund 187
local growth landscape 187–188
local housing allowances (LHAs) 221, 223
Local Resilience Forums (LRFs) 91–92,
    182
local taxes *103*
localism 163, 187
Localism Act 2011 163, 170, 341
lockdowns 2, 7, 8, 41, 47–48, 84, 125,
    127, 134, 135, 242, 264
London 105, 203
London Borough of Sutton 100–101
  Beddington Zero Energy Development
    (BedZED) 104
  central government funding 102
  'Transformation Programme' 274–275
  zero-carbon strategy
    active travel and air quality 107–109
    energy and buildings 106–107
    partnership working 109–110
London Recovery Board 105
Loraine, R.K. 357
'lost decade' 366–374
  background 368–369
  EU referendum 372–374
  rise and decline of austerity 369–372
  widening inequalities gap 366–368
Lovelace, B. 118
'low-traffic neighbourhoods' 108–109
Lowndes, V. 271

M

Macfarlane, R. 340
Mack, E. 44
Madani, D. 118
Maguire, N. 222, 287
Major administration 216

Major, L.E. 74
Majumdar, S. 126
Malachi Project 290, *291*
Malnick, E. 398
Mamouni-Limnios, E. 24
Manzanedo, R.D. 10
Māori population 145
Māori tribes 143
March, J. 24
Markard, J. 10
market pricing perspective 49
Marmor, T. 59
Marmot, M. 56, 70, 74
Marmot Review (2010) 1, 18, 104, 285,
    286, 396
Marmot Review (2020) 2, 18, 58, 70, 71,
    75, 285, 286, 392, 396
Marshall, K. 283
Marx, K. 42
Maslow, A.H. 245
Matheson, A. 145
Mattinson, D. 87
Matzopoulos, R. 125
May, T. 373
Mayer, C. 386
Mayor of London 105, 106
McGuire, M. 22
McMinn, S. 116
Meek, J. 212, 225
Menon, A. 88, 90
mental health 74–75, 237
Meynhardt, T. 161, 165
migrant workers 136, 296
    see also immigrants
Milbourne, L. 246
Ministry of Housing, Communities
    and Local Government
    (MHCLG) 216, 223
minority communities 115, 119
Mkise, V. 127, 128
modern methods of construction
    (MMC) *313*, 314–315, 316
modern slavery 135–139, 294–299
Modern Slavery Act 2015 297
Mohan, J. 259, 263, 264
Moore, A.D. 44
Moore, M. 158, 159, 165, 166
Moore, S. 261
moral imperative 29
Morales, A. 399
Morris, R. 381
mortality data 2
mortality rates 58, 75
'Most Advantageous Tender' (MAT) 321
'Most Economically Advantageous Tender'
    (MEAT) 321
Mulgan, G. 33
Mullins, D. 219
multinationals 372

Murphie, A. 173
Murray, C. 42
mutual accountability 45
mutuality 327
My, J. 125

N

Nakamura, D. 117
National Audit Office (NAO) 64, 224,
    358, 396
National Council for Voluntary
    Organisations (NCVO) 242, 259
National Economic Development Office
    (NEDO) 352
National Health Service (NHS) 292, 338
    austerity 63, 370
    Integrated Care Systems 381
    and local government 91, 92
        Collaborative Newcastle **95–96**
        Durham County Council **94–95**
    long-term plan 90–91
    reorganisation 66, 88
National Housing Federation 220, 221
National Referral Mechanism (NRM) 297
Navajo Nation 115
needs, hierarchy of 245
Nepal
    COVID-19 pandemic 133–135
    modern slavery and human
        trafficking 135–139
networks of relationships 380–381
Neupane, S.R. 137
New Deal 231
New Deal for Disabled People
    (NDDP) 231
New Economic Foundation (NEF) 164
new homes, 1969–2020 *213–215*
New Labour 383
New Philanthropic Capital (NPC) 263
New Public Governance (NPG) 158
New Public Management
    (NPM) 158, 166
New York School of Relational
    Sociology 44
New Zealand 143–148
Newcastle **95–96**
Nexon, D.H. 45
Nicholls, A. 248
Nifa, F.A.A. 356
Night-Time Accommodation Project
    291
Nightingale Hospitals 319–320
Nisar, T.M. 357
Njoku, A. 116
'no recourse to public funds' (NRPF) 224
Noack, R. 118
Nombembe, P. 126
'non-commercial considerations'
    legislation 339–340

non-communicative diseases 41, 143–144
North and North-East England
'levelling up' agenda 83, 87–98,
373–374
devolution 89–90
health and social care futures 92–97
impact of COVID-19 91–92
NHS long-term plan 90
quangos 90
social determinant of health 156
North East Local Enterprise Partnership
(NELEP) 90
Northern Ireland 289
Northern Powerhouse 87, 88
Nova, A. 115

O

objectivist values 44
O'Brien, N. 87
O'Donnell, G. 260
Office for Budget Responsibility 221
Office for National Statistics 369
O'Flynn, J. 158, 159, 166
older people 292–294
O'Leary, C. 258, 259, 260, 265
O'Neill, O. 383
online exploitation 136, 137–138
operational disconnect 66
operational work 30, 31
Osborne, S.P. 159–160, 270
Ottawa Charter for Health Promotion
(1986) 143
outsourcing 63–65, 162, 380
Outsourcing Playbook (Cabinet Office,
2020a) 378
Oxford COVID-19 Government
Response Tracker 7

P

Palm, S. 126, 127, 128, 129
Paris Agreement 194, 195
Parkin, E. 220
Parnham, A. 41, 166
Parsons, T. 26
partnering 352–354
complexities and challenges 354–357
public-private partnering (PPP) 357–361
relational 49–50, 167, 317, 324,
334, *336*
see also partnership working
partnering environment 334
partnering relationships 346–348
partnership framework xxvii–xxviii
partnership working 109–110, 138, 246,
270–273
see also partnering; 'Transformation
Programme', London Borough
of Sutton
partnerships 33–34, 279–280, 316

see also local governments: and
NHS; partnering; public-third-
private partnerships
Passivhaus Trust 104
Paswan, A. 49
Paten, R. 259
Pathare, S. 135
patterns of social relations 27–28
Payne, C. 387
peace building 44
Pearce, N. 261
Pearcey, S. 74
Peleg, N. 76
performance management 162–163
performance measurement 164
Peterman, A. 125, 126
Pfeffer, J. 59
Phillips, J. 269
Phua, F.T.T. 356
physical activity 74
Pickett, K. 73, 75
Pinch, P.L. 357
place-based initiatives 84, 285
place leadership 156, 167
policy discourse 24
policymaking 21–22, 26–27
political choices 59
political science 58
politics 58, 59, 395
Pollard, T. 235
polyrational imagination 28, 34
polyrationality 25
Poortinga, Y.H. 45
Pope, T. 368
population health management (PHM)
77
Porteous, D. 90, 91
Porter, M. 380
poverty 74, 238, 328
see also destitution
Powell, P. 205
Pozzoni Architecture 320
preference satisfaction theories 44
private sector 63–65, 202
government contracts 377–378
housing 212–216
procurement and tendering 320–324,
346–348
public-private partnering (PPP) 357–361
see also public-third-private partnerships
privatisation 157, 162
Pro Bono Economics (PBO) 242
problem orientation 21
procurement 162–163, 164, 166–167,
319–324, 333, 367–368
COVID-19 pandemic 396
and good governance 346–348
post-Brexit 343–346
relational 351–362

complexities and challenges of
partnering 354–357
construction industry 351–354
public-private partnering
(PPP) 357–361
relational contract 378–380
resource focused approach 348–349
social value in 339–343
wellbeing in 338–349
procurement functions xxviii
Procurement Reform (Scotland) Act
2014 342
productivity 188, 371
Productivity Commission, New
Zealand 145
'profit for purpose' businesses 323
'Project 13' 358
Provan, K.G. 381
Public Accounts Committee 201
public and social value 157–158, 159–
161, 162
in local governance 163–164
and social determinants of health 164–
165, 166
see also social value
Public Finance Initiative (PFI) 357, 358
public governance, changing context
of 158–159
Public Health England 57, 66
public-health ethics 18, 46
public policy 59
public-private partnering (PPP) 357–358
public sector 63
and relationalism 46–47
role in private sector procurement 323
Public Service Act 2020, New
Zealand 146
public service reform 156–158
public services 166
effect of funding reductions 177–182
users 382
Public Services (Social Value) Act
2012 84, 164, 202, 341
public-third-private partnerships 337

Q

quangos 90
questioning 26
questions, asking the right 23–24
Quinn, R. 26

R

racism 114–117, 119–120
rainbow model of health (Dahlgren and
Whitehead) 1, 18, 50, 165, 166
Ramaphosa, C. 125, 126
Rankin, K. 134
Real Junk Food project 255
recession 188, 368–369, 371

'Red Toryism' 368
'Red Wall' 60, 87, 156, 343, 373–374, 384
Rees, T. 97
Reeves, E. 357
reflection 29
reform 385–387
refrigeration gases 330–331
refugees 286
Regan, R. 395
Regional Growth Fund 187
regional variations 83
regionalism 44
rehabilitation projects 329–330
relational autonomy 46, 397
relational behaviour 18
relational capital 31, 34
relational commissioning 285
relational competence and commitment
35
relational contract 309, 316, 378–379
relational contracting 351–362
complexities and challenges of
partnering 354–357
construction industry 351–354
public-private partnering (PPP) 357–361
relational culture 307
relational deficits 35
relational dividend 17, 29, 32–34, 35, 285,
308, *310*, 334
relational dynamics 30, 47
relational efforts 31
relational environment 48–49
relational governance 158
relational imperative 29–30
relational leadership 46–47
relational marketing 49
relational omnipotence 47
relational overload 35
relational partnering 49–50, 167, 317,
324, 334, *336*
relational phenomena 30
relational procurement 351–362
complexities and challenges of
partnering 354–357
construction industry 351–354
public-private partnering (PPP) 357–361
relational rents 33
relational solidarity 46
relational support 284–285, 302
relational theory 18
relational theory of practice 42
relational tools 376–377
relational values 18, 44, 397
relational work 17, 29, 30–32, 34–35
and trust-based relationships *32*
relationalism xxvii, 18, 334, 376, 397
Central England Co-operative 330
and climate change 45–46, 200
constraints 383–385

and culture and business
    development 48–50
faith-based organisations (FBOs) 262
geopolitical and regional
    perspectives 44–45
and housing 314, 316
importance in addressing wicked
    problems 27–29
Kyoto Protocol and Paris Agreement 193
and public sector 46–47
reform required for adoption of 385–387
soft structures 284
theories 42–43
and third sector 47–48
as a 'value proposition' 29–34
and values 43–44
and wicked issues 393–394
relationalism knowledge base 337
relationality 27
relationships
    extra-organisational 381–382
    inter-organisational 377–381
religion see faith-based organisations
    (FBOs)
rescue politics 395
resident associations 147–148
residential home services 216
residualisation 219
resilience 396
Resolution Foundation 372
resource focused commissioning 348–349
Restart programme 233
retail crime 329–330
Rhodes, R. 22, 26
Riches, G. 254
Rittel, H. 1, 3, 17, 21, 22, 23, 24, 28, 151
Ritzer, G. 45
Robert Wood Johnson Foundation 116
Roberts, G. 212
Rocco, L. 261
Rochdale Pioneers 326
Rogers, T. 115
rough sleeping 221–224, 289, 380
Rowlinson, S. 50
Royal College of Paediatrics 71
Royal Town Planning Institute 156
Russell, P. 5
Russian invasion of Ukraine 10–11, 392
Ryan, M. 125

S

sales, fees and charges compensation
    scheme 186
sales, fees and charges income 173–174,
    184
Salvation Army, The (TSA) 139, 277,
    278–279, 282, 284–285, 286
  Anti-Trafficking and Modern Slavery
    (ATMS) unit 295, 297–299, 300

nationalities of potential victims *298*
Homelessness Services Unit (HSU)
    287–288, 290
  user satisfaction surveys **289**, **290**
Malachi Project 290, *291*
Night-Time Accommodation
    Project 291
Older People's Services 293–294
volunteering 299–301
work with central and local
    governments 289–291
Sanderson, I. 26–27, 27
Sarma, J. 134
Save the Children 73, 74, 75
Schoenfield Walker, A. 118
Schön, D. 29
school closures 74, 136–137
schools 322
Schumpeter, J.A. 248
Schwirtz, M. 115
Scotland 194, 224, 233, 289, 340, 342
Scott, E. 277, 278
Senge, P. 381
Seriot, P. 367
service users 382
Sethy, P. 135
Settersten, Jr, R.A. 73
Shah, F. 47
Sharma, G. 135
Shelter 223, 224
Sherratt, F. 358
Shutt, J. 89, 90
Simmons, R. 24, 28, 29, 31, 33
Simon, H. 21
single-loop learning 27, 35
Skills for Every Young Person (House of
    Lords, 2021) 235
slavery 135–139
Sloan, L. 379
Small Charities Coalition 264
Smith, D. 118
Smith, R. 49, 167
Smith-Schoenwalder, C. 119
Smyth, H. 358
Smythe, E. 26
Snape, D. 270
social capital 260–261, 283
social care demand 177, *178*, 182
social care spending 70, 173, 177–181
social contract 382
social determinant of health 17, 396, 399
  Commission on Social Determinant of
    Health 143
  Policy Press publications *12*
  and public and social value 164–165
  rainbow model (Dahlgren and
    Whitehead) 1, 18, 50, 165, 166
  role of charities 259, 260
  and social capital 261

Social Determinant of Health (Bonner) 1
social epidemics 41
social evils 282–283, 284, 302
Social Finance 233
social housing 152
  housing associations 220–225
  local authorities 219–220
Social Housing Decarbonisation Fund
    (SHDF) 221
social innovation 248, *249*
social justice 286–287
social justice solidarity 397
social media 137–138
social movements 253, 255
social outcomes 311
social policy perspective 152–153
social relations, patterns of 27–28
social relationships 42
social responsibility 43
social value 33, 43, 157–158, 159–161,
    162, 202, 393–394
  Central England Co-operative 326–327
  environmental, social and governance
    (ESG) factors 322–323
  in local governance 163–164
  in projects appraisal 343–346
  in public procurement 339–343
  and social determinants of health
    164–165, 166
social value purpose 394
social welfare 245–246
soft market testing 324
soft structures 284
Solar, O. 261
Solent Jobs Programme 238
soup kitchens 249–250
South Africa 125–130
South African Council of Churches 129
South London Skills and Employment
    Board 107
Southby, K. 260, 261, 262
Spanish Flu 3
spending power 171, *172*
  debt servicing costs as share of *176*
Spending Reviews 155, 170, 187
Spiranovic, C. 126
Sport England 74
Springford, J. 398
Srivastava, R. 136
St James Settlement 254
stakeholders 28
Standing Together Against Domestic
    Abuse *272*
Starter Homes Scheme 217
Stellenbosch University 129
Stewart, J. 28, 33–34
stigma 135
Stoker, G. 159
Stop AAPI Hate 117

strategic offense 24
strategic planning 334
Strategic Value Triangle (SVT) 159
structural racism 114–117, 119–120
structural work 30, 31
Stuttgart model 254
subjectivist values 44
substantialism 42
Sullivan, H. 270
Sumberg, J. 24
Sunak, R. 7
Sunday Times 61
Sundquist, V. 353, 354
supernormal value 33
Supplementary Nutrition Assistance
    Program (SNAP) 251
supply chain integration 352
supply chain partners 320
supported employment 230–231
sustainability *see* financial sustainability
Sustainable Development Goals
    (SDGs) 194, 210, 225, 341
sustainable housing land 212
Sustainable Procurement Task Force 341
Sutton Borough Council 100–101
  Beddington Zero Energy Development
    (BedZED) 104
  central government funding 102
  'Transformation Programme' 274–275
  zero-carbon strategy
    active travel and air quality 107–109
    energy and buildings 106–107
    partnership working 109–110
Sutton Plan 110, 274
syndemic 72
syphilis 116
system change 402–403
systemic racism 119

T

Tafel 254
tame problems 23, 151
tax losses 186–187, 190
taxes *103*
  see also council tax
Taylor, B. 118
Taylor, I. 380
Taylor, J. 42
technologies 204–205
Tees Valley 89
Teesside hospitals **96**
temporary accommodation 223
tendering 321–324, 352
  see also compulsory competitive tendering
    (CCT)
Territorial Local Authorities (TLAs) 146
Test and Trace system 64–65, 182
Thatcher, M. 212, 225, 383, 385,
    386, 395

third sector 127–129, 241–243
  collaboration 245–247
  Exemplar Projects Initiative 311
  and relationalism 47–48
  see also charities; food banks; Link
    Cafe, Merton; public-third-private
    partnerships; Salvation Army, The
    (TSA); voluntary sector
Third Way 283
Thomas, A. 97
Thompson, M. 28
Thornton, P. 26, 27
Time Like No Other, A (Hadebe) 129
Toogood, S. 329
Total Place initiative (2010) 163
training 75
'Transformation Programme', London
  Borough of Sutton 274–275
Transforming Public Procurement (HMG,
  2020) 345–346, 367, 374
transparency 346, 377
transport 203–204
  see also active travel
Trump, D. 117, 118, 119, 195
Trussell Trust 247, 249, 250, 253
trust xxvii, 31, 49, 109, 116–117, 271,
  333, 352, 355, 377
trust-based partnering 50
trust-based relationships and relational
  work *32*
truth 43, 49
Turnbull, N. 21, 22, 23, 24
'Tuskegee Study of Untreated Syphilis in
  the Negro Male' 116

U

Uhl-Bien, M. 47
UK
  carbon emissions 197–198, 203
  Christian church 284
  communities 147
  deaths from COVID-19 393
  general election 2019 60–61, 87,
    156, 384
  health inequalities 57–58
  key risk areas from climate
    change 199–200
    flooding 200–201
    heatwaves 201
  'lost decade' 366–374
    background 368–369
    EU referendum 372–374
    rise and decline of austerity 369–372
    widening inequalities gap 366–368
  Modern Slavery Act 2015 297
  National Economic Development Office
    (NEDO) 352
  National Infrastructure Commission
    155

National Referral Mechanism
  (NRM) 297
nominal house prices *313*
regional variations 83
retail industry 330
share of gross domestic product by
  region *156*
Sustainable Development Goals
  (SDGs) 194
UK COVID-19 Inquiry 65
UK government
  COVID-19 response 7–8, 42, 56–57,
    59–61
    agenda for reform 65–67
    assessment framework *9*
    policy failures 61–65
  external contracts 377–378
  fiscal centralisation 102
  infrastructure strategy 358
  'Kickstart' scheme 236
  'levelling up' agenda 83, 87–98, 238,
    241, 285, 373–374, 384, 398
  devolution 89–90
  health and social care futures 92–97
  impact of COVID-19 91–92
  NHS long-term plan 90
  quangos 90
  social determinant of health 156
  and third sector 311
  local government funding 102, 171,
    184–187
    effect of funding reductions 177–182
  procurement 319–324
  Rough Sleeping Strategy 223
  Spending Reviews 155, 170, 187
  Starter Homes Scheme 217
  work with The Salvation Army 289
UK Shared Prosperity Fund
  (UKSPF) 237–239
Ukraine invasion 10–11, 392
unemployment 75, 84, 115, 188, 236,
  237
  see also employment support
UNICEF 136, 137
Union of Concerned Scientists 192–193
United Nations 144
United Nations Framework
  Convention on Climate Change
    (UNFCCC) 193, 200
  Convention of the Parties 194
United Nations Paris Agreement 194,
  195
United Nations Sustainable Development
  Goals (SDGs) 194, 210, 225, 341
United States 114–120
  Business Roundtable 380
  carbon emissions 394
  and China 398
  Construction Industry Institute 352, 353

Feeding America 250
food banks 251, 252, 253
Kyoto Protocol 194
political landscape during
    COVID-19 117–119
resident associations 147–148
structural racism 114–117, 119–120
Supplementary Nutrition Assistance
    Program (SNAP) 251
unringfenced grants 184

V

vaccination programmes 134, 367
vaccination rates 3, 7, 116–117
vaccinations 5, 319
value 34, 320–321
    see also environmental value; public and
        social value; social value
value conflict resolution 159
value for money assessments 155
value proposition, relationalism as
    29–34
values 22, 34
    and partnership working 270
    relational 18, 44, 397
    and relationalism 43–44
van den Bree, B.M. 396
Van Ess Coeling, H. 26
Veenstra, G. 43
Venkatraman, S. 117
vertical farming 254
Verweij, M. 25, 28
Vibert, S. 300
Victor, D. 118
Villineuve-Smith, F. 379
violence against women and children
    (VAW/C) 125–127
    third sector collaboration 127–130
voluntary sector 277
    see also charities
volunteering 242, 251, 259, 260–265,
    299–301, 382, 387
voters 387

W

Wales 343, 373
Walker, M. 115
wealth 166
Weick, K. 27
Welfare Reform and Work Act 2016
    221
welfare state 383
welfarism 220
Well-being of Future Generations (Wales)
    Act 2015 343
wellbeing 274
    in commissioning and
        procurement 338–349
    see also health and wellbeing

wellbeing indices 160
Welwyn 205
West Midlands Combined Authority
    (WMCA) 204
Wexler, M. 270
Whānau Ora 145
What Works Wellbeing 274
White, C. 341
Whole Health Approach 273
wicked issues / problems xxvii, 1, **3**,
    10–11, 17, 34, 46, 151
    collaboration and innovation 246–247
    criteria **4–5**
    importance of relationalism in
        addressing 27–29
    nature and governance 22–27
    need for novel solutions to 161–163
    partnering as 354
    partnership working 270–271
    and politics 395
    and relationalism 393–394
    sources of suboptimality in addressing 35
wicked policy problems 21
Wildavsky, A. 23
Wilkinson, R. 222
Williams, G. 255
Williams, P. 271
Wilson, T. 230, 235, 238
women
    domestic abuse 269, 277, 278
    human trafficking 137, 296
    violence against women and children
        (VAW/C) 125–127
Women's Aid 270
Wood, C. 33
Wood, L. 259
Work and Health programme 232
Work Choice programme 232
Work programme 232
Workprep programme 231
Workstep programme 231
World Bank 160
World Economic Forum 367
World Health Organization (WHO) 3, 83
    1978 Alma Ata 143
    Commission on Social Determinant of
        Health 143
    deaths in WHO regions 6
    gender-based violence 125
    health equity status report 57
    Independent Panel for Pandemic
        Preparedness and Response
        (IPPPR) 57

Y

Yeung, J.W.K. 260
Young, J.A. 48–49
young people *see* children / children and
    young people (CYP)

Youth Hubs 236
youth unemployment 236

Z

Zaharna, R.S. 50
zero-carbon strategy, Sutton Council

active travel and air quality 107–109
energy and buildings 106–107
partnership working 109–110
Zimmer, C. 49